© Copyright 2022 - Jasmine T Williams. All rights reserved.

The content contained within this book may not be reproduced, duplicated or transmitted without direct written permission from the author or the publisher.
Under no circumstances will any blame or legal responsibility be held against the publisher, or author, for any damages, reparation, or monetary loss due to the information contained within this book. Either directly or indirectly.

Legal notice:

This book is copyright protected. This book is only for personal use. You cannot amend, distribute, sell, use, quote or paraphrase any part, or the content within this book, without the consent of the author or publisher.

Disclaimer Notice:

Please note the information contained within this document is for educational and entertainment purposes only. All effort has been executed to present accurate, up-to-date, and reliable, complete information, No warranties of any kind are declared or implied. Readers acknowledge that the author is not engaging in the rendering of legal, financial, medical, or professional advice. The content within this book has been derived from various sources. Please consult a licensed professional before attempting any techniques outlined in this book.

By reading this document, the reader agrees that under no circumstances is the author responsible for any loss, direct or indirect, which are incurred as a result of the use of the information contained within this document, including, but not limited to, errors, omissions, or inaccuracies.

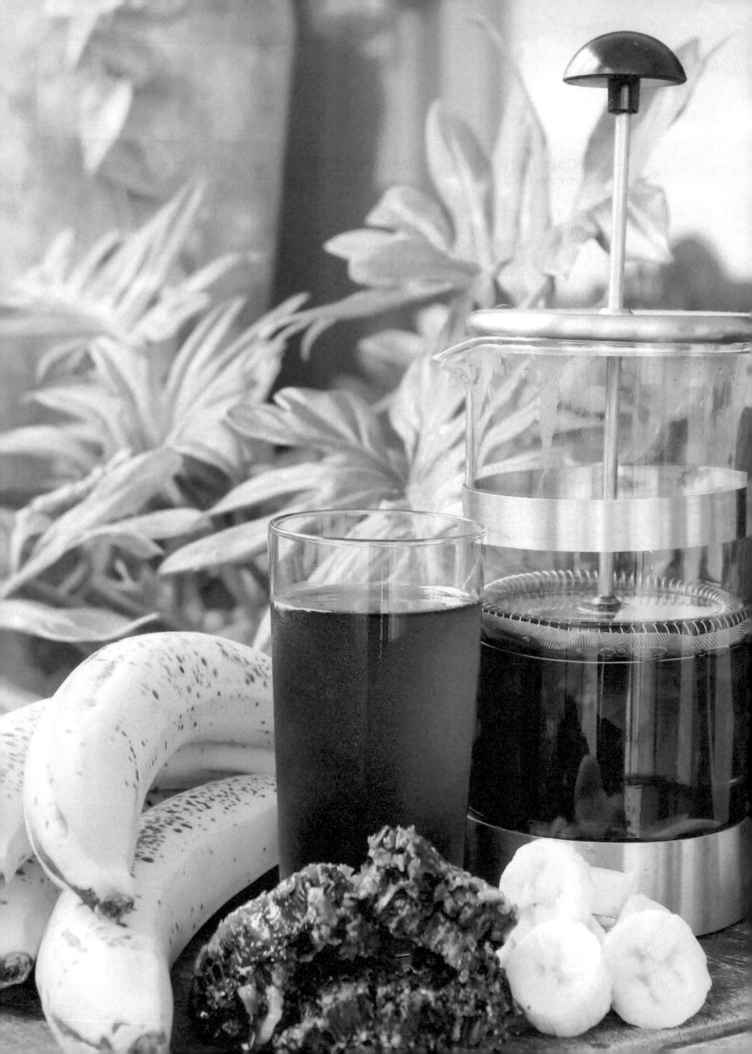

CONTENTS

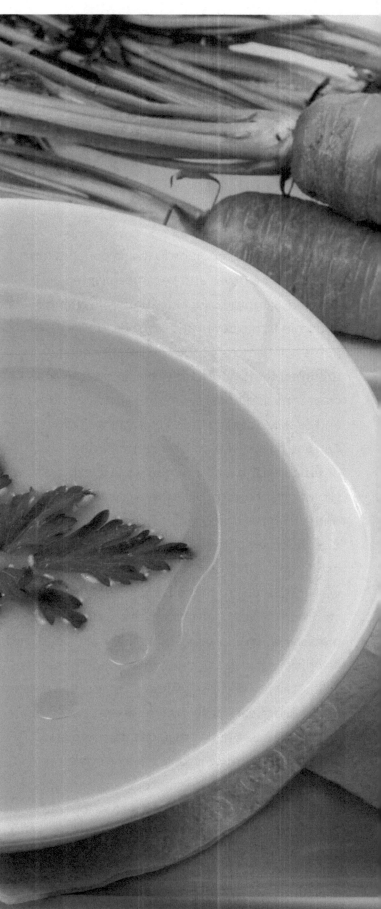

Diverticulitis Causes and Symptoms   5

Taking care of diverticulitis   9

Diverticulitis Diet Basics   11

- Foods to Avoid
- Foods to Eat

Steps of Diverticulitis Diet   12

Stage 1: The Clear Liquid Diet
Stage 2: Low-Fiber, Low-Residue Diet
Stage 3: The High-Fiber Diet

Foodchart   17

Recipes   18

Clear Liquid Diet   18

- Breakfast   18
- Lunch   28
- Dinner   38

Low Fiber, Low Residue Diet   45

- Breakfast   46
- Lunch   53
- Dinner   68

High Fiber Diet   81

- Breakfast   82
- Lunch   99
- Dinner   118

Meal Plans   136

Conclusion   142

Appendix 1: Recipe Index   144

Appendix 2: Measurement Conversion Chart   150

Introduction

Diverticulitis is a condition in which pouches form out of the colon wall and become inflamed or infected. Symptoms include sudden, lo crampswer abdominal pain, fever, and diarrhea. Unlike other forms of inflammatory bowel disease, such as Crohn's disease or ulcerative colitis, diverticulosis creates no additional symptoms such as weight loss and usually does not cause rectal bleeding.

Can you have diverticulitis without having diverticulosis? In order for someone to exhibit symptoms of diverticulitis there must first be an underlying medical condition known as diverticular disease. Diverticulosis is a term used to refer to the condition in which pouches form out of the colon wall and become inflamed or infected. The most common causes of diverticulosis are: diverticular disease (which can cause right-sided, left-sided, and colonic diverticula), Crohn's disease, and ulcerative colitis. Diverticular disease, however, is not necessary for people to exhibit symptoms of diverticulitis. In fact, some cases of diverticulosis go completely undetected because people have no symptoms other than having loose stool or being constipated. Diverticulitis, therefore, is not a disease but rather a complication of the medical condition known as diverticulosis.

There are two main forms of diverticulitis: left-sided and right-sided. Left-sided diverticulitis is usually caused by fecal matter moving through the colon and getting trapped in a pouch located near the spleen. This can cause pressure to build up in the area surrounding this pouch which causes pain or swelling. Additionally, when bacteria enters that pouch, it can cause an infection that can also cause pain or swelling around this area. Right-sided diverticulitis, on the other hand, is usually caused by fecal matter being trapped in a pouch located near where the colon and small intestine meet. This can cause pressure to build up near these pouches which also causes pain or swelling. Additionally, when bacteria enters this pouch it can cause an infection that can also cause pain or swelling around this area. Left-sided and right-sided diverticulitis are treated with dosages of antibiotics that are different depending on which side of the colon is affected.

Although diverticulitis is not life threatening, it does affect one's quality of life because it causes chronic abdominal discomfort and diarrhea (sometimes bloody). People with diverticular disease often have a hiatus hernia, which is an abnormal protrusion of the intestine through the abdominal wall or a weak spot in the abdominal wall. This condition can cause prolapse of organs such as the spleen, colon, bowel, and bladder into the abdominal cavity. These organs can then get stuck or become strangulated if they are not removed through surgery.

Although many people with diverticular disease do not exhibit symptoms that are severe enough to warrant medical attention, they still need to be treated as soon as possible due to them having a higher risk of developing other problems including colon cancer and diverticulitis.

When a diverticulitis diet is structured properly, it can help to reduce the risk of recurrence, prevent further inflammation and provide benefit to the gastrointestinal tract. This type of diet plan is usually very restrictive in nature; however, there are some exceptions. The key components to a diverticulitis diet include:

Surprisingly, the guidelines for healthy eating do not include much information on how to minimize the risk of conditions such as diverticulitis. The general recommendation is that individuals should eat a balanced diet that includes high fiber foods such as whole grains (e.g. bran cereal) and vegetables (e.g.,

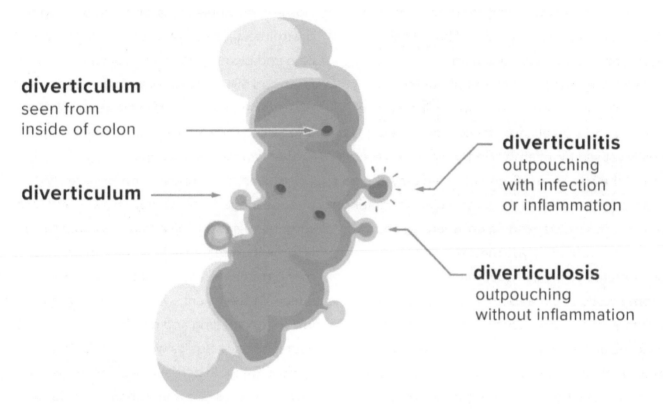

kale). These foods are recommended to help to relieve constipation and improve bowel movements. Eating a high fiber diet also helps to reduce carbohydrate cravings, which is important because most carbohydrates stimulate the production of gas in the large intestine. Individuals who experience significant gas production should cut down on their intake of beans, corn, and other grains that are difficult for the body to digest. However, whole grains are considered healthy for most people, even individuals with diverticulitis.

Diverticulitis Causes and Symptoms

Diverticula are tiny, bulging pockets that develop around the lining of the digestive system. They usually form around the regions of the lower large intestine, known as the colon. Diverticula is a common condition, especially among those over the age of 40. But they are rarely known to be problematic. Having diverticula means that you suffer from diverticulosis. When diverticulitis occurs, you become susceptible to symptoms, such as a substantial change in your typical bowel habits, nausea, fever, and abdominal pain.

In many cases, the pain brought about by diverticulitis is not extreme. However, it may be a nuisance and a great cause for concern. The pain is usually caused by inflammation, which often occurs around the area of the diverticula. Pain may also be induced by pressure on the diverticula or migrating enzyme pockets. Depending on where and how severe the problem is, you may experience concentrated or general abdominal pain.

In some cases, you may demonstrate alternate symptoms that are associated with diverticulitis. These include vomiting, diarrhea, nausea, and fever. Unfortunately, this condition is not evenly distributed among those who suffer from diverticulosis. Although diverticulitis does not automatically mean that you are prone to infection, it is possible. While this condition may be an isolated occurrence, it can also develop into a recurrent problem that will need treatment from time to time.

A sudden change in bowel movements often characterizes attacks that are brought about by diverticulitis.

Different Types of Diverticulitis
Diverticulosis

Diverticulosis is the several small pockets or bulges in the colon known as diverticula. These bulges are pretty harmless and do not require any form of treatment. Neither do they present symptoms. But, if care is not taken, diverticulosis could spiral into a more dangerous condition. Put, if diverticula are neither inflamed nor infected, the condition is known as diverticulosis. Research reveals that 80 percent of patients with diverticulosis present with no symptoms (Persons, 2019). Thus, since there is no symptom, treatments are unnecessary. However, in worse cases, diverticulosis triggers gastrointestinal symptoms such as abdominal pain and bloating. When this occurs, the condition is termed SUDD (symptomatic uncomplicated diverticular disease). When diverticulosis develops into SUDD, there's a 4% chance that it might further worsen diverticulitis.

Once diverticula appear, they never really disappear again unless they are removed through surgery. As a result, diverticulosis could last a lifetime if untreated. Albeit, the condition is manageable with some dietary adjustments. With adequate treatment, symptoms of diverticulosis, including bleeding and pain, could lessen within a couple of days. But it's worth noting that symptoms could persist or worsen in the event of severe illnesses or complications. People who consume lots of fiber in their day-to-day diets have a lower susceptibility to developing diverticular diseases. The American Dietetic Association posits that the daily recommended intake of fiber borders between 20 to 35 grams. But not all fibers are suitable for the body. For diverticulosis, you are better off getting your fiber from grains, fruits, and veggies. Your physician or dietician could also place you on a diet with unprocessed bran or specific fiber products. To improve your daily intake of fiber, undergo the process gradually. Additionally, it would help if you took lots of water to help bowel movements by improving bulk.

Doing this will help to reduce pressure when passing the bowel.

Diverticulitis

Diverticulitis only occurs due to infection and inflammation (swelling) in one or multiple diverticula. Meaning, for diverticulitis to occur, one must already have diverticulosis. Fever, nausea, and pain are some of the common symptoms of diverticulitis, among others. Unlike diverticulosis, diverticulitis is a graver condition with the potential to become dangerous over time. This condition, however, is treatable. For mild diverticulitis, antibiotics, changes in diet, and enough rest can help to cure symptoms. But recurring or severe diverticulitis may require surgical procedures.

These perforations stem from the constant strain and pressure caused by the movement of stool via the colon. Ruptures could also arise from abscesses, which are infected diverticula with pus, which could grow and ruin the tissues of the colon. If the bumps that appear on the colon are tiny and do not exceed the region, they could be cleared up with some antibiotic treatment. Otherwise, they might have to be drained to prevent further complications. However, large abscesses present even more significant problems and could worsen the condition due to the infection leaking out and contaminating the outer region of the colon.

An Infected Diverticula could also lead to scarring, resulting in total or partial blockage of the large intestine. When such intestinal obstruction occurs, it becomes difficult for the colon to manage bowel movement effectively. Hence, emergency surgical interventions are imperative.

Symptoms of Diverticulitis

There are many diverticulitis patients that do not experience daily symptoms outside of a flare. This, as you can imagine, makes diagnosis in difficult outside of routine tests for general digestive issues. This isn't the reality for all patients; however, some experience warning signs or symptoms including:

Severe Constipation

Constipation can become so severe in diverticulitis patients that it prevents the passage of both gas and stool through the large intestine, and hence, a person is unable to pass the unwanted nitrogenous wastes out of the body.

Severe Pain in the Abdomen

Some may argue that abdominal pain is the most frequent symptom as over 95% of patients experience cramps in the left lower portion of the abdomen. These cramps can vary from person to person, but has been generally described as an achy, dull, or even sharp pain in some cases. At times, this pain may radiate to the lower back. The pain is sudden and severe in most cases, but it can also be mild in some cases.

Fever

Many patients experience a light fever in the early stages of diverticulitis and though it isn't a defining factor it does suggest the presence of an underlying infection. It is often associated with altered bowel habits, chills or both.

Diverticular Bleeding

Though bleeding isn't common, it does occur in some patients. On the off chance that you have bleeding, it can be serious. Luckily, the bleeding in some cases may also stop on its own without requiring any form of treatment. Be that as it may, if you begin to experience any form of bleeding form your rectum, regardless of the amount, you should see a medical professional immediately.

To discover the site of the bleeding and stop it, a specialist may play out a colonoscopy. Your specialist may likewise utilize an automated tomography (CT) check or an angiogram to discover the bleeding site. An angiogram is a unique sort of x-beam in which your specialist strings a dainty, adaptable tube through an extensive corridor, frequently from your crotch, to the bleeding region.

Urinary Symptoms

Another symptom that is not as widely linked to diverticulitis is urinary tract issues. These can vary from a burning sensation during urination, frequent urination, and other urinary related issues due to the position of the bladder and colon in the body.

Nausea & Vomiting

Diverticulitis patients often suffer from indigestion related symptoms such nausea, vomiting and heart burn.

Diverticulitis when controlled often times doesn't severely affect your life outside of a flare. On the flip side, however, when the symptoms are left uncontrolled until it's too late, several more serious complications can pop up as a result. Including, but not limited to, intestinal perforation, fistula or abscess formation, peritonitis, bleeding and stricture (blockade).

These complications, however, are often rare and mainly in patients who already have a compromised or weak immune system, for example, those with previous underlying autoimmune or chronic illnesses such as AIDs, cancer, heart disease, and also diabetes. Or some patients who have been taking steroids for a long period.

Diverticular Disease Causes

A majority of the time, diverticulitis is caused by a large amount of waste in the lower part of your bowel due to disease, bacterial infection, physical trauma, or major change in diet. The enlarged pouch becomes inflamed and this can cause inflammation and bleeding into other organs within your abdomen. Diverticulitis can occur anywhere in the large intestine but causes symptoms such as gas pain under the ribs, fever, diarrhea that lasts for more than two weeks without improvement, and abdominal tenderness.

Causes of Diverticulitis

Diet and Intestinal Bacteria

About 90% of people with diverticulitis suffer from chronic constipation. For otherwise healthy patients, it is nearly always caused by a diet low in fiber, which can make the stool too large for the intestine to handle. Also, it's important to know that a large number of people have developed diverticulosis-like symptoms on an all-meat diet. This condition is known as "rabbit starvation" and has been documented throughout history in areas where rabbits are the primary food source.

Past Medical History

People who have had an intestinal perforation or surgery for colorectal cancer are also at a higher risk of developing diverticulosis and diverticulitis.

Age

People under the age of 60 have a higher risk of developing diverticulitis than people over the age of 60.

Hemorrhoids and Clogged Pouches

The development of the condition is in part caused by hemorrhoids, also known as piles, which are enlarged veins in the bottom chamber of your rectum. People with these conditions may have lower levels of internal pressure that can lead to pouching or squeezing off small sacs from within the large intestine. It's also possible for a blockage to form when blood collects inside a small blood vein or artery and leaks into that sac and causes it to swell.

Family History

If your family has been affected by diverticulosis or diverticulitis, you're at a higher risk for developing it than someone who doesn't have this history. It is important to mention that most people with this condition will never develop diverticulitis.

Pregnancy

During pregnancy, a woman's body releases a hormone that causes the colon to relax and allows even small particles to travel more easily through it. This can cause a pouching effect within the large intestine, which can lead to diverticulitis.

Physical Trauma

Fecal matter can become trapped in partial obstruction and this can cause an inflammatory reaction.

Symptoms of Diverticulitis

Abdominal Pain

Diverticulitis pain is often located near the belly button and can sometimes move to either side of the belly. It may resemble a tummy ache, but unlike an upset stomach, it comes and goes.

Fever

You may also experience a fever, which can be mild or high. Your doctor will need to understand if you have ever been diagnosed with diverticulitis, as this condition requires immediate medical attention.

Bleeding

Diverticula can rupture and bleed into neighboring organs like the colon or bladder, or into the abdominal cavity itself. It's not uncommon for some people to pass blood in their stools without knowing that it came from their intestines. Throbbing pain, fever, and nausea can point to an intestinal rupture.

Diarrhea

Diverticulitis can cause diarrhea that is sometimes watery with mucus or blood, according to the National Digestive Diseases Information Clearinghouse (NDDIC). You should see your doctor if you have diarrhea that lasts for more than two weeks without improvement.

Weight Loss

Weight loss and eating a low-fiber diet can lead to diverticulosis and many people may not know until there's a complication like diverticulitis. You need to bring any of these symptoms to your doctor's attention as soon as you notice them because they may be pointing to another serious disease.

Stool Changes

You may notice fluctuations in your stools, such as more than usual mucus, which may indicate a buildup of bacteria or inflammatory material. It is also possible to have a blockage in your intestines that can lead to constipation and cause this extra mucus.

Other symptoms include abdominal swelling that persists after you've passed stool, difficulty breathing or swallowing, the urge to defecate but not being able to do so, and blood in your stool.

Taking care of diverticulitis

By now you know that changing your diet is one of the best preventive measures you can take to avoid further flare-ups. However, there are nondietary steps to take in combination with changes to your current eating habits. Keep in mind that you should always consult your doctor before pursuing any new tactics that may affect your digestive and overall health.

Probiotics

These supplements contain certain strains of bacteria that have been proven to alleviate abdominal pain, bloating, constipation, and diarrhea and can help improve the function of your gut's natural microorganisms. However, it's important to talk to your doctor when choosing a probiotic, as they're not all made the same. For example, most probiotics contain lactose, which is not a good choice if you're sensitive to dairy. Studies on diverticulitis and probiotics have shown promising outcomes, but more research is needed before the relationship is considered clinically significant.

Prebiotics

Prebiotics are a type of dietary fiber that helps feed healthy bacteria in the large intestine. They occur naturally in many foods, such as bananas, barley, apples, leeks, asparagus, chicory, Jerusalem artichokes, garlic, onions, wheat, oats, flaxseed, oat bran, jicama root, seaweed, and soybeans.

Antibiotics

Though antibiotics have often been used to help reduce pain, infection, and fever in moderate to severe cases of diverticulitis, newer research is leaning toward reducing the length of antibiotic usage. A 2014 study published in Drug, Healthcare and Patient Safety comparing four- and seven-day courses of antibiotics found that they had equivalent outcomes, implying that diverticulitis sufferers do not need to be on antibiotics for extended periods of time.

Surgery

If you've had many flare-ups, the damage to your colon may be too advanced to see improvement from medication or diet, and your doctor may recommend surgery to remove the affected area. There are a few options they may consider:

Simple colostomy: During this procedure, the surgeon pulls a small section of the colon out through an incision in the abdomen and attaches a pouch that will collect waste. This allows your bowel an extended period to heal without any stool moving through it. If your colon heals well from the surgery, the colostomy may be only temporary.

Bowel resection: This is the removal of the infected part of the colon, followed by reconnection of the bowel. The surgeon cuts away the damaged area and reconnects the intestine, sometimes to the rectum.

Both a bowel resection and a simple colostomy can be done open or closed.

Open: The surgeon makes a 6- to 8-inch incision in your abdomen to see a full view of the affected digestive tract.

Closed (or laparoscopic): The surgeon makes a very small incision (typically less than 1 centimeter) and inserts a small tube with a camera and surgical instruments through it to perform the surgery.

Lifestyle Changes

One reason diverticulitis may be so common in North America is because many North Americans eat a fairly low-fiber diet and lead more sedentary lifestyles. Diverticulitis is unheard of in Africa or the Middle East, where the typical diet relies heavily on high-fiber foods such as whole grains and legumes. It's no surprise then that increasing your fiber intake (when you are not experiencing a flare-up) is a good way to keep diverticulitis symptoms at bay. But it's not the only lifestyle change that can help.

Physical Activity

For adults age 18 or older, doctors recommend getting at least 150 minutes of moderate to vigorous aerobic physical activity per week, in increments of at least 10 minutes at a time. They also suggest including muscle- and bone-strengthening exercises one to two days per week. Not only does regular physical activity help reduce your weight and increase muscle formation, it has proven to be beneficial in helping the bowels move stool through the body.

Hydration

As you increase your fiber intake, it's also important to stay hydrated to aid digestion. The average recommended water consumption per day is 2 to 2½ liters for women and 2½ to 3 liters for men. Increasing your fluid intake will help prevent dehydration, which can be a problem if you are having frequent loose bowel movements. It also protects against constipation, which is a side effect of increased fiber without proper hydration.

Losing Weight

Obesity has been shown to increase complications with diverticulitis, namely because of its link to chronic inflammation. It also can contribute to your risk of developing several other digestive diseases, such as liver scarring (cirrhosis), gallstone disease, gastroesophageal reflux disease (GERD), colon cancer, esophageal cancer, and pancreatic cancer. But there's good news: Losing just 5 to 10 percent of your body weight can decrease your risk of complications.

Quitting Tobacco Products

Along with increasing your risk of lung cancer, tobacco products have been shown to decrease blood flow to vital organs, which can cause tissues to die and raise your risk for infection. But quitting can have immediate benefits: Studies have shown that the stomach and lining of the small intestine will return to normal within a few hours of quitting tobacco use. Foregoing tobacco products for the long term can reverse some of the more serious harmful effects tobacco has on the digestive system as well.

Diverticulitis Diet Basics

Some Mild cases of diverticulitis are treated with antibiotics but those suffering from severe diverticulitis may have to rest eating by mouth and may adopt a special type of diet until the bleeding and pain subside. The Diverticulitis Diet is a highly recommended diet that can help alleviate acute diverticulitis. Although this diet is supposed to be short-term, it can bring about huge relief among individuals who suffer from diverticulitis. Moreover, it can also be used by people who have a sensitive digestive system.

While the Diverticulitis Diet is designed for people who suffer from diverticulitis, people who suffer from other digestive distress can benefit from the Diverticulitis diet. Moreover, normal healthy individuals who also want to give their digestive tract enough rest can benefit from this diet.

Foods to Avoid

Red and processed meat

Eating a diet strong in red and processed meats may increase your chance of having diverticulitis. A diet very rich in fruits, vegetables, and whole grains may help to lower the risk of heart disease.

High-sugar and high-fat foods

The typical Western diet is high in fat, sugar, but low in fiber. As a result, a person's risk of having diverticulitis may increase.

Foods high in FODMAPs

Some persons with irritable bowel syndrome benefit from following a low FODMAP diet (IBS). Some persons with diverticulitis may benefit from following a low FODMAP diet (IBS)..

FODMAPs are carbohydrate types. Fermentable oligosaccharides, disaccharides, monosaccharide's, and polyols are all included.

People that are following this type of diet avoid foods that are rich in FODMAPS. This includes, for example, the following foods:

- Apples, pears, and plums are examples of fruits.
- Fermented foods, such as sauerkraut or kimchi beans dairy foods, such as milk, yogurt, and ice cream
- Legumes
- Meals with a lot of Trans fats
- Cabbage with soy sauce
- Brussels sprouts

- Garlic and onions

Foods to Eat

Clear liquid diet for diverticulitis

A clear liquid diet may be recommended if a diverticulitis flare-up is severe or necessitates surgery. "You graduate from clear liquids to a low-fiber diet after a day or two.

You can eat the following foods on a clear liquid diet:

- Broths that are clear (not soup).
- Juices that are clear and pulp-free (such as apple and cranberry juice)
- Popsicles
- Water

Low-fiber diet for diverticulitis

Eat a low-fiber, or GI soft, diet for milder forms of diverticulitis. Depending on the severity of the flare-up, a low-fiber diet restricts fiber consumption to 8 to 1/2 grams per day.

Low-fiber foods to consider include:

Grains: Lovers of white spaghetti and white bread, delight! Low-fiber alternatives include these, as well as white rice and white crackers.

Starches with low fiber content: Remove your peeler from the drawer. Skinless potatoes are one alternative. You can mash, roast, or bake them. Low-fiber cereals like corn flakes and puffed rice cereal receive a thumbs up.

Protein can be found in eggs and egg whites, tofu, beef, and seafood. The best options are shredded chicken, lean ground beef, and soft baked salmon.

Fruits: Fruits contain a lot of fiber, so be cautious when eating them. Soft, ripe cantaloupe and honeydew, as well as canned fruits like peaches and pears, applesauce, ripe bananas, and soft, ripe cantaloupe and honeydew, are also wonderful options. Because you don't eat the skin, there isn't a lot of fiber. The skins contain insoluble fiber, which can irritate irritated polyps.

Cottage cheese and Greek yogurt are major winners if you're recovering from a flare-up: They're high in protein, calcium, and other minerals, but they're also deficient in fiber. If you're unwell, they're also soft, wet, and easier to swallow. There's also milk and cheese to choose from.

Steps of Diverticulitis Diet

The diverticulitis diet is a special diet meant to heal any existing diverticulitis in the digestive system and prevent it from coming back.

The first step in healing diverticulitis is to eliminate all inflammatory foods from your diet. This means that you should no longer drink milk. If you are already lactose intolerant, reintroduce dairy foods such as plain yogurt, but do not consume cow's milk for the rest of your life. This will dramatically improve your digestive health and lead to a higher quality of life after diverticulitis is gone.

Dairy products can also be reintroduced one at a time into your diet in small amounts to see how well you tolerate them. If you can accept it, go for it. If not, skip it.

Sugar is another inflammatory food that should be removed from your diet. Sugar can be institute in so many foods that you will have to start reading labels and learn how to spot it independently. It is also disguised under many names, including corn syrup, high fructose corn syrup, sucrose, and dextrose. However, if you stick with fresh fruits and vegetables, your sugar intake should be minimal or nonexistent.

Refined grains are a category of food that should also be tossed out of your diet for a while. This means that you should conduct clear white bread, rice, pasta, and pastries for as long as it takes to heal the inflammation in your digestive tract. If you are unable to wean yourself off these foods for now, at least cut out all of the grains from your diet until the diverticulitis is gone.

Dairy, sugar, and refined grains are inflammatory foods that must be eliminated from your diet to get rid of diverticulitis.

Fiber, which is institute in foods like fruits, vegetables, and whole grains, is an integral part of staying healthy and can help protect the digestive tract from further attacks of diverticulitis. It has been shown to significantly reduce the severity of inflammatory bowel diseases such as Crohn's disease and ulcerative colitis.

Stage 1: The Clear Liquid Diet

Just as the name implies, a clear liquid diet is a diet that consists entirely of clear liquids.

These liquids include broth, water, juices with no pulp, and gelatin (the plain one). The liquid may be colored, but they're clear once you can see through them.

A clear liquid diet is usually prescribed by the doctor when the patient has to undergo certain medical procedures involving the gastrointestinal tract, like colonoscopies.

A clear liquid diet may also be recommended to relieve you of some digestive disorders, such as diarrhea, diverticulitis, and Crohn's disease. It is also recommended after some types of surgery. Why? Because your digestive system can easily digest this diet, and because they're mostly liquid, they help to clean out your digestive tract.

A clear liquid diet for the treatment of diverticulitis is advised post-surgery or a stage exceeding acute complicated diverticulitis. Post-surgery, the abdominal region, particularly the intestinal region and any area that has been operated in and around the colon experience a strong meltdown in their ability to function. This slowdown in bodily functions and the existing wounds make it difficult for them to digest food and process it as they normally do. Any added pressure on these areas because of any kinds of heavy foods may cause an outbreak of infection and lead to the persistence of the condition.

The liquid phases of diverticulitis diet last for 8 to 10 days. The liquid phases of the diverticulitis diet are only recommended when patients have had their ileostomy bags removed. If you have not had your ileostomy bags removed, speak with a doctor about the best course of action.

Goals

The following are the goals of adhering to a clear liquid diet:

- Giving proper rest to the intestinal region.
- By intake of cleared liquid foods, the abdomen is saved from so much stress. The digestion becomes quicker and smoother. This allows the intestine to be at rest while the operated region steps back to its original functioning.
- Strengthen the intestines for digestion.

A clear liquid diet acts as a cleanser that washes the abdominal and intestinal region of any undesired bacteria and enzymes that are causing the condition to persist. Regular intake of clear liquid diets will flush off all the toxicities and create a healing environment more acceptable to nutrition intake.

Easy Excretion

After the diverticulitis surgery, the colon and rectum are usually in bad shape. The pouches in the colon are still in recovery mode and hence passing of the stool becomes a problem. A clear liquid diet ensures the passing of excreta in the most painless way possible. Since most of it is liquid part and contains water, a substantial amount of excretion occurs through mostly effortless urination. And hence protects the patient from further damage.

Maintenance of Hydration

Most surgical treatments rely on heavy antibiotics post-treatment. These drain the hydration out of the body making it highly deficient in water content. One of the aims of liquid diets is to replenish the body of all the lost water content. Along with the water content, such diets also replenish the electrolyte and vitamin levels in the body bringing back sodium, potassium levels to the required ranges.

Clear liquid diets also improve overall body health particularly targeting the gut region that may be prone to leaky gut syndrome. The cellulite levels may also be reduced significantly. All of this eventually helps the digestive tract to heal faster and function better.

What to Eat and Avoid on the Clear Fluids Diet

What to Eat

- Clear, fat-free broth
- Dairy-free coffee or tea (no creamer or milk)
- Boost clear or boost juice
- Gelatin
- Pulp-free juice
- Sports drinks
- Pulp-free fruit ice pops

What to Avoid

- All solid foods
- Soda
- Fruit skins, seeds, or pulp
- Peanut butter

Stage 2: Low-Fiber, Low-Residue Diet

Diets that are low in fiber and residue may be recommended for patients who have ulcerative colitis, diverticulitis, bowel inflammation, and Crohn's disease. You may also use these diets when you experiencing a narrowing of the bowel, before or after surgery of the digestive system. Low-residue and low-fiber diets cause stool to move slowly down the intestines. It also decreases the amount of stool in the intestines. By so doing, it prevents blockage.

Plants are the major source of dietary fiber. Humans cannot digest fiber. Residue refers to the fiber, and other substances, present in the colon after digestion. A low-fiber diet does not contain up to 15 grams of fiber per day. It also does not contain foods that bulk your stool. Basically, a low-residue diet is a low-fiber diet with some restrictions.

You can get the Recommended Dietary Allowances from both low-residue and low-fiber diets if you choose the right foods. But note that long-term use of a low-residue or low-fiber diet may cause a folic acid or vitamin C deficiency.

A low-residue (or low-fiber) diet acts as the reintroduction phase, after your flare-up symptoms have mostly passed but before your body is ready for high-fiber foods. "Residue"

The low fiber phases are also known as hunger periods in which you abstain from eating any food that contains a lot of fiber as well as high-fiber foods. The low fiber diet is usually recommended for 10 to 20 days,

What to Eat

- Coffee, tea; decaffeinated coffee; cereal beverage; carbonated beverage.
- Any tender meat, fish, or fowl; eggs; cottage cheese; mild cheese; cream-style peanut butter.
- Butter; margarine; cream; vegetable oil; crisp bacon; avocado; gravy; cream sauce; mildly seasoned salad dressings.
- Milk and milk beverages; yogurt made with allowed fruits.
- All juices, cooked or canned fruits: applesauce, apricots, cherries, peaches, pears, pineapple;

raw fruit: banana and citrus fruit only without membrane.
- Cooked mild-flavored vegetables: asparagus, green or wax beans, beets, peas, carrots, spinach, mushrooms, pumpkin, tomato juice, squash.
- Broth; bouillon; cream or canned soups made with foods allowed.
- Gelatin, sherbet; ice cream; custard; pudding; cake; cookies; pastry, Sugar; honey; jelly; candy. Any with coconut, nuts, or disallowed fruit, all others.

What to Avoid
- Fried; highly seasoned meats (such as cold cuts); strong cheese.
- All other soups.
- All other cooked vegetables; all raw vegetables.
- All other cooked fruits; all other fresh fruit; dried fruits.
- Olives; nuts, highly seasoned salad dressings.

Stage 3: The High-Fiber Diet

This is the final stage where the diverticulitis condition has almost healed and the patient is on track to adopt a normal eating lifestyle. Though the diverticulitis condition has healed, it is still important that the patient monitors his diet for days to come. This will eliminate any possibility of reoccurrence of the disease.

Goals

Goals of a high fiber diet are to bring back a patient in his normal and healthy eating routine. It aims at enabling the patient to resume his daily life post-treatment of diverticulitis. The fiber intake is advised to be monitored carefully to not overburden the intestine all of a sudden. Only when a low residue diet shows positive results, does a patient shift to a high fiber diet.

Guidelines for High-Fiber Diet

A high-fiber diet should be started only after the body adapts to fiber intake through a low residue diet.

High-fiber diets should be well complemented by the intake of water and other fluids. The water makes absorption of fiber easier and hence aids digestion. The fibrous intake should be controlled in portion size. Just because the patient is allowed to take up an increased amount of foods, does not mean the portion size does not matter. High-fiber diets should be well calculated in portions and only about 25-30 grams of fiber should be eaten on daily basis. Anything more than this will again cause problems of constipation and poor digestion.

Since most of the diverticulitis condition is cured by this stage, it is quite likely that a patient will fall back to his previous eating habits. It is strongly advised that patients keep off anything that got them to have the disease in the first place.

The general consensus is that this phase should last between two and six weeks. This will typically equate to something like 30 grams of fiber per day.

Foods to Include and Exclude in High-Fiber Diet
- **Bread and starches**: High-fiber diets may include finely grounded whole grains like wheat, barley, etc. Pasta, noodles, and rice can be eaten normally as well starches from potatoes, wheat, graham, and rye can be included in the diet. It is still desirable to keep off refined flours that may cause indigestion.
- **Meat and protein**: Soft tender meats like fish and slightly stiffer meats like chicken, eggs, proteins in the form of lentils, cheese particularly cottage cheese are advised to be eaten regularly. Red meat is to be avoided at all costs since it is very high in fat and causes severe indigestion.

- **Vegetables**: All vegetables can be included in the diet especially the green leafy ones that have adequate fiber. However, avoid gas-inducing vegetables like cauliflower, broccoli, cabbage, radish, and kale.
- **Fruits**: A high-fiber diet may include all fruits like apples, oranges, peaches, pears, grapes, watermelon, melon, and papaya. Almost all fruits work pretty well since there is no restriction on fiber intake. Dried fruits, whether cooked or raw still remain an exception.
- **Dairy products**: Milk and milk products, especially yogurt is very good for the cure of diverticulitis. Yogurts blended with fruits are a good way to keep the gut function under control.
- **Fats**: Fats from red meats pose serious issues in a diverticulitis diet. Olive oils are denser forms of oil that again should be avoided until complete recovery. Any other kinds of fat like butter, margarine, cream fat, etc. are all fine to be used in a high-fiber diverticulitis guide.
- **Sweets and desserts**: All sweets can be eaten normally with a condition that they are free from nuts and dried fruits. Honey and sugar can be used for sweetness. Candies and fruit jellies are another way to satiate the sweet tooth while recovering from diverticulitis disease.

It is important to note, however, that you do not want to jump directly from a significantly low-fiber diet (such as a clear fluid diet) to a high-fiber diet, as this will do more harm to your colon than good. It is always best to ease into any stage of the plan that requires an increase in your fiber intake. Aim to increase your fiber intake by 2 to 4 grams per week until you reach the recommended amount for your age and biology. Bear in mind that as you increase your fiber, you also need to increase your water intake to help move the fiber through your intestinal tract.

Phases	Days	What to Avoid	What to Eat
Clear Liquid Diet	8-10 days	• All solid foods • Soda • Fruit skins, seeds, or pulp • Peanut butter	• Clear, fat-free broth • Dairy-free coffee or tea (no creamer or milk) • Boost clear or boost juice • Gelatin • Pulp-free juice • Sports drinks • Pulp-free fruit ice pops
Low-Fiber, Low-Residue Diet	10 - 20 days	• Coffee, tea; decaffeinated coffee; cereal beverage; carbonated beverage. • Any tender meat, fish, or fowl; eggs; cottage cheese; mild cheese; cream-style peanut butter. • Butter; margarine; cream; vegetable oil; crisp bacon; avocado; gravy; cream sauce; mildly seasoned salad dressings. • Milk and milk beverages; yogurt made with allowed fruits. • All juices, cooked or canned fruits: applesauce, apricots, cherries, peaches, pears, pineapple; raw fruit: banana and citrus fruit only without membrane. • Cooked mild-flavored vegetables: asparagus, green or wax beans, beets, peas, carrots, spinach, mushrooms, pumpkin, tomato juice, squash. • Broth; bouillon; cream or canned soups made with foods allowed. • Gelatin, sherbet; ice cream; custard; pudding; cake; cookies; pastry, Sugar; honey; jelly; candy. Any with coconut, nuts, or disallowed fruit, all others.	• Fried; highly seasoned meats (such as cold cuts); strong cheese. • All other soups. • All other cooked vegetables; all raw vegetables. • All other cooked fruits; all other fresh fruit; dried fruits. • Olives; nuts, highly seasoned salad dressings.
High-Fiber Diet	2 - 6 weeks	• Refined flours • Red meat • Cauliflower, broccoli, cabbage, radish, and kale. • Dried fruits	• Whole grains like wheat, barley, pasta, noodles, and rice, potato • Soft tender meats like fish and slightly stiffer meats like chicken, eggs, proteins in the form of lentils • All vegetables, especially the green leafy ones that have adequate fiber • All fruits like apples, oranges, peaches, pears, grapes, watermelon, melon, and papaya. • Milk and milk products

CLEAR LIQUID DIET

BREAKFAST

1. GINGER PEACH SMOOTHIE

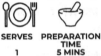

SERVES 1 | **PREPARATION TIME** 5 MINS | **COOKING TIME** 5 MINS | **TOTAL TIME** 10 MINS

INGREDIENTS:
- 2 ripe, juicy peaches, (you can use frozen peaches, but if you do, use a fresh banana and not a frozen one)
- 1 medium frozen banana (fresh or frozen)
- ¾ cup (180 mls) non-dairy milk
- 1 tablespoon maple syrup (optional - add to taste or not at all)
- 1 approx 2½ inches long stick fresh ginger, roughly x ½inch wide
- Or ¼ to ½ teaspoon ground ginger

DIRECTIONS:
1. Remove the pits from the peaches and combine them with the remaining ingredients in a blender. I recommend using only half of the fresh ginger or 14 teaspoons of ground ginger to begin.
2. Blend until smooth, then taste it. If you want a stronger flavor, add a little more ginger.
3. Serve right away.

NUTRITION FACTS:
calories: 337 |carbs: 72 g | protein: 9 g | fat: 4 g | cholesterol: 186 mg

2. PERSIMMON SMOOTHIE

SERVES 1 | **PREPARATION TIME** 5 MINS | **COOKING TIME** 0 MINS | **TOTAL TIME** 5 MINS

INGREDIENTS:
- 2 medium ripe persimmon
- 1 medium frozen banana
- 1 cup dairy-free milk
- About 10 cashews; if you don't have a high-powered blender, soak the cashew in hot water for 5 minutes before adding to the blender. See notes for cashew alternatives.
- ¼ teaspoon cinnamon, add a little more if you prefer a stronger cinnamon taste
- 1 tablespoon maple syrup

DIRECTIONS:
1. Remove and discard the persimmon leaves, then chop each fruit into a few pieces. Blend them, together with the remaining ingredients except for the maple syrup, in a blender until smooth.
2. Use the blender to give it a brief taste and, if required, add the maple syrup. After adding it, give it a brisk 5-second mix before serving.

NUTRITION FACTS:
calories: 298 |carbs: 41 g | protein: 11 g | fat: 12 g | cholesterol: 121 mg

3. CRANBERRY SMOOTHIE

SERVES 1 | **PREPARATION TIME** 5 MINS | **COOKING TIME** 5 MINS | **TOTAL TIME** 10 MINS

INGREDIENTS:
- 2 large kale leaves, washed with stems removed. Use a couple of handfuls of baby kale instead for a milder kale flavor
- 1 large apple, cored (no need to peel unless you want to).
- 1 tablespoon chia
- 2 teaspoons ground flax or whole flax
- 1 - 2 tablespoons maple syrup
- ½ medium lemon, juice only
- 180mls / ¾ cup plant-based milk, add up to a ¼ cup more to thin if you prefer it that way
- 5 ice cubes, optional but will make it colder and a bit thicker
- 1 tablespoon almond butter, optional - it's great with or without

DIRECTIONS:
1. Blend all of the ingredients in a blender until smooth. On my blendtec, I use the smoothie option.
2. Check the sweetness and, if required, add a bit more maple syrup.
3. Serve right away.

NUTRITION FACTS:
calories: 319 |carbs: 63 g | protein: 9 g | fat: 7 g | cholesterol: 266 mg

4. KALE APPLE SMOOTHIE

Serves: 2 | Preparation Time: 5 mins | Cooking Time: 5 mins | Total Time: 10 mins

INGREDIENTS:
- 2 large kale leaves, washed with stems removed. Use a couple of handfuls of baby kale instead for a milder kale flavor
- 1 large apple, cored (no need to peel unless you want to).
- 1 tablespoon chia
- 2 teaspoons ground flax or whole flax
- 1 - 2 tablespoons maple syrup
- ½ medium lemon, juice only
- 180mls / ¾ cup plant-based milk, add up to a ¼ cup more to thin if you prefer it that way
- 5 ice cubes, optional but will make it colder and a bit thicker
- 1 tablespoon almond butter, optional - it's great with or without

DIRECTIONS:
1. Blend all of the ingredients in a blender until smooth. On my blendtec, I use the smoothie option.
2. Check the sweetness and, if required, add a bit more maple syrup.
3. Serve right away.

NUTRITION FACTS:
calories: 319 |carbs: 63 g | protein: 9 g | fat: 7 g | cholesterol: 266 mg

5. GLOWING SKIN SMOOTHIE

Serves: 2 | Preparation Time: 5 mins | Cooking Time: 5 mins | Total Time: 10 mins

INGREDIENTS:
- ¼ cup cashew pieces or 1 very heaping ¼ cup of whole ones about 38g
- 1 cup | 240mls water or coconut water for an extra skin boost!
- 1 medium banana
- 1 very heaping cup frozen mango pieces around 140g, see recipe notes if you only have fresh mango
- 1 tablespoon chia, optional
- ⅛ teaspoon vanilla bean powder or ½ teaspoon vanilla extract
- ½ teaspoon ground cardamon
- ¼ teaspoon ground turmeric
- ⅛ teaspoon ground ginger or a small piece of fresh ginger
- 1 tablespoon of maple syrup or 1 large medjool date

DIRECTIONS:
1. If you don't have a high-powered blender, soak the cashew in boiling water for 15 minutes or cold water for 2 hours (this technique will maintain the nutrients), then drain.
2. Blend the cashew with the water in a blender until smooth. You've just created cashew milk!
3. Add the other ingredients and mix until smooth.
4. Serve with a decorative sprinkling of cardamon and turmeric if desired.

NUTRITION FACTS:
calories: 342 |carbs: 70 g | protein: 8 g | fat: 15 g | cholesterol: 82 mg

6. CRANBERRY SAUCE

Serves: 16 | Preparation Time: 5 mins | Cooking Time: 15 mins | Total Time: 20 mins

INGREDIENTS:
- 24 oz / 680 g fresh or frozen cranberries
- ½ cup / 100 g sugar, granulated white or cane sugar is best
- ½ cup / 120 ml maple syrup (real, natural maple syrup, not pancake syrup)
- ⅓ cup / 80 mls vegan red wine or port, or orange juice for an alcohol-free alternative
- 1 large orange, zest and juice of
- 1 medium cinnamon stick
- 1 approx 3-inch piece of fresh rosemary

DIRECTIONS:

To make on the stovetop
1. 1Wash the cranberries and remove any that are soft. 1 cup of them should be set aside, and the rest should be combined with everything else in a medium saucepan. Cook, frequently stirring, over medium heat until the sauce thickens and becomes jammy and the cranberries break down. Usually, it takes approximately 15 minutes.
2. Remove the rosemary and cinnamon stick from the pan and set aside. Take a quick taste, but be careful because it will be extremely hot. If you want to add more sugar, do so now because it will dissolve in the heat. But keep in mind that it's intended to taste tart. Its purpose is to cut through the richness of your holiday fare.
3. Stir in the cranberries that have been set aside. The residual heat will cook them sufficiently before the sauce cools, giving them a good texture.
4. Allow cooling completely before transferring to sterilized jars or freezer-safe containers.

To make in an instant pot
1. Wash the cranberries and remove any that are soft. Scoop out approximately 1 cup and set aside till the end. Place the remaining ingredients in the instant pot.
2. Stir in the sugar, maple syrup, red wine, orange juice, and zest. On top, place the cinnamon stick and rosemary.
3. Close the vent and replace the cover on the instant pot. Cook for 3 minutes on high pressure before allowing the pressure to naturally release. Open the lid once the pin has dropped. Don't be alarmed if it appears frothy and unappealing. Remove the cinnamon stick and rosemary, and then stir in the saved cranberries. The remaining heat is sufficient to cook them. Stir everything together thoroughly. It now appears to be in good condition. Take a short sip. Take cautious since it will be quite hot. If you find it too sour, add a bit of extra sugar now since it will dissolve in the heat. But keep in mind that a little acidity is excellent since it pairs well with your rich holiday meals.
4. Allow cooling completely before using. At this stage, the lid can be on or off, although it will cool faster with the cover off. Decant into jars or freezer-safe containers once cold.

NUTRITION FACTS:
calories: 74 |carbs: 18 g | protein: 1 g | fat: 1 g | cholesterol: 80 mg

7. CHOCOLATE TAHINI PUMPKIN SMOOTHIE

Serves: 1 | Preparation Time: 5 mins | Cooking Time: 0 mins | Total Time: 5 mins

INGREDIENTS:
- 1 frozen banana
- 1 tablespoon cocoa
- 8 tablespoons | ½ cup pumpkin puree canned or fresh
- 1 slightly heaping tablespoon tahini
- 2 tablespoons maple syrup
- 180mls | ¾ cup non-dairy milk

DIRECTIONS:
1. Add all ingredients to a blender.
2. Blend until completely smooth.
3. Serve immediately.

8. CARAMEL SAUCE

SERVES: 2 | PREPARATION TIME: 5 MINS | COOKING TIME: 5 MINS | TOTAL TIME: 10 MINS

INGREDIENTS:
- 100g | 1/2 cup coconut sugar (sometimes called coconut palm sugar (i have not tried this with any other sugar, so i can't guarantee it will work as well if you make a sub)
- 2 tablespoons water
- 2 tablespoons tahini (see recipe note)
- 2 tablespoons vegan butter or coconut oil (solid measurement)
- 1/8 - 1/4 teaspoon salt (add to taste)

DIRECTIONS:
1. In a saucepan, combine the coconut sugar and water.
2. Cook over medium heat until the sugar has fully dissolved and the mixture is just beginning to bubble. Don't stir!! Swirl the pan a little if necessary. It will take no more than two to three minutes. If you leave it unattended for too long, it will quickly burn.
3. Take the pan off the heat and stir in the tahini, salt, and vegan butter or coconut oil. Stir vigorously until everything is fully incorporated. It's natural to see a few bright specks through it. If you're having problems getting it to come together, place it back over low heat for 30 seconds or so.

NUTRITION FACTS:
calories: 195 |carbs: 25 g | protein: 1 g | fat: 10 g | cholesterol: 156 mg

9. LEMON CHEESECAKE SMOOTHIE

SERVES: 4 | PREPARATION TIME: 3 MINS | COOKING TIME: 2 MINS | TOTAL TIME: 5 MINS

INGREDIENTS:
- 1 medium juicy lemon
- 1 cup (240 mls) light canned coconut milk
- 1/4 heaping cup (50 grams) cooked chickpeas
- 1 to 2 medjool dates
- 1/4 cup (25 grams) chopped pecan measured in pieces, not whole
- 1 cup (150 grams) frozen mango pieces
- 1/4 teaspoon ground turmeric
- 1/4 teaspoon salt
- 1/2 teaspoon apple cider vinegar
- 1 tablespoon maple syrup optional

DIRECTIONS:
1. To begin, zest the lemon. Blend the lemon zest, then remove the remaining peel and pith (the white stuff) from the lemon. I do this by cutting both sharp ends of the lemon and then standing it up on the board. Then, with a sharp knife, i sliced all the way around it, just deep enough to remove the pith while leaving the flesh intact.
2. After that, place the entire lemon in the blender and remove the pith and peel.
3. Except for the maple syrup, combine all of the remaining ingredients in a mixing bowl.
4. Blend until the mixture is totally smooth. It yields a thick smoothie. If you like it a little thinner, add a little extra coconut milk or a drop of water to thin it out.
5. If you want a little extra sweetness, add a little more maple syrup. It goes well with maple syrup. Blend for a second on low to disperse, then pour into a glass and serve.

NUTRITION FACTS:
calories: 549 |carbs: 68 g | protein: 6 g | fat: 39 g | cholesterol: 140 mg

10. BRANDY JAVA ICE

SERVES: 2 | PREPARATION TIME: 2 MINS | COOKING TIME: 0 MINS | TOTAL TIME: 2 MINS

INGREDIENTS:
- Four scoops of vanilla ice cream large
- 2 oz brandy
- Two teaspoons of ground coffee, not instant granules

DIRECTIONS:
1. In a blender, combine all of the ingredients and blend until smooth. Enjoy!

NUTRITION FACTS:
calories: 339 |carbs: 21 g | protein: 5 g | fat: 15 g | cholesterol: 100 mg

11. CHOCOLATE SMOOTHIE

SERVES: 2 | PREPARATION TIME: 5 MINS | COOKING TIME: 0 MINS | TOTAL TIME: 5 MINS

INGREDIENTS:
- Two scoops of chocolate-flavored whey protein
- Two cups of ice
- Two tablespoons southern comfort® liqueur (optional)
- 1/2 cup evaporated milk
- 1/4 cup condensed milk
- 1/4 teaspoon ground cinnamon
- Pinch of nutmeg

DIRECTIONS:
1. In a neat blender, combine all ingredients except the cinnamon and mix on high for 1–2 minutes, or until smooth.
2. To serve, top with whipped cream and sprinkle with cinnamon.

NUTRITION FACTS:
calories: 142 |carbs: 17 g | protein: 10 g | fat: 4 g | cholesterol: 120 mg

12. BANANA BREAKFAST SMOOTHIE

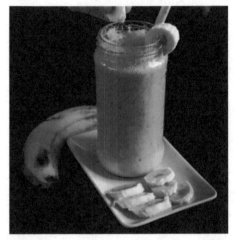

SERVES: 1 | PREPARATION TIME: 10 MINS | COOKING TIME: 5 MINS | TOTAL TIME: 15 MINS

INGREDIENTS:
- One medium banana
- 1 cup milk, almond or regular
- 1/2 cup plain yogurt
- 1/4 cup 100% bran flakes
- One teaspoon vanilla extract
- Two teaspoons honey or agave syrup
- 1/2 cup ice
- One pinch cinnamon
- One pinch nutmeg

DIRECTIONS:
1. In a neat blender, combine all of the ingredients and mix on medium speed until smooth.
2. Garnish with cinnamon and/or nutmeg if desired.

NUTRITION FACTS:
calories: 58 |carbs: 2 g | protein: 3 g | fat: 5 g | cholesterol: 16 mg

CLEAR LIQUID DIET - BREAKFAST

13. SPINACH VEGETABLE BARLEY BEAN SOUP

- SERVES: 6
- PREPARATION TIME: 20 MINS
- COOKING TIME: 60 MINS
- TOTAL TIME: 80 MINS

INGREDIENTS:
- One tablespoon extra-virgin olive oil
- Two stalks of celery chopped
- One medium onion diced
- Two carrots chopped
- One medium leek white and pale green parts only washed thoroughly and thinly sliced
- One cup quick-cooking barley
- One tablespoon tomato paste
- 8 cups low sodium vegetable broth
- 15 oz cannellini beans or other beans rinsed and drained
- Two teaspoon sprigs of fresh thyme or one dried thyme
- One teaspoon stem fresh basil or one dried thyme
- Four handfuls of baby spinach

DIRECTIONS:
1. In a soup saucepan, heat the oil. Cook until the celery, onion, carrots, and leeks are cooked, about 5 minutes, over medium heat. Cook, constantly tossing, until the barley and tomato paste are covered and glossy, approximately 30 seconds. Bring the broth, beans, thyme, and basil to a boil. Simmer for 1 hour on low heat.
2. Cook until the spinach is barely wilted (if you use Swiss chard or kale, it will take slightly longer to cook). Take off the thyme branch and the wilted basil. Season with salt and taste.

NUTRITION FACTS:
calories: 277 |carbs: 47 g | protein: 14 g | fat: 5 g | cholesterol: 221 mg

14. CHOCOLATE NICE CREAM

- SERVES: 4
- PREPARATION TIME: 5 MINS
- COOKING TIME: 1 MINS
- TOTAL TIME: 6 MINS

INGREDIENTS:
- 4 bananas ripened and frozen
- ¼ cup organic cocoa powder
- 1 tablespoon organic vanilla extract
- 1 tablespoon coconut milk or another dairy-free milk (optional)

DIRECTIONS:
1. Frozen bananas should be cut into pieces. Put everything in a food processor or blender. Blend until the mixture is crumbly.
2. Mix in the chocolate powder and vanilla extract. Blend until everything is properly blended. In the food processor, it will form a ball.
3. If the mixture needs additional liquid to blend effectively, add coconut milk or another dairy-free milk.

NUTRITION FACTS:
calories: 128 |carbs: 30 g | protein: 2 g | fat: 1 g | cholesterol: 13 mg

15. HEALTHY WATERMELON POPSICLES

- SERVES: 4
- PREPARATION TIME: 10 MINS
- COOKING TIME: 180 MINS
- TOTAL TIME: 190 MINS

INGREDIENTS:
- 2 cups watermelon cubed
- 1 cup strawberries hulled and halved
- 2 tablespoon vegan chocolate chips or raisins
- ¼ cup coconut milk (full fat) plus 2 tablespoon
- 2 kiwi peeled and cubed

DIRECTIONS:
1. Watermelon should be cut and cubed. Strawberries should be de-stemmed and sliced into quarters. Blend the 2 cups of watermelon and 1 cup of strawberries in a large mixing bowl until smooth. Fill four popsicle molds about 3/4 full with the mixture.
2. Divide the chocolate chips equally between the four molds. Gently press the chocolate chips into the molds with a popsicle stick, spreading them evenly. Raisins can also be used.
3. Freeze for one hour or until frozen.
4. While the first is frozen, combine 14 cups coconut milk and 1 teaspoon maple syrup. After the initial layer has hardened, equally distribute the coconut milk among the four molds, about 1 tablespoon each mold.
5. Freeze for one further hour or until set.
6. While the second layer is freezing, remove the kiwi's outer covering and slice it into tiny bits. Combine with 2 tablespoons coconut milk.
7. Pour the kiwi layer on top of the coconut layer after it has set. Freeze for another hour or until set. Serve and have fun!

NUTRITION FACTS:
calories: 174 |carbs: 26 g | protein: 3 g | fat: 9 g | cholesterol: 356 mg

16. SPINACH MANGO VEGAN POPSICLES

- SERVES: 4
- PREPARATION TIME: 10 MINS
- COOKING TIME: 180 MINS
- TOTAL TIME: 190 MINS

INGREDIENTS:
- 1 cup unsweetened almond milk
- 1 ½ cups fresh spinach
- ⅓ cup unsweetened coconut milk yogurt
- ½ cup frozen mango
- ½ cup frozen banana optional
- 2 tablespoon maple syrup optional

DIRECTIONS:
1. Blend almond milk and spinach in a blender. Blend on medium-high until the spinach is thoroughly broken down and incorporated.
2. Combine the coconut milk, mango, banana (optional), and maple syrup in a mixing bowl. Blend until completely smooth.
3. Fill popsicle molds with the mixture. Popsicle sticks should be inserted. If they don't stand straight in the molds, place them in the freezer for an hour before inserting them.
4. For best results, freeze for at least 3 hours, preferably overnight.

NUTRITION FACTS:
calories: 81 |carbs: 15 g | protein: 1 g | fat: 1 g | cholesterol: 253 mg

17. MANGO BANANA SMOOTHIE

- SERVES: 2
- PREPARATION TIME: 5 MINS
- COOKING TIME: 0 MINS
- TOTAL TIME: 5 MINS

INGREDIENTS:
- 1 cup frozen cubed mango
- 1 frozen banana chopped
- 1 cup unsweetened almond milk
- ¼ cup dairy-free coconut milk yogurt plain unsweetened
- 1 scoop pea protein powder optional

DIRECTIONS:
1. Fill your blender or smoothie cup with almond milk, coconut yogurt, protein powder, fresh mangoes, and chopped frozen banana in the following order: almond milk, coconut yogurt, protein powder, fresh mangoes, and chopped frozen banana.
2. Connect the blender lid or the smoothie attachment blade. Begin on low and gradually increase speed until all items are thoroughly mixed.
3. Pour the mixture into two glasses.

Serve with fresh mango, chia, and coconut flakes on top (optional)

NUTRITION FACTS:
calories: 193 | carbs: 30 g | protein: 14 g | fat: 1 g | cholesterol: 318 mg

18. SPINACH BLUEBERRY SMOOTHIE

SERVES	PREPARATION TIME	COOKING TIME	TOTAL TIME
1	3 MINS	2 MINS	5 MINS

INGREDIENTS:
- 1 cup almond milk unsweetened vanilla or regular
- 1 cup raw spinach loosely packed
- 1 frozen banana chopped into chunks
- ½ cup frozen blueberries
- 1 tablespoon chia

DIRECTIONS:
1. In a blender, combine the ingredients in the sequence listed in the recipe, beginning with the almond milk and working your way up to the spinach, frozen banana, frozen blueberries, and chia. Blend until completely smooth.

NUTRITION FACTS:
calories: 247 | carbs: 45 g | protein: 6 g | fat: 1 g | cholesterol: 261 mg

19. SNOWMAN CHRISTMAS SMOOTHIE

SERVES	PREPARATION TIME	COOKING TIME	TOTAL TIME
2	5 MINS	0 MINS	5 MINS

INGREDIENTS:
- 1 banana frozen and chopped
- 1 cup unsweetened almond milk
- ¼ cup desiccated coconut shredded, unsweetened
- ½ cup coconut whipped cream optional
- Blue sugar sprinkles optional

DIRECTIONS:
1. Assemble the snowman cups. To construct the mouth, draw two circular eyes, one triangular nose, and 5-6 tiny circles in a curved shape.
2. In a blender, combine the almond milk, banana, and coconut.
3. Blend until completely smooth. Approximately 5-10 seconds.
4. Pour the smoothie into the glasses. Sprinkle with blue sugar sprinkles and top with coconut whipped cream.

NUTRITION FACTS:
calories: 51 | carbs: 17 g | protein: 8 g | fat: 6 g | cholesterol: 201 mg

20. CLEAN GREEN SHAMROCK SHAKE

SERVES	PREPARATION TIME	COOKING TIME	TOTAL TIME
1	5 MINS	0 MINS	5 MINS

INGREDIENTS:
- 1 cup light coconut milk
- ¼ avocado
- 1 banana frozen
- ½ cup fresh leaf spinach
- ⅛ tablespoon peppermint extract
- 1 tablespoon dairy-free chocolate chips optional

DIRECTIONS:
1. In a blender, combine the frozen banana, coconut milk, avocado, spinach, and peppermint essence. Blend until smooth and well blended.
2. Fill a glass halfway with ice and top with chocolate chunks.

NUTRITION FACTS:
calories: 382 | carbs: 41 g | protein: 3 g | fat: 23 g | cholesterol: 183 mg

21. PUMPKIN SMOOTHIEPUMPKIN SMOOTHIE

SERVES	PREPARATION TIME	COOKING TIME	TOTAL TIME
1	5 MINS	0 MINS	5 MINS

INGREDIENTS:
- 1 banana frozen
- ½ cup pumpkin puree
- 1 cup almond milk unsweetened
- ½ tablespoon pumpkin pie spice
- 1 tablespoon maple syrup optional
- ½ cup ice cubes

DIRECTIONS:
1. In a blender, combine the frozen banana, pumpkin purée, almond milk, pumpkin pie spice, and maple syrup.
2. Blend until the mixture is smooth and creamy. If using a high-speed blender, start at the lowest level and gradually increase to 5 or 6 until all components are incorporated. Blend in the ice until well mixed.
3. Pour the mixture into two glasses. Serve with a sprinkling of pumpkin pie spice on top.

NUTRITION FACTS:
calories: 119 | carbs: 26 g | protein: 2 g | fat: 1 g | cholesterol: 19 mg

22. CITRUS SPORTS DRINK

SERVES	PREPARATION TIME	COOKING TIME	TOTAL TIME
1	5 MINS	0 MINS	5 MINS

INGREDIENTS:
- 4 cups coconut water
- 4 large oranges juice (about 1 ½ cup), strained
- 2 tablespoons lemon juice, strained
- 2 tablespoons honey or maple syrup
- 1 teaspoon sea salt

DIRECTIONS:
1. Place the coconut water, orange juice, lemon juice, honey, and salt in a jug or pitcher.
2. Stir until the salt is dissolved.
3. Serve cold.

NUTRITION FACTS:
calories: 59 | fat: 1 g | carbs: 14 g | fiber: 1 g | protein: 1 g | sodium: 304 mg

23. HOMEMADE ORANGE GELATIN

SERVES	PREPARATION TIME	COOKING TIME	TOTAL TIME
4	4 HRS - 10 MINS	3 MINS	4 HRS - 13 MINS

INGREDIENTS:
- 8 large oranges juice (about 3 cups), strained and divided
- 2 tablespoons unflavored gelatin
- 2 tablespoons honey or maple syrup

DIRECTIONS:
1. In a large bowl, pour in 1/2 cup of orange juice and sprinkle with gelatin. Whisk well and let sit until the gelatin begins to set but is not quite smooth.
2. In a saucepan over low heat, pour in the remaining 2 ½ cups of orange juice and cook until just before boiling, 2-3 minutes.
3. Remove from the heat and pour the hot juice into the gelatin mixture. Attach the honey or maple syrup and stir until the gelatin is dissolved.
4. Pour into an 8 x 8 inches baking dish and transfer to the refrigerator.
5. Cool for 4 hours to set. Serve cold.

NUTRITION FACTS:
calories: 127 | fat: 1 g | carbs: 28 g | fiber: 1 g | protein: 6 g | sodium: 2 mg

24. RASPBERRY LEMONADE ICE POPS

SERVES	PREPARATION TIME	COOKING TIME	TOTAL TIME
4	4 HRS - 10 MINS	0 MINS	4 HRS - 10 MINS

INGREDIENTS:
- 3 cups frozen raspberries
- 1 teaspoon lemon juice, strained
- 1/4 cup coconut water
- 1/4 cup honey or maple syrup

DIRECTIONS:
1. In a blender, puree the raspberries, lemon juice, and coconut water until smooth.
2. Set the mixture through a fine-mesh strainer into a bowl to remove the seeds. Stir in the honey until well mixed.
3. Divide the mixture equally among 4 popsicle molds and freeze until solid, 3-4 hours.

NUTRITION FACTS:
calories: 120 |fat: 0 g | carbs: 31 g | fiber: 7 g | protein: 1 g | sodium: 2 mg

25. HOMEMADE NO PULP ORANGE JUICE

   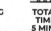

SERVES	PREPARATION TIME	COOKING TIME	TOTAL TIME
1	5 MINS	0 MINS	5 MINS

INGREDIENTS:
- 4 oranges

DIRECTIONS:
- Lightly squeeze the oranges on a hard surface to soften the exterior. Slice each in half.
- Squeeze each orange over a fine-mesh strainer.
- Gently, press the pulp to extract all possible liquid.
- Serve over ice. Enjoy!

NUTRITION FACTS:
calories: 50 |fat: 0 g | carbs: 11 g | fiber: 7 g | protein: 1 g | sodium: 2 mg

26. APPLE ORANGE JUICE

SERVES	PREPARATION TIME	COOKING TIME	TOTAL TIME
2	5 MINS	0 MINS	5 MINS

INGREDIENTS:
- 1 Gala apple, peeled, cored and sliced
- 2 oranges, peeled, halved and seeded
- 2 teaspoons honey (optional)
- 3/4 cup water

DIRECTIONS:
1. Squeeze each orange over a fine-mesh strainer.
2. Gently, press the pulp to extract as much liquid as possible.
3. Add in the apple, water, and orange juice in your blender and pulse.
4. Set a fine-mesh strainer in a bowl. Before transferring your juice into the strainer.
5. Once again, gently press the pulp to remove all possible liquid then discard it.
6. Stir in your honey then serve over ice.

NUTRITION FACTS:
calories: 180 |fat: 1 g | carbs: 43 g | fiber: 1 g | protein: 2 g

27. PINEAPPLE MINT JUICE

SERVES	PREPARATION TIME	COOKING TIME	TOTAL TIME
4	5 MINS	0 MINS	5 MINS

INGREDIENTS:
- 3 cups pineapple, cored, sliced and chunks
- 10-12 mint leaves, or to taste
- 2 tablespoons sugar, or to taste (optional)
- 1 ½ cup water
- 1 cup ice cubes

DIRECTIONS:
1. Set all the ingredients into your blender, and pulse.
2. Set a fine-mesh strainer in a bowl. Before transferring your juice into the strainer.
3. Gently, press the pulp to extract all possible liquid then discard it.
4. Serve over ice. Enjoy!

NUTRITION FACTS:
calories: 78 |fat: 1 g | carbs: 22 g | fiber: 2 g | protein: 1 g |

28. CELERY APPLE JUICE

SERVES	PREPARATION TIME	COOKING TIME	TOTAL TIME
2	5 MINS	0 MINS	5 MINS

INGREDIENTS:
- 12 celery stalks, peeled and chopped
- 3 Apple, peeled, cored, seeded and sliced
- 1 inch ginger root, peeled and chopped
- 1/4 lemon juice
- 2 cups water

DIRECTIONS:
1. Set all the ingredients into your blender, and pulse.
2. Set a fine-mesh strainer in a bowl. Before transferring your juice into the strainer.
3. Gently, press the pulp to extract all possible liquid then discard it.
4. Serve over ice. Enjoy!

NUTRITION FACTS:
calories: 119 |fat: 1 g | carbs: 29 g | fiber: 7 g | protein: 2 g

29. HOMEMADE BANANA APPLE JUICE

SERVES	PREPARATION TIME	COOKING TIME	TOTAL TIME
2	10 MINS	0 MINS	10 MINS

INGREDIENTS:
- 2 bananas, peeled and sliced
- 1/2 apple, peeled, cored and chopped
- 1 tablespoon honey
- 1 ½ cup water

DIRECTIONS:
1. Set all the ingredients into your blender, and pulse.
2. Set a fine-mesh strainer in a bowl. Before transferring your juice into the strainer.
3. Gently, press the pulp to extract all possible liquid then discard it.
4. Serve over ice. Enjoy!

NUTRITION FACTS:
calories: 132 |fat: 2 g | carbs: 27 g | fiber: 3 g | protein: 4 g

30. SWEET DETOX JUICE

SERVES	PREPARATION TIME	COOKING TIME	TOTAL TIME
2	10 MINS	0 MINS	10 MINS

INGREDIENTS:
- 2 cups baby spinach, chopped
- 1 handful parsley, chopped
- 1 green apple, peeled, cored, seeded and sliced
- 1 large English cucumber, seeded and chopped
- 1 inch ginger, peeled
- 1 lemon, juiced

DIRECTIONS:
1. Set all the ingredients into your blender, and pulse.
2. Set a fine-mesh strainer in a bowl. Before transferring your juice into the strainer.
3. Gently, press the pulp to extract all possible liquid then discard it.
4. Serve over ice. Enjoy!

NUTRITION FACTS:
calories: 209 |fat: 2 g | carbs: 48 g | fiber: 17 g | protein: 12 g

31. PINEAPPLE GINGER JUICE

SERVES 7 | PREPARATION TIME 35 MINS | COOKING TIME 0 MINS | TOTAL TIME 35 MINS

INGREDIENTS:
- 10 cups pineapple, chopped
- 6 cups water
- 3 Fuji apples, chopped
- 4-inch ginger root, peeled and chopped
- 1/4 cup lemon juice
- 1/4 cup sugar

DIRECTIONS:
1. Set all the ingredients into your blender, and pulse.
2. Set a fine-mesh strainer in a bowl. Before transferring your juice into the strainer.
3. Gently, press the pulp to extract all possible liquid then discard it.
4. Serve over ice. Enjoy!

NUTRITION FACTS:
calories: 71 |fat: 1 g | carbs: 20 g | fiber: 3 g | protein: 1 g

32. CARROT ORANGE JUICE

SERVES 2 | PREPARATION TIME 15 MINS | COOKING TIME 0 MINS | TOTAL TIME 15 MINS

INGREDIENTS:
- 1 medium yellow tomato, cut into wedges

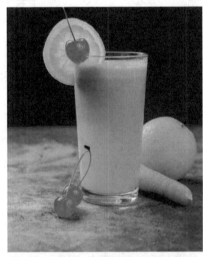

- 1 orange, peeled and quartered
- 1 apple, peeled, cored and chopped
- 4 jumbo carrots, peeled and chopped
- 2 cups water

DIRECTIONS:
1. Set all the ingredients into your blender, and pulse.
2. Set a fine-mesh strainer in a bowl. Before transferring your juice into the strainer.
3. Gently, press the pulp to extract all possible liquid then discard it.
4. Serve over ice. Enjoy!

NUTRITION FACTS:
calories: 111 |fat: 2 g | carbs: 24 g | fiber: 1 g | protein: 2 g

33. STRAWBERRY APPLE JUICE

SERVES 8 | PREPARATION TIME 5 MINS | COOKING TIME 0 MINS | TOTAL TIME 5 MINS

INGREDIENTS:
- 2 cups strawberries (tops removed)
- 1 red apple, peeled, seeded, cored and chopped
- 1 tablespoon chia seeds
- 1 cup water

DIRECTIONS:
1. Set all the ingredients into your blender, and pulse.
2. Set a fine-mesh strainer in a bowl. Before transferring your juice into the strainer.
3. Gently, press the pulp to extract all possible liquid then discard it.
4. Add in your chia seeds then leave to sit for at least 5 minutes.
5. Serve over ice. Enjoy!

NUTRITION FACTS:
calories: 245 |fat: 5 g | carbs: 52 g | fiber: 7 g | protein: 4 g

34. AUTUMN ENERGIZER JUICE

SERVES 2 | PREPARATION TIME 10 MINS | COOKING TIME 0 MINS | TOTAL TIME 10 MINS

INGREDIENTS:
- 2 pears, peeled, seeded and chopped
- 2 Ambrosia apples, peeled, cored and chopped
- 2 Granny Smith apples, peeled, cored, chopped
- 2 mandarins, juiced
- 2 cups sweet potato, peeled and chopped
- 1 pint cape gooseberries
- 2 inches ginger root, peeled

DIRECTIONS:
1. Set all the ingredients into your blender, and pulse.
2. Set a fine-mesh strainer in a bowl. Before transferring your juice into the strainer.
3. Gently, press the pulp to extract all possible liquid then discard it.
4. Serve over ice. Enjoy!

NUTRITION FACTS:
calories: 170 |fat: 3 g | carbs: 33 g | fiber: 9 g | protein: 4 g

35. ASIAN INSPIRED WONTON BROTH

SERVES 2 | PREPARATION TIME 5 MINS | COOKING TIME 95 MINS | TOTAL TIME 100 MINS

INGREDIENTS:
- 1 chicken thigh, skin on
- 1 carrot, coarsely chopped
- 1 celery stalk, coarsely chopped
- 1 small onion, quartered
- 3 dime-sized ginger pieces
- 2 tablespoons kosher salt
- 1/4 teaspoon turmeric
- 1/8 teaspoon MSG (don't leave it out)
- 5 white peppercorns (can be substituted with black)
- 1 liter water

DIRECTIONS:
1. Transfer all the ingredients to your stockpot. Top with enough water to cover then allow to slowly come to a boil on high heat.
2. Switch to low heat and simmer for at least 1 hour and 30 minutes.
3. Set and pour the mixture through a fine-mesh strainer into a large bowl.
4. Taste and season with salt.
5. Serve hot.

NUTRITION FACTS:
calories: 181 |fat: 7 g | carbs: 14 g | fiber: 1 g | protein: 14 g

36. MUSHROOM, CAULIFLOWER AND CABBAGE BROTH

SERVES 2 | PREPARATION TIME 10 MINS | COOKING TIME 50 MINS | TOTAL TIME 60 MINS

INGREDIENTS:
- 1 large yellow onion
- 1 cup celery stalks, chopped
- 2 carrots, diced or cubed
- 10 French beans
- 1/2 cabbage, diced
- 1-2 stalks celery leaves
- 1 ½ cup mushrooms, sliced
- 8 florets cauliflower
- 1 teaspoon garlic, chopped
- 1 teaspoon ginger, chopped
- 1 tablespoon oil
- 1 scallion stalk
- 1/2 teaspoon pepper, crushed

DIRECTIONS:

1. Transfer all the ingredients to your stockpot. Top with enough water to cover then allow to slowly come to a boil on high heat.
2. Switch to low heat and simmer for 50 minutes.
3. Set and pour the mixture through a fine-mesh strainer into a large bowl. Mash the vegetables well to extract all their juices.
4. Taste and season with salt. Enjoy.

NUTRITION FACTS:

calories: 141 |fat: 5 g | carbs: 22 g | fiber: 7 g | protein: 5 g

37. INDIAN INSPIRED VEGETABLE STOCK

 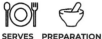

SERVES	PREPARATION TIME	COOKING TIME	TOTAL TIME
3	10 MINS	11 MINS	21 MINS

INGREDIENTS:

- 3/4 cup onions, roughly chopped
- 3/4 cup carrot, roughly chopped
- 3/4 cup tomatoes, roughly chopped
- 3/4 cup potatoes, roughly chopped
- 1 teaspoon turmeric
- Salt to taste

DIRECTIONS:

1. Transfer all the ingredients to your stockpot. Top with enough water to cover then allow to slowly come to a boil on high heat.
2. Switch to low heat and simmer for 11 minutes.
3. Set and pour the mixture through a fine-mesh strainer into a large bowl. Taste and season with salt.
4. Serve hot. Enjoy!

NUTRITION FACTS:

calories: 103 |fat: 1 g | carbs: 24 g | fiber: 3 g | protein: 2 g

38. BEEF BONE BROTH

SERVES	PREPARATION TIME	COOKING TIME	TOTAL TIME
8	10 MINS	12 HRS	12 HRS

INGREDIENTS:

- 2 pounds beef bones
- 1 onion, chopped in quarters
- 2 celery stalks, chopped in half
- 2 carrots, chopped in half
- 3 whole garlic cloves
- 2 bay leaves
- 1 tablespoon salt
- Filtered water (enough to cover bones)

DIRECTIONS:

1. Transfer the bones and vegetables to your stockpot. Top with enough water to cover then allow to slowly come to a boil on high heat.
2. Switch to low heat and simmer for at least 2 hours and up to 12 hours.
3. Set and pour the mixture through a fine-mesh strainer into a large bowl. Taste and season with salt.
4. Serve hot.

NUTRITION FACTS:

calories: 69 |fat: 4 g | carbs: 1 g | fiber: 0 g | protein: 6 g

39. GINGER, MUSHROOM AND CAULIFLOWER BROTH

 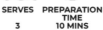

SERVES	PREPARATION TIME	COOKING TIME	TOTAL TIME
3	10 MINS	50 MINS	60 MINS

INGREDIENTS:

- 1 large yellow onion
- 1 cup celery stalks, chopped
- 2 carrots, diced or cubed
- 10 French beans
- 1 ginger root, peeled, diced or grated
- 1-2 stalks celery leaves or coriander leaves
- 1 ½ cup mushrooms, sliced
- 8 florets cauliflower
- 1 teaspoon garlic, chopped
- 1 tablespoon oil
- 1 stalk spring onion greens or scallions
- 1/2 teaspoon crushed pepper or ground pepper

DIRECTIONS:

1. Transfer all the ingredients to your stockpot. Top with enough water to cover then allow to slowly come to a boil on high heat.
2. Switch to low heat and simmer for at least 50 minutes.
3. Set and pour the mixture through a fine-mesh strainer into a large bowl. Taste and season with salt.
4. Serve hot. Enjoy!

NUTRITION FACTS:

calories: 141 |fat: 5 g | carbs: 22 g | fiber: 7 g | protein: 5 g

40. FISH BROTH

 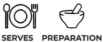

SERVES	PREPARATION TIME	COOKING TIME	TOTAL TIME
3	15 MINS	45 MINS	60 MINS

INGREDIENTS:

- 1 large onion, chopped
- 1 large carrot chopped
- 1 fennel bulb and fronds, chopped (optional)
- 3 celery stalks, chopped
- Salt
- 2-5 pounds fish bones and heads
- 1 handful dried mushrooms (optional)
- 2-4 bay leaves
- 1 star anise pod (optional)
- 1-2 teaspoons thyme, dried or fresh
- 3-4 pieces dried kombu kelp (optional)

DIRECTIONS:

1. Transfer the bones and vegetables to your stockpot. Top with enough water to cover then allow to slowly come to a boil on high heat.
2. Set to low heat and simmer for 45 minutes.
3. Set and pour the mixture through a fine-mesh strainer into a large bowl. Taste and season with salt.
4. Serve hot. Enjoy!

NUTRITION FACTS:

calories: 29 |fat: 1 g | carbs: 2 g | fiber: 1 g | protein: 1 g

41. CLEAR PUMPKIN BROTH

SERVES	PREPARATION TIME	COOKING TIME	TOTAL TIME
6	15 MINS	30 MINS	45 MINS

INGREDIENTS:

- 6 cups water
- 2 tablespoons ginger, minced
- 2 cups potatoes, peeled and diced
- 3 cups kabocha, peeled and diced
- 1 carrot, peeled and diced
- 1 onion, diced
- 1/2 cup scallions, chopped

DIRECTIONS:

1. Transfer the bones and vegetables to your stockpot. Top with enough water to cover then allow to slowly come to a boil on high heat.
2. Switch to low heat and simmer for at least 30 minutes.
3. Set and pour the mixture through a fine-mesh strainer into a large bowl. Taste and season with salt.
4. Serve hot. Enjoy!

NUTRITION FACTS:

calories: 215 |fat: 1 g | carbs: 37 g | fiber: 4 g | protein: 8 g

42. PORK STOCK

SERVES	PREPARATION TIME	COOKING TIME	TOTAL TIME
8	15 MINS	12 HRS	12 HRS

INGREDIENTS:

- 2 Pounds pork bones, roasted
- 1 onion, chopped in quarters
- 2 celery stalks, chopped in half
- 2 carrots, chopped in half
- 3 whole garlic cloves
- 2 bay leaves
- 1 tablespoon salt
- Filtered water (enough to cover bones)

DIRECTIONS:

1. Transfer the bones and vegetables to your stockpot. Top with enough water to cover then allow to slowly come to a boil on high heat.
2. Set to low heat and simmer for 12 hours.
3. Set and pour the mixture through a fine-mesh strainer into a large bowl. Taste and season with salt.
4. Serve hot. Enjoy!

NUTRITION FACTS:

calories: 69 |fat: 4 g | carbs: 1 g | fiber: 0 g | protein: 6 g

43. SLOW COOKER PORK BONE BROTH

SERVES	PREPARATION TIME	COOKING TIME	TOTAL TIME
12	15 MINS	24 HRS	12 HRS

INGREDIENTS:

- 2 pounds pork bones, roasted
- 1/2 onion, chopped
- 2 medium carrots, chopped
- 1 stalk celery, chopped
- 2 whole garlic cloves
- 1 bay leaf
- 1 tablespoon sea salt
- 1 teaspoon peppercorns
- 1/4 cup apple cider vinegar
- Filtered water (enough to cover bones)

DIRECTIONS:

1. Transfer all the ingredients to your slow cooker. Top with enough water to cover then allow to slowly come to a boil on high heat.
2. Switch to low heat and simmer for at least 24 hours.
3. Set and pour the mixture through a fine-mesh strainer into a large bowl. Taste and season with salt.
4. Serve hot. Enjoy!

NUTRITION FACTS:

calories: 65 |fat: 2 g | carbs: 7 g | fiber: 4 g | protein: 6 g

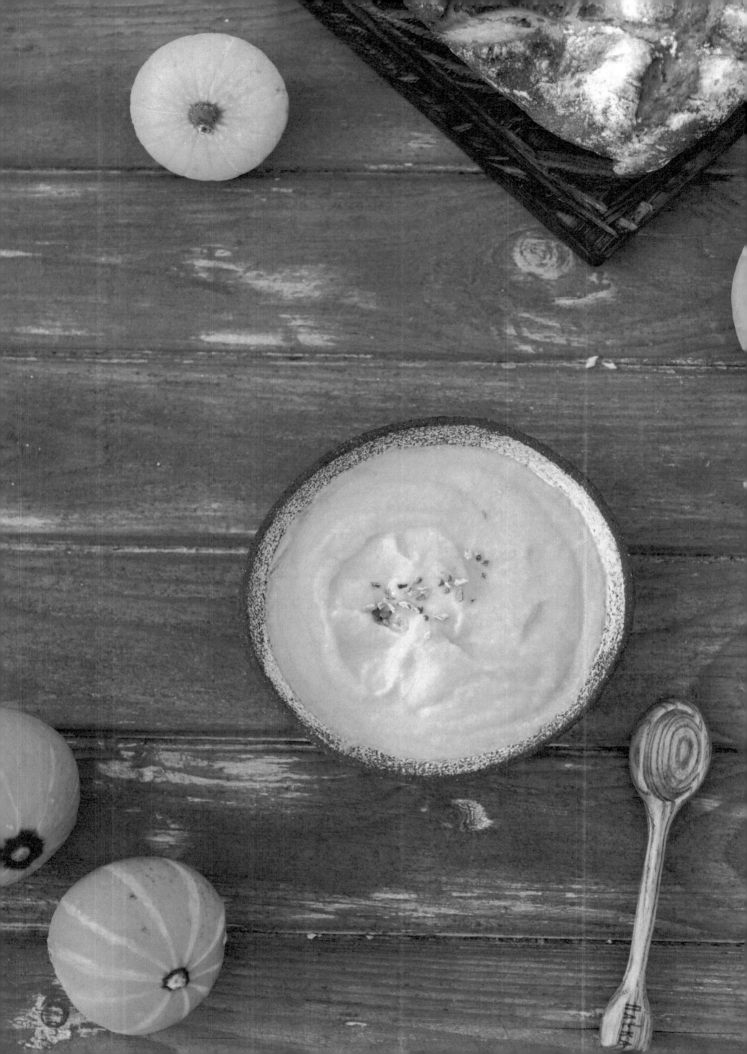

CLEAR LIQUID DIET

LUNCH

44. HEALTHIER APPLE JUICE

SERVES: 2 | PREPARATION TIME: 5 MINS | COOKING TIME: 0 MINS | TOTAL TIME: 5 MINS

INGREDIENTS:
- 8 medium apples, cored and quartered

DIRECTIONS:
1. Add the apples into a juicer and extract the juice according to the manufacturer's method.
2. Through a cheesecloth-lined sieve, strain the juice and transfer it into 2 glasses.
3. Serve immediately.

NUTRITION FACTS:
calories: 164 |fat: 2 g | carbs: 124 g | fiber: 21 g | protein: 3 g | sodium 123 mg

45. CITRUS APPLE JUICE

SERVES: 2 | PREPARATION TIME: 5 MINS | COOKING TIME: 0 MINS | TOTAL TIME: 5 MINS

INGREDIENTS:
- 5 large apples, cored and chopped
- 1 small lemon
- 1 cup fresh orange juice

DIRECTIONS:
1. Attach all the ingredients in a blender and pulse until well combined.
2. Through a cheesecloth-lined sieve, strain the juice and transfer it into 2 glasses.
3. Serve immediately.

NUTRITION FACTS:
calories: 148 |fat: 2 g | carbs: 90 g | fiber: 14 g | protein: 3 g | sodium 6 mg

46. RICHLY FRUITY JUICE

SERVES: 2 | PREPARATION TIME: 5 MINS | COOKING TIME: 0 MINS | TOTAL TIME: 5 MINS

INGREDIENTS:
- 5 large green apples, cored and sliced
- 2 cups seedless white grapes
- 2 teaspoon fresh lime juice

DIRECTIONS:
1. Set all ingredients into a juicer and extract the juice according to the manufacturer's method.
2. Through a cheesecloth-lined sieve, strain the juice and transfer it into 2 glasses.
3. Serve immediately.

NUTRITION FACTS:
calories: 152 |fat: 2 g | carbs: 93 g | fiber: 14 g | protein: 2 g | sodium 7 mg

47. DELISH GRAPE JUICE

SERVES: 3 | PREPARATION TIME: 15 MINS | COOKING TIME: 0 MINS | TOTAL TIME: 15 MINS

INGREDIENTS:
- 2 cups white seedless grapes
- 1 ½ cup filtered water
- 6-8 ice cubes

DIRECTIONS:
1. Attach all the ingredients in a blender and pulse until well combined.
2. Through a cheesecloth-lined sieve, strain the juice and transfer it into 3 glasses.
3. Serve immediately.

NUTRITION FACTS:
calories: 41 |fat: 0 g | carbs: 11 g | fiber: 10 g | protein: 1 g | sodium 1 mg

48. LEMONY GRAPE JUICE

SERVES: 3 | PREPARATION TIME: 15 MINS | COOKING TIME: 0 MINS | TOTAL TIME: 15 MINS

INGREDIENTS:
- 4 cups seedless white grapes
- 2 tablespoons fresh lemon juice

DIRECTIONS:
1. Attach all the ingredients in a blender and pulse until well combined.
2. Through a cheesecloth-lined sieve, strain the juice and transfer it into 3 glasses.
3. Serve immediately.

NUTRITION FACTS:
calories: 85 |fat: 0 g | carbs: 21 g | fiber: 1 g | protein: 1 g | sodium 4 mg

49. HOLIDAY SPECIAL JUICE

SERVES	PREPARATION TIME	COOKING TIME	TOTAL TIME
4	15 MINS	0 MINS	15 MINS

INGREDIENTS:
- 4 cups fresh cranberries
- 1 tablespoon fresh lemon juice
- 2 cups filtered water
- 1 teaspoon raw honey

DIRECTIONS:
1. Attach all the ingredients in a blender and pulse until well combined.
2. Through a cheesecloth-lined sieve, strain the juice and transfer it into 4 glasses.
3. Serve immediately.

NUTRITION FACTS:
calories: 66 |fat: 0 g | carbs: 12 g | fiber: 4 g | protein: 0 g | sodium 1 mg

50. VITAMIN C RICH JUICE

SERVES	PREPARATION TIME	COOKING TIME	TOTAL TIME
2	15 MINS	0 MINS	15 MINS

INGREDIENTS:
- 8 oranges, peeled and sectioned

DIRECTIONS:
1. Add the orange sections into a juicer and extract the juice according to the manufacturer's method.
2. Through a cheesecloth-lined sieve, strain the juice and transfer it into 2 glasses.
3. Serve immediately.

NUTRITION FACTS:
calories: 146 |fat: 1 g | carbs: 87 g | fiber: 18 g | protein: 7 g | sodium 1 mg

51. INCREDIBLE FRESH JUICE

SERVES	PREPARATION TIME	COOKING TIME	TOTAL TIME
4	15 MINS	0 MINS	15 MINS

INGREDIENTS:
- 2 pounds carrots, trimmed and scrubbed
- 6 small oranges, peeled and sectioned

DIRECTIONS:
1. Add the carrots and orange sections into a juicer and extract the juice according to the manufacturer's method.
2. Through a cheesecloth-lined sieve, strain the juice and transfer it into 4 glasses.
3. Serve immediately.

NUTRITION FACTS:
calories: 183 |fat: 0 g | carbs: 45 g | fiber: 10 g | protein: 4 g | sodium 156 mg

52. FAVORITE SUMMER LEMONADE

SERVES	PREPARATION TIME	COOKING TIME	TOTAL TIME
8	15 MINS	0 MINS	15 MINS

INGREDIENTS:
- 8 cups filtered water
- 1/2 cup fresh lemon juice
- 1/4 teaspoon pure stevia extract
- Ice cubes, as required

DIRECTIONS:
- In a pitcher, place the water, lemon juice and stevia. Mix well.
- Through a cheesecloth-lined sieve, strain the lemonade in another pitcher.
- Refrigerate for 30-40 minutes.
- Set ice cubes in serving glasses and fill with lemonade.
- Serve chilled.

NUTRITION FACTS:
calories: 4 |fat: 0 g | carbs: 0 g | fiber:0 g | protein: 4 g | sodium 3 mg

53. ULTIMATE FRUITY PUNCH

SERVES	PREPARATION TIME	COOKING TIME	TOTAL TIME
12	15 MINS	0 MINS	15 MINS

INGREDIENTS:
- 3 cups fresh pineapple juice
- 2 cups fresh orange juice
- 1 cup fresh ruby red grapefruit juice
- 1/4 cup fresh lime juice
- 2 cups seedless watermelon, cut into bite-sized chunks
- 2 cups fresh pineapple, cut into bite-sized chunks
- 2 oranges, peeled and cut into wedges
- 2 limes, quartered
- 1 lemon, sliced
- 2 (12 ounces) cans diet lemon-lime soda
- Crushed ice, as required

DIRECTIONS:
1. In a large pitcher, add all ingredients except for soda cans and ice. Stir to combine.
2. Set aside for 30 minutes.
3. Through a cheesecloth-lined sieve, strain the punch into another large pitcher.
4. Set the glasses with ice and top with punch about 3/4 of the mixture.
5. Add a splash of the soda and serve.

NUTRITION FACTS:
calories: 95 |fat: 0 g | carbs: 24 g | fiber: 2 g | protein: 2 g | sodium 156 mg

54. THIRST QUENCHER SPORTS DRINK

SERVES	PREPARATION TIME	COOKING TIME	TOTAL TIME
8	15 MINS	0 MINS	15 MINS

INGREDIENTS:
- 7 cups spring water
- 1 cup fresh apple juice
- 2-3 teaspoons fresh lime juice
- 2 tablespoons honey
- 1/4 teaspoon sea salt

DIRECTIONS:
1. In a large pitcher, add all ingredients and stir to combine.
2. Through a cheesecloth-lined sieve, strain the punch into another large pitcher.
3. Refrigerate to chill before serving.

NUTRITION FACTS:
calories: 30 |fat: 0 g | carbs: 28 g | fiber: 0 g | protein: 0 g | sodium 60 mg

55. REFRESHING SPORTS DRINK

SERVES	PREPARATION TIME	COOKING TIME	TOTAL TIME
9	15 MINS	0 MINS	15 MINS

INGREDIENTS:
- 8 cups fresh cold water, divided
- 3/4 cup fresh orange juice
- 1/4 cup fresh lemon juice
- 1/4 cup fresh limes juice
- 3 tablespoons honey
- 1/2 teaspoon salt

DIRECTIONS:
1. In a large pitcher, add all ingredients and stir to combine.
2. Through a cheesecloth-lined sieve, strain the punch into another large pitcher.
3. Refrigerate to chill before serving.

NUTRITION FACTS:
calories: 33 |fat: 0 g | carbs: 8 g | fiber: 0 g | protein: 0 g | sodium 130 mg

56. PERFECT SUNNY DAY TEA

DIVERTICULITIS COOKBOOK

SERVES 6 | **PREPARATION TIME** 15 MINS | **COOKING TIME** 3 MINS | **TOTAL TIME** 18 MINS

INGREDIENTS:
- 5 cups filtered water
- 5 green tea bags
- 1/4 cup fresh lemon juice, strained
- 1/4 cup fresh lime juice, strained
- 1/4 cup honey
- Ice cubes, as required

DIRECTIONS:
1. In a medium pan, add 2 cups of water and bring to a boil.
2. Set in the tea bags and turn off the heat.
3. Immediately, cover the pan and steep for 3-4 minutes.
4. With a large spoon, gently press the tea bags against the pan to extract the tea completely.
5. Detach the tea bags from the pan and discard them.
6. Set honey and stir until dissolved.
7. In a large pitcher, place the tea, lemon and lime juice and stir to combine.
8. Add the remaining cold water and stir to combine.
9. Refrigerate to chill before serving.
10. Attach ice cubes in serving glasses and fill with tea.
11. Serve chilled.

NUTRITION FACTS:
calories: 46 |fat: 0 g | carbs: 12 g | fiber: 0 g | protein: 0 g | sodium 3 mg

57. NUTRITIOUS GREEN TEA

SERVES 4 | **PREPARATION TIME** 15 MINS | **COOKING TIME** 3 MINS | **TOTAL TIME** 18 MINS

INGREDIENTS:
- 4 cups filtered water
- 4 orange peel strips
- 4 lemon peel strips
- 4 green tea bags
- 2 teaspoons honey

DIRECTIONS:
1. In a medium pan, add the water, orange, and lemon peel strips over medium-high heat and bring to a boil.
2. Set the heat to low and stir, uncovered, for about 10 minutes.
3. With a slotted spoon, remove the orange and lemon peel strips and discard them.
4. Attach in the tea bags and turn off the heat.
5. Immediately, cover the pan and steep for 3 minutes.
6. With a large spoon, gently press the tea bags against the pan to extract the tea completely.
7. Detach the tea bags from the pan and discard them.
8. Add honey and stir until dissolved.
9. Strain the tea in mugs and serve immediately.

NUTRITION FACTS:
calories: 11 |fat: 0 g | carbs: 3 g | fiber: 0 g | protein: 0 g | sodium 30mg

58. SIMPLE BLACK TEA

SERVES 2 | **PREPARATION TIME** 15 MINS | **COOKING TIME** 3 MINS | **TOTAL TIME** 18 MINS

INGREDIENTS:
- 2 cups filtered water
- 1/2 teaspoon black tea leaves
- 1 teaspoon honey

DIRECTIONS:
1. In a pan, add the water and bring to a boil.
2. Stir in the tea leaves and turn off the heat.
3. Immediately, cover the pan and steep for 3 minutes.
4. Add honey and stir until dissolved.
5. Strain the tea in mugs and serve immediately.

NUTRITION FACTS:
calories: 11 |fat: 0 g | carbs: 3 g | fiber: 0 g | protein: 0 g | sodium 123mg

59. LEMONY BLACK TEA

SERVES 6 | **PREPARATION TIME** 10 MINS | **COOKING TIME** 3 MINS | **TOTAL TIME** 13 MINS

INGREDIENTS:
- 1 tablespoon black tea leaves
- 1 lemon, sliced thinly
- 1 cinnamon stick
- 6 cups boiling water

DIRECTIONS:
1. In a large teapot, place the tea leaves, lemon slices and cinnamon stick.
2. Pour hot water over the ingredients and immediately cover the teapot.
3. Set aside for about 5 minutes to steep.
4. Strain the tea in mugs and serve immediately.

NUTRITION FACTS:
calories: 1 |fat: 0 g | carbs: 3 g | fiber: 0 g | protein: 0 g | sodium 1 mg

60. METABOLISM BOOSTER COFFEE

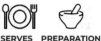

SERVES 1 | **PREPARATION TIME** 5 MINS | **COOKING TIME** 4 MINS | **TOTAL TIME** 9 MINS

INGREDIENTS:
- 1/4 teaspoon coffee powder
- 1 ¼ cup filtered water
- 1 teaspoon fresh lemon juice
- 1 teaspoon honey

DIRECTIONS:
1. In a small pan, attach the water and coffee powder. Bring it to boil.
2. Cook for about 1 minute.
3. Detach from the heat and pour into a serving mug.
4. Add the honey and lemon juice then stir until dissolved
5. Serve hot.

NUTRITION FACTS:
calories: 23 |fat: 0 g | carbs: 6 g | fiber: 0 g | protein: 0 g | sodium 1mg

61. BEST HOMEMADE BROTH

SERVES 8 | **PREPARATION TIME** 15 MINS | **COOKING TIME** 2 HRS + 5MINS | **TOTAL TIME** 2 HRS + 20MINS

INGREDIENTS:
- 1 (3 pounds) chicken, cut into pieces
- 5 medium carrots
- 4 celery stalks with leaves
- 6 fresh thyme sprigs
- 6 fresh parsley sprigs
- Salt to taste
- 9 cups cold water

DIRECTIONS:
1. In a large pan, attach all the ingredients over medium-high heat and bring to a boil.
2. Set the heat to medium-low and stir, covered for about 2 hours, skimming the foam from the surface occasionally.
3. Through a fine-mesh sieve, strain the broth into a large bowl.
4. Serve hot.

NUTRITION FACTS:
calories: 275 |fat: 5 g | carbs: 4 g | fiber: 1 g | protein: 50 g | sodium 160 mg

62. CLEAN TESTING BROTH

SERVES 10 | **PREPARATION TIME** 10 MINS | **COOKING TIME** 6 HRS | **TOTAL TIME** 6 HRS

INGREDIENTS:
- 4 pounds chicken bones
- Salt to taste

- 10 cups filtered water
- 2 tablespoons apple cider vinegar
- 1 lemon, quartered
- 3 bay leaves
- 3 teaspoons ground turmeric
- 2 tablespoons peppercorns

DIRECTIONS:

1. Preheat the oven to 400°F.
2. Arrange the bones onto a large baking sheet and sprinkle with salt.
3. Roast for about 45 minutes.
4. Detach from the oven and transfer the bones into a large pan.
5. Add the remaining ingredients and stir to combine.
6. Put the pan over medium-high heat and bring to a boil.
7. Set the heat to low and stir, covered for about 4-5 hours, skimming the foam from the surface occasionally.
8. Through a fine-mesh sieve, strain the broth into a large bowl.
9. Serve hot.

NUTRITION FACTS:

calories: 140 |fat: 3 g | carbs: 1 g | fiber: 0 g | protein: 25 g | sodium 73 mg

63. HEALING BROTH

SERVES	PREPARATION TIME	COOKING TIME	TOTAL TIME
12	10 MINS	8-10 HRS	8-10 HRS

INGREDIENTS:

- 3 tablespoons extra-virgin olive oil
- 2 ½ pounds chicken bones
- 4 celery stalks, chopped roughly
- 3 large carrots, peeled and chopped roughly
- 1 bay leaf
- 1 tablespoon black peppercorns
- 2 whole cloves
- 1 tablespoon apple cider vinegar
- Warm water, as required

DIRECTIONS:

1. In a Dutch oven, heat the oil over medium-high heat and sear the bones for about 3-5 minutes or until browned.
2. With a slotted spoon, transfer the bones into a bowl.
3. In the same pan, add the celery stalks and carrots. Cook for about 15 minutes, stirring occasionally.
4. Add browned bones, bay leaf, black peppercorns, cloves and vinegar. Stir to combine.
5. Add enough warm water to cover the bones mixture completely and bring to a gentle boil.
6. Set the heat to low and stir, covered for about 8-10 hours, skimming the foam from the surface occasionally.
7. Through a fine-mesh sieve, strain the broth into a large bowl.
8. Serve hot.

NUTRITION FACTS:

calories: 67 |fat: 4 g | carbs: 2 g | fiber: 0 g | protein: 6 g | sodium 29 mg

64. VEGGIE LOVER'S BROTH

SERVES	PREPARATION TIME	COOKING TIME	TOTAL TIME
10	10 MINS	2-3 HRS	2-3 HRS

INGREDIENTS:

- 4 carrots, peeled and chopped roughly
- 4 celery stalks, chopped roughly
- 3 parsnips, peeled and chopped roughly
- 2 large potatoes, peeled and chopped roughly
- 1 medium beet, trimmed and chopped roughly
- 1 large bunch fresh parsley
- 1 (1 inch) piece fresh ginger, sliced
- Filtered water, as required

DIRECTIONS:

1. In a pan, add all the ingredients over medium-high heat.
2. Add enough water to cover the veggie mixture and bring to a boil.
3. Set the heat to low and simmer, covered for about 2-3 hours.
4. Through a fine-mesh sieve, strain the broth into a large bowl.
5. Serve hot.

NUTRITION FACTS:

calories: 82 |fat: 0 g | carbs: 19 g | fiber: 4 g | protein: 2 g | sodium 37 mg

65. BRAIN HEALTHY BROTH

SERVES	PREPARATION TIME	COOKING TIME	TOTAL TIME
16	10 MINS	10-12 HRS	10-12 HRS

INGREDIENTS:

- 12 cups filtered water
- 2 pounds non-oily fish heads and bones
- 1/4 cup apple cider vinegar
- Sea salt to taste

DIRECTIONS:

1. In a large pan, attach all the ingredients over medium-high heat.
2. Add enough water to cover the veggie mixture and bring to a boil.
3. Set the heat to low and simmer, covered for about 10-12 hours, skimming the foam from the surface occasionally.
4. Through a fine-mesh sieve, strain the broth into a large bowl.
5. Serve hot.

NUTRITION FACTS:

calories: 75 |fat: 2 g | carbs: 1 g | fiber: 0 g | protein: 14 g | sodium 253 mg

66. MINERALS RICH BROTH

SERVES	PREPARATION TIME	COOKING TIME	TOTAL TIME
8	10 MINS	2-3 HRS	2-3 HRS

INGREDIENTS:

- 5-7 pounds non-oily fish carcasses and heads
- 2 tablespoons olive oil
- 3 carrots, scrubbed and chopped roughly
- 2 celery stalks, chopped roughly

DIRECTIONS:

1. In a pan, heat the oil over medium-low heat and cook the carrots and celery for about 20 minutes, stirring occasionally.
2. Add the fish bones and enough water to cover by 1-inch and stir to combine.
3. Set the heat to medium-high and bring to a boil.
4. Set the heat to low, covered, for about 1-2 hours, skimming the foam from the surface occasionally.
5. Through a fine-mesh sieve, strain the broth into a large bowl.
6. Serve hot.

NUTRITION FACTS:

calories: 113 |fat: 5 g | carbs: 1 g | fiber: 1 g | protein: 14 g | sodium 234 mg

67. HOLIDAY FAVORITE GELATIN

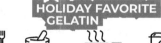

SERVES	PREPARATION TIME	COOKING TIME	TOTAL TIME
6	2-3 HRS	20 MINS	2-3 HRS

INGREDIENTS:

- 1 tablespoon grass-fed gelatin powder
- 1 ¾ cup fresh apple juice, warmed
- 1/4 cup boiling water
- 1-2 drops fresh lemon juice

DIRECTIONS:

1. In a medium bowl, pour in the tablespoon of gelatin powder.
2. Add just enough warm apple juice to cover the gelatin and stir well.
3. Set aside for about 2-3 minutes or until it forms a thick syrup.
4. Add 1/4 cup of the boiling water and stir until gelatin is dissolved completely.
5. Add the remaining juice and lemon juice then stir well.
6. Transfer the mixture into a parchment paper-lined baking

dish and refrigerate for 2 hours or until the top is firm before serving.

NUTRITION FACTS:

calories: 40 |fat: 0 g | carbs: 8 g | fiber: 0 g | protein: 2 g | sodium 5 mg

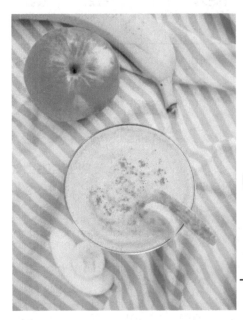

68. BANANA-APPLE SMOOTHIE

SERVES 1 | PREPARATION TIME 15 MINS | COOKING TIME 0 MINS | TOTAL TIME 15 MINS

INGREDIENTS:

- 1/2 banana, peeled & cut into chunks
- 1/2 cup plain yogurt
- 1/2 cup unsweetened applesauce
- 1/4 cup skim milk
- 1 tablespoon honey
- 2 tablespoons oat bran

DIRECTIONS:

1. In a blender, combine the banana, yogurt, applesauce, milk, and honey.
2. Blend until completely smooth.
3. Blend in the oat bran until it is thickened.

NUTRITION FACTS:

calories: 292 |carbs: 61 g | protein: 9 g | fat: 17 g | cholesterol: 103 mg

69. BERRYLICIOUS SMOOTHIE

SERVES 2 | PREPARATION TIME 15 MINS | COOKING TIME 0 MINS | TOTAL TIME 15 MINS

INGREDIENTS:

- 1/4 cup cranberry juice cocktail
- 2/3 cup silken tofu, firm
- 1/2 cup raspberries, frozen, unsweetened
- 1/2 cup blueberries, frozen, unsweetened
- 1 teaspoon vanilla extract
- 1/2 teaspoon powdered lemonade, such as country time

DIRECTIONS:

1. Fill a blender halfway with juice.
2. Combine the remaining ingredients.
3. Blend until completely smooth.
4. Serve right away and enjoy!

NUTRITION FACTS:

calories: 115 |carbs: 18 g | protein: 6 g | fat: 3 g | cholesterol: 223 mg

70. BUTTERMILK HERB RANCH DRESSING

SERVES 2 | PREPARATION TIME 15 MINS | COOKING TIME 0 MINS | TOTAL TIME 15 MINS

INGREDIENTS:

- 1/2 cup mayonnaise
- 1/2 cup milk
- 2 tablespoons vinegar
- 1 tablespoon fresh chives, chopped
- 1 tablespoon dill
- 1 tablespoon oregano leaves, chopped
- 1/4 teaspoon garlic powder

DIRECTIONS:

1. In a medium mixing dish, combine mayonnaise, milk, and vinegar.
2. Then, with 1/4 teaspoon garlic powder, add fresh chives, dill, and oregano leaves.
3. Combine everything.
4. Allow at least one hour for flavors to emerge.
5. Before serving, thoroughly mix the dressing.

NUTRITION FACTS:

calories: 83 |carbs: 1 g | protein: 1 g | fat: 6 g | cholesterol: 64 mg

71. CITRUS RELISH

SERVES 8 | PREPARATION TIME 10 MINS | COOKING TIME 10 MINS | TOTAL TIME 20 MINS

INGREDIENTS:

- 2 pounds small lemons, limes, kumquats or oranges
- 1-quart white vinegar
- 1/4 cup mustard
- Glass jars
- 2-4 tablespoons sugar

DIRECTIONS:

Pickled fruit

1. At the stem end of each fruit, make a cross. Quarter the oranges if using.
2. Fill glass jars halfway with vinegar.
3. To each jar, add 2 tablespoons of mustard. Put on the lids.
4. Allow it to sit at room temperature for about a month before preparing the relish listed below and serving.

Citrus relish

1. In a small frying pan, combine the fruit and sugar; add additional sugar to taste.
2. 5-10 minutes, shake the pan often over medium heat until the mixture boils and the fruit turns glossy and transparent.
3. Serve hot or cold.
4. The vinegar left over from the pickled fruit can be used to make salad dressing or to marinade chicken or seafood.

NUTRITION FACTS:

calories: 26 |carbs: 7 g | protein: 0 g | fat: 0 g | cholesterol: 37 mg

72. RED WINE SANGRIA RECIPE

SERVES 8 | PREPARATION TIME 2 HRS | COOKING TIME 0 MINS | TOTAL TIME 2 HRS

INGREDIENTS:

- 750 ml rioja wine
- 3/4 cup solerno blood orange liqueur
- 3/4 cup leblon cachaca brazilian rum
- 1 1/2 cup orange juice
- 3/4 cup cherry juice
- 3/4 cup simple syrup sugar syrup
- 1/2 cup fresh lime juice
- 1 1/2 cups watermelon balls
- 1 cup raspberries
- 1 cup blackberries
- 2 mandarin oranges sliced
- 1 lime sliced
- 1 bunch basil leaves

DIRECTIONS:

1. Stir together all of the liquid ingredients in a large pitcher. Then, to the pitcher, add the fresh fruit.
2. Refrigerate for at least 2 hours, covered. Pour into glasses and garnish with fresh basil leaves when ready to serve.

NUTRITION FACTS:

calories: 360 |carbs: 51 g | protein: 1 g | fat: 1 g | cholesterol: 423 mg

73. SALTY DOG COCKTAIL RECIPE

SERVES: 2 | **PREPARATION TIME:** 3 MINS | **COOKING TIME:** 10 MINS | **TOTAL TIME:** 13 MINS

INGREDIENTS:
- Four oz ruby red grapefruit juice
- Two oz vodka
- One ounce club soda or sparkling grapefruit-flavored water
- 1-2 teaspoons simple syrup
- Ice
- For garnish: kosher salt or fleur de sel agave syrup, grapefruit wedges

DIRECTIONS:
1. Set out two tiny shallow plates for the salt rim. In one plate, spread salt, and in the other, spread a thin layer of agave syrup (or just syrup). Dip the edge of a highball glass in the syrup before dipping it in the salt.
2. Fill the glass three-quarters full of ice for each cocktail. Combine the grapefruit juice, vodka, club soda, and 1 teaspoon simple syrup in a mixing bowl.
3. Use a cocktail swizzle stick to stir. If desired, add a bit extra simple syrup to taste. Serve with a fresh grapefruit slice on the rim.

Notes: add a sprinkle of cayenne to the salt before dipping for a fiery salty dog.

NUTRITION FACTS:
calories: 202 | carbs: 18 g | protein: 1 g | fat: 11 g | cholesterol: 26 mg

74. SIMPLE SYRUP

SERVES: 8 | **PREPARATION TIME:** 2 MINS | **COOKING TIME:** 3 MINS | **TOTAL TIME:** 5 MINS

INGREDIENTS:
- 1 cup water
- 1 cup granulated sugar or turbinado, demerara

DIRECTIONS:
1. Heat a small saucepot on high. Fill the saucepan halfway with water and sugar.
2. Bring to a boil, stirring constantly. Once boiling, remove from heat and stir. (if using herbs for infusion, add them to the simple boiling syrup.)
3. Allow cooling to room temperature before storing in an airtight container.

NUTRITION FACTS:
calories: 97 | carbs: 25 g | protein: 2 g | fat: 12 g | cholesterol: 44 mg

75. ROSE SANGRIA RECIPE

SERVES: 8 | **PREPARATION TIME:** 2 HRS | **COOKING TIME:** 0 MINS | **TOTAL TIME:** 2 HRS

INGREDIENTS:
- 750 ml french rosé wine (1 bottle)
- 1 cup pink grapefruit juice
- 3/4 cup bourbon
- 1/2 cup honey
- 1/4 cup chambord (raspberry liqueur)
- 2 cups watermelon balls
- 1 1/2 cups fresh sliced strawberries
- 6 oz fresh raspberries

Directions:
1. Scoop 2 cups of watermelon balls from a big piece of fresh watermelon using a melon baller. Strawberries, sliced
2. In a large pitcher, combine the rosé wine, grapefruit juice, whiskey, honey, and chambord. Stir the honey into the mixture until it melts. (if your honey is particularly thick, reheat it first to thin it up before adding to the recipe.) After that, toss in the watermelon balls and strawberries. Refrigerate for at least 2 hours, covered.
3. Stir and taste for sweetness after at least two hours. If you want your sangria sweeter, add a bit, extra honey. If the sangria is too powerful, serve it over ice. When ready to serve, mix in the fresh raspberries and divide among glasses.

NUTRITION FACTS:
calories: 209 | carbs: 26 g | protein: 0 g | fat: 0 g | cholesterol: 180 mg

76. CHAMPAGNE HOLIDAY PUNCH

SERVES: 16 | **PREPARATION TIME:** 5 MINS | **COOKING TIME:** 0 MINS | **TOTAL TIME:** 5 MINS

INGREDIENTS:
- 750 ml of champagne (1 bottle)
- 24 oz ginger beer (2 bottles)
- Three cups of cranberry juice cocktail (or juice blend)
- Two cups of ruby red grapefruit juice
- One cup of spiced rum, optional
- Possible garnishes: fresh cranberries, grapefruit slices, cinnamon sticks

DIRECTIONS:
1. All ingredients should be chilled. When ready to serve, combine all of the ingredients in a punch bowl.
2. Serve with cranberries, grapefruit slices, and cinnamon sticks as garnish.

NUTRITION FACTS:
calories: 107 | carbs: 13 g | protein: 0 g | fat: 0 g | cholesterol: 0 mg

77. WHITE SANGRIA

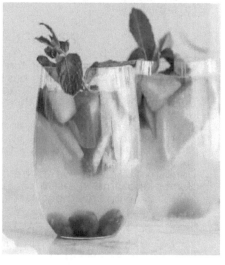

SERVES: 8 | **PREPARATION TIME:** 2 MINS | **COOKING TIME:** 3 MINS | **TOTAL TIME:** 5 MINS

INGREDIENTS:
- 750 ml moscato wine riesling is my second choice
- 1 1/2 cups orange-pineapple juice
- 1 cup domaine de canton ginger liqueur
- 1/2 cup midori melon liqueur
- 1 cup cantaloupe balls
- 1 cup sliced strawberries
- 2 mandarin oranges sliced
- 1 lime sliced
- 1-liter club soda chilled

DIRECTIONS:
1. In a large pitcher, combine the wine, juice, and liqueurs. Refrigerate for at least 2 hours after adding the fruit.
2. Pour into glasses 2/3 full (scoop in some fruit) and top with club soda when ready to serve. Serve chilled.

NUTRITION FACTS:
calories: 218 | carbs: 27 g | protein: 1 g | fat: 1 g | cholesterol: 18 mg

78. RASPBERRY MOJITOS WITH BASIL

SERVES: 8 | **PREPARATION TIME:** 10 MINS | **COOKING TIME:** 0 MINS | **TOTAL TIME:** 10 MINS

INGREDIENTS:

- One cup simple syrup 3/4 cup sugar + 3/4 cup water, heated to dissolve
- 1/2 cup torn basil leaves
- One cup fresh key lime juice use regular limes for slightly less acidity
- One cup white rum
- 1/4 cup chambord raspberry liquor
- 1-liter club soda
- Ice
- Fresh raspberries and lime slices to garnish

DIRECTIONS:

1. In a large pitcher, combine the simple cooled syrup and the torn basil leaves. Muddle the basil leaves with a big spoon/ladle to unleash their flavor—beat them up quite hard.
2. Combine the lime juice, rum, and chambord in a mixing glass. Stir. Stir in the club soda and top with ice if the pitcher permits.
3. Garnish each glass with fresh berries and lime slices to serve. Serve cold with or without ice.

NUTRITION FACTS:

calories: 283 |carbs: 36 g | protein: 1 g | fat: 1 g | cholesterol: 53 mg

79. MARGARITA

 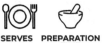

SERVES	PREPARATION TIME	COOKING TIME	TOTAL TIME
8	20 MINS	0 MINS	20 MINS

INGREDIENTS:

- 18 oz tequila blanco
- 18 oz fresh-squeezed lime juice (could be fresh bottled lime juice from the refrigerated section, but not the concentrated kind. Fresh)
- Nine oz la belle or grand marnier
- Eight oz simple syrup + a little extra for glass rims
- Three oz orange juice
- Three oz triple sec
- Coarse or flake sea salt for glass rims
- Sliced lime and orange for garnish

DIRECTIONS:

1. If you don't have any on hand, start by preparing some simple syrup. 7 oz sugar and 7 oz water microwave until the sugar is completely dissolved. You should have around 9-10 oz left over for rimming the glasses.
2. Combine all of the margarita ingredients in a big pitcher. Chill after thoroughly stirring.
3. Pour the simple leftover syrup into a shallow dish when ready to serve. In a second shallow dish, add sea salt (or flake salt). Then, dip the rims of the glasses in simple syrup, followed by salt.
4. If preferred, add ice to the glasses, and fill a shaker halfway with ice. Shake the margarita mix for 10-15 seconds in a shaker. Pour into serving glasses. Serve the cups garnished with cut limes or oranges. Ole'!

NUTRITION FACTS:

calories: 300 |carbs: 32 g | protein: 0 g | fat: 0 g | cholesterol: 29 mg

80. GRAPEFRUIT BASIL SORBET

SERVES	PREPARATION TIME	COOKING TIME	TOTAL TIME
6	3 HRS	30 MINS	3.5 HRS

INGREDIENTS:

- Four large ruby red grapefruits, juiced
- Two cups of water
- 1 3/4 cups of organic cane sugar or palm sugar
- Two lemons, zested and juiced
- One cup of basil leaves, packed
- Pinch salt

DIRECTIONS:

1. In a small saucepan, bring the water and sugar to a boil. When the water is boiling, add the lemon zest, basil leaves, and salt. Remove from the heat and cover with a lid. For at least 20 minutes, steep the basil leaves in the simple syrup.
2. Meanwhile, fill a 4-cup measuring pitcher halfway with lemon juice. Juice the grapefruits into the pitcher until 3 glasses of combined juices are measured.
3. Remove the basil leaves and strain the simple syrup. Then combine the syrup and the juice. Refrigerate for at least 2-3 hours (or to speed up, put in the freezer for 1 hour.)
4. Fill an electric ice cream maker halfway with the sorbet mixture. Turn on and mix for at least 20 minutes, or until the mixture achieves a "soft-serve" consistency.
5. Sorbet may be eaten right away or frozen in an airtight container. Allow the sorbet to soften for 10-15 minutes after it has been frozen before serving.

Note: to achieve the brightest, freshest flavor, use freshly squeezed grapefruits

NUTRITION FACTS:

calories: 272 |carbs: 70 g | protein: 1 g | fat: 1 g | cholesterol: 38 mg

81. BRULEED GRAPEFRUIT (PAMPLEMOUSSE BRÛLÉ)

Preparation Time: 5 minutes

Cooking Time: 8 minutes

Servings: 8

INGREDIENTS:

- 4 large ripe ruby red grapefruits
- 8 teaspoons granulated sugar
- Brulee torch

DIRECTIONS:

1. Place your index finger on the top of a grapefruit stem and cup your palm around it from top to bottom. Then, cut it in half in the middle. (if you don't notice a floral pattern, you've chopped the grapefruit the incorrect way.) Cut each grapefruit in this manner.
2. I am using a tiny serrated knife cut along the inside rim of each grapefruit half to separate the fruit from the skin. Then, cut along the membrane between each small triangle section so that each mouthful comes out easily with a spoon. Keep everything intact.
3. Sprinkle 1 teaspoon of granulated sugar over the top of each grapefruit half, one at a time. Then, hold the flame over the grapefruit and brulee the top until the sugar turns golden and has candied the top of each half. This should take 30-60 seconds per half. Serve immediately and repeat.

NUTRITION FACTS:

calories: 67 |carbs: 12 g | protein: 2 g | fat: 2 g | cholesterol: 86 mg

82. FROZEN BEERITAS RECIPE

 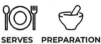

SERVES	PREPARATION TIME	COOKING TIME	TOTAL TIME
2	5 MINS	0 MINS	5 MINS

INGREDIENTS:

- 3 oz tequila blanco
- Oz triple sec (orange liqueur)
- 3 oz fresh lime juice
- 3 oz simple syrup
- 2 oz orange juice
- 14 oz mexican beer, such as two 7-ounce coronitas or one 12-ounce can any mexican beer
- 3-4 cups ice

DIRECTIONS:

Self-serve method

- In a blender, combine tequila, triple sec, lime juice, simple syrup, and orange juice. Pour with 3 glasses of ice. Puree the mixture until it is smooth and foamy. Serve the margaritas in two big tumblers, with a coronita on the

CLEAR LIQUID DIET - LUNCH

side. As they sip their margarita, each individual can add beer to it.

Mixed batch method

- In a blender, combine the tequila, triple sec, lime juice, simple syrup, orange juice, and a 12-ounce lager. Pour with 4 glasses of ice. Puree the mixture until it is smooth and foamy. Pour into serving glasses and serve.

NUTRITION FACTS:

calories: 386 |carbs: 51 g | protein: 1 g | fat: 0 g | cholesterol: 55 mg

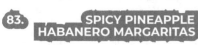

83. SPICY PINEAPPLE HABANERO MARGARITAS

 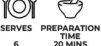

SERVES	PREPARATION TIME	COOKING TIME	TOTAL TIME
6	20 MINS	10 MINS	30 MINS

INGREDIENTS:

- 1 cup tequila silver
- 1 cup triple sec
- 1 cup fresh-squeezed lime juice
- 2 1/2 cups pineapple juice
- 4 habanero chiles
- Optional garnishes: salt, limes, habaneros, pineapple slices

DIRECTIONS:

1. Melt the butter in a small pan over medium heat. Remove the from the habaneros by cutting them in half. Place the chiles in the skillet and cook until they are blistered on both sides. Remove from the heat.
2. In a pitcher, combine the tequila, triple sec, lime juice, and pineapple juice. Stir everything together thoroughly.
3. Toss in the blistered habaneros. Allow them to soak in the margarita mix for 15 minutes to overnight. The longer they soak in the mixture, the hotter it will get. After 15 minutes, taste the mixture to see how long you want to soak them. When the heat level is to your taste, remove the habaneros.
4. Pour the margaritas into glasses with ice when ready to serve. Garnish with lime wedges, pineapple slices, or more habaneros if desired.

NUTRITION FACTS:

calories: 287 |carbs: 31 g | protein: 1 g | fat: 0 g | cholesterol: 65 mg

84. CRANBERRY POMEGRANATE MARGARITA WITH SPICED RIM

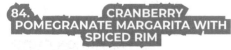

Preparation Time: 5 minutes

Cooking Time: 0 minutes

Servings: 4

INGREDIENTS:

- 2 cups cranberry pomegranate juice blend
- 2 cups tequila blanco
- 1 cup fresh squeezed lime juice
- 1/2 cup triple sec
- 2 tablespoons coarse sea salt
- 1 teaspoon old el paso taco seasoning
- 2 tablespoons agave syrup

DIRECTIONS:

1. Put 1 tablespoon water and 1 tablespoon agave syrup on a dish, gently mix everything together.
2. On a separate dish, combine the salt and old el paso taco seasoning.
3. Using the agave syrup, coat the rims of 4-6 glasses. Then, dip the rims in the seasoned salt. Fill the cups halfway with ice.
4. In a large ice-filled shaker or pitcher, combine the cranberry pomegranate juice, tequila, lime juice, and triple sec. Shake or mix before pouring into glasses and serving!

NUTRITION FACTS:

calories: 483 |carbs: 38 g | protein: 0 g | fat: 0 g | cholesterol: 346 mg

85. PEACH MILKSHAKE (COPYCAT CHIK-FIL-A PEACH SHAKE RECIPE!)

 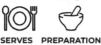

SERVES	PREPARATION TIME	COOKING TIME	TOTAL TIME
4	5 MINS	0 MINS	5 MINS

INGREDIENTS:

- 6 ripe peaches pitted, skins on
- 7 scoops of vanilla ice cream
- 3 tablespoons granulated sugar
- ½ teaspoon vanilla extract
- 1 pinch salt
- Optional: whipped cream and maraschino cherries

DIRECTIONS:

1. Remove the pits from the peaches and cut them in half.
2. Combine the peaches, ice cream, sugar, vanilla, and salt in a large blender.
3. Puree till smooth, covered.

NUTRITION FACTS:

calories: 397 |carbs: 62 g | protein: 7 g | fat: 9 g | cholesterol: 14 mg

86. JUGO VERDE (GREEN JUICE)

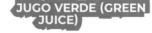

Preparation Time: 5 minutes

Cooking Time: 0 minutes

Servings: 4

INGREDIENTS:

- 2 cups orange juice
- 1 1/2 cups fresh pineapple chunks
- 1/2 nopal cactus paddle chopped (or substitute 1 celery stalk)
- 1 large cucumber with peel, cut into chunks
- 1/4 cup packed parsley or cilantro

DIRECTIONS:

1. In a blender, combine all of the ingredients. Add a bit of salt, close the lid tightly, and puree until smooth.
2. When the mixture is green and frothy, serve immediately or strain over a screen to remove the pulp.

NUTRITION FACTS:

calories: 67 |carbs: 12 g | protein: 2 g | fat: 2 g | cholesterol: 86 mg

87. PERFECT MANHATTAN RECIPE

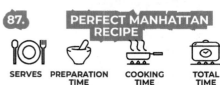

SERVES	PREPARATION TIME	COOKING TIME	TOTAL TIME
1	5 MINS	0 MINS	5 MINS

INGREDIENTS:

- 2 oz bourbon or rye whiskey
- 1-ounce sweet vermouth like antica
- 2 dashes of angostura bitters
- Garnishes: twist of lemon rind, orange rind, or a maraschino cherry

DIRECTIONS:

1. Fill a cocktail shaker halfway with ice for each manhattan cocktail. Combine the bourbon, sweet vermouth, and bitters in a mixing glass.
2. Using a bar spoon, stir everything together. Don't jiggle. Then strain into a coupe cocktail glass or a low ball glass filled with ice.
3. Serve with a maraschino cherry, lemon peel twist, or orange rind twist as a garnish.

NUTRITION FACTS:

calories: 190 |carbs: 2 g | protein: 1 g | fat: 16 g | cholesterol: 293 mg

88. FROZEN COCONUT MOJITO

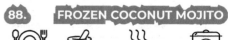

 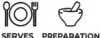

SERVES	PREPARATION TIME	COOKING TIME	TOTAL TIME
2	5 MINS	0 MINS	5 MINS

INGREDIENTS:

- 4 oz cream of coconut
- 4 oz coconut rum
- 2 oz fresh lime juice
- 8 fresh mint leaves
- 4 cups ice

DIRECTIONS:
1. In a high-powered blender, combine all of the ingredients with 4 cups of ice. Pour into glasses after blending until totally smooth.
2. If desired, garnish with mint and lime slices.

NUTRITION FACTS:
calories: 386 |carbs: 43 g | protein: 1 g | fat: 9 g | cholesterol: 182 mg

89. MULLED LEMONADE RECIPE

 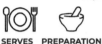

SERVES 8 | PREPARATION TIME 20 MINS | COOKING TIME 10 MINS | TOTAL TIME 30 MINS

INGREDIENTS:
- 5 cups water divided
- 1 cup granulated sugar
- 1 cup fresh lemon juice
- 3 cinnamon sticks
- 6 whole star anise
- 4 slices fresh ginger
- 4 pieces orange peel large
- 20 whole cloves
- 6 cracked green cardamom pods
- 1/2 teaspoon pink peppercorns

DIRECTIONS:
1. 2 cups of water, brought to a boil mix in the sugar and all of the pieces. Allow the simple syrup to steep for at least 20 minutes, covered. (the more time you have, the better.)
2. Fill a big pitcher halfway with syrup. Then add the remaining three cups of water and lemon juice. Fill the pitcher halfway with ice and swirl well.

Notes: if you don't want "floaties" in your drinks, drain the spices out of the simple syrup.

NUTRITION FACTS:
calories: 117 |carbs: 30 g | protein: 1 g | fat: 1 g | cholesterol: 70 mg

90. CUCUMBER ROSE APEROL SPRITZ

 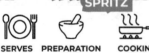

SERVES 1 | PREPARATION TIME 5 MINS | COOKING TIME 0 MINS | TOTAL TIME 5 MINS

INGREDIENTS:
- Oz rose-infused aperol
- 2 oz sparkling wine such as prosecco
- 2 slices cucumber about an inch thick
- Splash club soda

DIRECTIONS:
1. To make rose-infused aperol, mix one 750ml bottle aperol with one ounce dried rose petals (these can be found in the bulk section of most specialty food stores). Shake everything together and set it aside for a few hours or overnight. After straining off the rose petals, the aperol is ready to use.
2. In a cocktail shaker, combine the rose aperol and cucumber with ice. Fill a tall collins glass halfway with ice and strain it into it. Pour in the sparkling wine and ice. Garnish with fresh cucumber and a dash of club soda.

NUTRITION FACTS:
calories: 143 |carbs: 12 g | protein: 1 g | fat: 1 g | cholesterol: 50 mg

91. PINK GRAPEFRUIT MARGARITA

SERVES 2 | PREPARATION TIME 5 MINS | COOKING TIME 0 MINS | TOTAL TIME 5 MINS

INGREDIENTS:
- Five oz of freshly squeezed ruby red grapefruit juice
- Four oz of white tequila
- 1 1/2 oz of triple sec orange liquor
- 1/2 ounce of agave syrup + extra for glass rims
- Fresh grapefruit slices for garnish
- Salt for rim

DIRECTIONS:
1. Put a little quantity of agave syrup on one plate and salt on another. Dip the rims of the glasses first in the syrup, then in the salt. Fill the cups halfway with ice and set them aside.
2. Fill an ice-filled cocktail shaker halfway with ice. Fill the shaker halfway with fresh grapefruit juice, tequila, triple sec, and agave.
3. Cover and vigorously shake for 30 seconds. After that, pour into the glasses. Enjoy with fresh grapefruit slices as a garnish!

NUTRITION FACTS:
calories: 251 |carbs: 20 g | protein: 1 g | fat: 1 g | cholesterol: 192 mg

92. STRAWBERRY MARGARITA

INGREDIENTS:
- 1 pound fresh strawberries, trimmed
- 1 cup tequila
- 3/4 cup fresh lime juice
- 2/3 cup strawberry jam
- 1/4 cup triple sec
- 10 mint leaves
- 3-4 cups ice
- Optional garnish: margarita salt, lime slices, extra strawberries

DIRECTIONS:
1. Prepare a big blender. Add the fresh-cut strawberries, tequila, lime juice, strawberry jam, triple sec, mint leaves, and ice to the container.
2. Blend until smooth.
3. Toppings: paint additional strawberry jam around the rims of four glasses using a pastry brush. Dip the rims of the glasses in margarita salt. Fill the glass halfway with cold margaritas.
4. Serve with a fresh lime slice and a strawberry on top.

NUTRITION FACTS:
calories: 391 |carbs: 57 g | protein: 1 g | fat: 1 g | cholesterol: 142 mg

93. LARGE-BATCH GOOMBAY SMASH CARIBBEAN COCKTAILS

 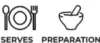

SERVES 40 | PREPARATION TIME 5 MINS | COOKING TIME 3 MINS | TOTAL TIME 8 MINS

INGREDIENTS:
- 14 cups 100% pineapple juice
- 2 bottles of dark caribbean rum (750 ml each - i used pusser's)
- 1 bottle coconut rum (750 ml - cruzan)
- 2 cups fresh-squeezed lime juice
- 1 1/2 cups simple syrup
- 1 cup orange liqueur (cointreau)
- 1/2 teaspoon bitters, optional
- Fresh pineapple slices for garnish

DIRECTIONS:
1. If you're creating your own simple syrup, mix 1 cup granulated sugar and 1 cup water. Cook until the

SERVES 9 | PREPARATION TIME 15 MINS | COOKING TIME 30 MINS | TOTAL TIME 45 MINS

sugar melts on the burner. Allow cooling fully.
2. Fill a big beverage dispenser halfway with all of the ingredients. Stir everything together thoroughly. Chill until ready to serve, then top with cut pineapples.
3. Serve with ice.

NUTRITION FACTS:
calories: 222 |carbs: 22 g | protein: 0 g | fat: 0 g | cholesterol: 11 mg

94. GREEN CHICKEN SOUP

SERVES	PREPARATION TIME	COOKING TIME	TOTAL TIME
12	15 MINS	25 MINS	40 MINS

INGREDIENTS:

- Two quarts of chicken broth or stock
- 1 ½ pound boneless, skinless chicken breast
- Two celery stalks, chopped
- Two cups of green beans, cut into

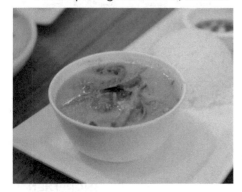

1-inch pieces
- One and a half cups peas, fresh or frozen
- Two cups asparagus, cut into 1-inch pieces, tops and middles (avoid tough ends)
- One cup of diced green onions
- 4-6 cloves garlic, minced
- Two cups of fresh spinach leaves, chopped and packed
- One bunch watercress, chopped with large stems removed
- 1/2 cup of fresh parsley leaves, chopped
- 1/3 cup of fresh basil leaves, chopped
- One teaspoon salt

DIRECTIONS:

1. In a large saucepan, boil the chicken broth over medium-high heat. Bring the chicken breasts to a simmer in the sauce. The cooking time is 15 minutes.
2. Combine the celery, green beans, peas, asparagus, onions, garlic, salt in a mixing bowl. Simmer for 5-10 minutes, or until the vegetables are soft, then remove from the heat.
3. Remove the chicken breasts and shred or cut them into bite-sized pieces with two forks. Back to the pot.
4. Combine the spinach, watercress, parsley, and basil in a mixing bowl. Season with salt to taste.

NUTRITION FACTS:

calories: 105 |carbs: 7 g | protein: 15 g | fat: 2 g | cholesterol: 134 mg

95. VEGETABLE BEEF STOCK

Preparation Time: 10 minutes

Cooking Time: 55 minutes

Servings: 12

INGREDIENTS:

- 1 pound lean beef shank, dice
- 2 slices fresh ginger
- 7 cups water
- ½ radish, chopped
- 2 carrots, chopped
- Salt, to taste

DIRECTIONS:

1. In a big pot, cook the onion until it is translucent. Bring the beef and water to a boil.
2. Turn the heat down to low, cover, and let it cook for 40 minutes. Remove the layer of fat that will rise to the top.
3. Add salt, carrots, and radishes. Keep cooking for 10 more minutes.
4. Strain to get rid of all the solids and keep just the broth.
5. Keep stock in the fridge overnight. Take off the layer of fat before using.

NUTRITION FACTS:

calories: 87 |carbs: 5 g | protein: 12 g | fat: 13g | cholesterol: 172 mg

96. FISHY TOMATO BROTH

Preparation Time: 15 minutes

Cooking Time: 50 minutes

Servings: 12

INGREDIENTS:

- 1 lb. fish bones
- 1 block silken tofu, cubed
- 7 cups water
- 2 cups tomatoes, finely chopped
- Salt, to taste
- 4 slices ginger root

DIRECTIONS:

1. Put water in a big pot and bring it to a boil. Boil the water with the fish bones and ginger for 10 minutes.
2. Put in the tomatoes and tofu. Turn the heat down to low and cover. Simmer for 40 minutes.
3. Strain to get rid of all the solids and keep just the broth.
4. Refrigerate stock overnight. Take off the layer of fat before using.

NUTRITION FACTS:

calories: 99 |carbs: 8 g | protein: 1 8g | fat: 6 g | cholesterol: 53 mg

CLEAR LIQUID DIET

DINNER

97. CHICKEN BONE BROTH

SERVES 8 | PREPARATION TIME 30 MINS | COOKING TIME 90 MINS | TOTAL TIME 120 MINS

INGREDIENTS:
- 3-4 pounds bones (from 1 chicken)
- 4 cups water
- 2 large carrots, cut into chunks
- 2 large stalks celery
- 1 large onion
- 2 cups Fresh rosemary sprigs
- 3 fresh thyme sprigs
- 2 tablespoons apple cider vinegar
- 1 teaspoon kosher salt

DIRECTIONS:
1. Put all the ingredients in your pot and allow to sit for 30 minutes.
2. Pressure cook and adjust the time to 90 minutes.
3. Set the release naturally until the float valve drops and then unlock the lid.
4. Strain the broth and transfer it into a storage container. The broth can be refrigerated for 3-5 days or frozen for up to 6 months.

NUTRITION FACTS:
calories: 140 |carbs: 0 g | protein: 25 g | fat: 0 g | Sodium: 73 mg | fiber 0 g

98. HOMEMADE BEEF STOCK

SERVES 6 | PREPARATION TIME 10 MINS | COOKING TIME 2-12 HRS | TOTAL TIME 2-12 HRS

INGREDIENTS:
- 2 pounds beef bones (preferably with marrow)
- 5 celery stalks, chopped
- 4 carrots, chopped
- 1 white or Spanish onion, chopped
- 2 garlic cloves, crushed
- 2 bay leaves
- 1 teaspoon dried thyme
- 1 teaspoon dried sage
- 1 teaspoon black peppercorns
- Salt

DIRECTIONS:
1. Preheat the oven to 425°F.
2. On a baking sheet, spread out the beef bones, celery, carrots, onion, garlic, and bay leaves. Sprinkle the thyme, sage, and peppercorns over the top.
3. Roast until the vegetables and bones have a rich brown color.
4. Transfer the roasted bones and vegetables to a large stockpot. Cover with water and slowly bring to a boil over high heat.
5. Set the heat to medium-low for at least 2 hours and up to 12 hours.
6. Pour the mixture through a fine-mesh strainer into a large bowl.
7. Taste and season with salt. Serve hot.

NUTRITION FACTS:
calories: 37 |carbs: 3 g | protein: 4 g | fat: 1 g | Sodium: 58 mg | fiber 0 g

99. THREE-INGREDIENT SUGAR-FREE GELATIN

SERVES 8 | PREPARATION TIME 5 MINS | COOKING TIME 0 MINS | TOTAL TIME 5 MINS

INGREDIENTS:
- 1/4 cup room temperature water
- 1/4 cup hot water
- 1 tablespoon gelatin
- 1 cup orange juice, unsweetened

DIRECTIONS:
1. Combine your gelatin and room temperature water, stirring until fully dissolved.
2. Stir in hot water then leave to rest for about 2 minutes.
3. Add in the juice and stir until combined.
4. Transfer to serving size containers then place on a tray in the refrigerator to set for about 4 hours.
5. Enjoy!

NUTRITION FACTS:
calories: 17 |carbs: 4 g | protein: 0 g | fat: 1 g | fiber 0 g

100. CRANBERRY-KOMBUCHA JELL-O

SERVES 8 | PREPARATION TIME 5 MINS | COOKING TIME 0 MINS | TOTAL TIME 5 MINS

INGREDIENTS:
- 1/4 cup room temperature water
- 1/4 cup hot water
- 1 tablespoon gelatin
- 1 cup cranberry kombucha, unsweetened

DIRECTIONS:
1. Combine your gelatin and room temperature water, stirring until fully dissolved.
2. Stir in hot water then leave to rest

for about 2 minutes.
3. Add in the kombucha and stir until combined.
4. Transfer to serving size containers then place on a tray in the refrigerator to set for about 4 hours.
5. Enjoy!

NUTRITION FACTS:
calories: 13 |carbs: 1 g | protein: 0 g | fat: 1 g | fiber 0 g

101. STRAWBERRY GUMMIES

 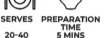

SERVES 20-40 | PREPARATION TIME 5 MINS | COOKING TIME 5 MINS | TOTAL TIME 10 MINS

INGREDIENTS:
- 1 cup strawberries, hulled and chopped
- 3/4 cup water
- 2 tablespoons gelatin

DIRECTIONS:
1. Bring your water and berries to a boil on high heat. Detach from the heat as soon as the mixture begins to boil.
2. Transfer to the blender and pulse. Add in your gelatin then blend once more.
3. Pour the mixture into a silicone gummy mold.
4. Place on a tray in the refrigerator to set for about 4 hours.
5. Enjoy!

NUTRITION FACTS:
calories: 3 |carbs: 1 g | protein: 0 g | fat: 1 g | fiber 0 g

102. FRUITY JELL-O STARS

 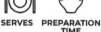

SERVES 4 | PREPARATION TIME 4 HRS | COOKING TIME 0 MINS | TOTAL TIME 4 HRS

INGREDIENTS:
- 1 tablespoon gelatin, powdered
- 3/4 cup boiling water
- 3 ½ cups fruit
- 1 tablespoon honey
- 1 teaspoon lemon juice

DIRECTIONS:
1. Attach all your ingredients into a blender and pulse.
2. Add in the gelatin then blend once more.
3. Pour the mixture into a silicone gummy mold.
4. Place on a tray in the refrigerator to set for about 4 hours.
5. Enjoy!

NUTRITION FACTS:
calories: 4 |carbs: 1 g | protein: 0 g | fat: 1 g | fiber 0 g

103. SUGAR-FREE CINNAMON JELLY

SERVES 2 | PREPARATION TIME 5 MINS | COOKING TIME 0 MINS | TOTAL TIME 5 MINS

INGREDIENTS:
- 1 cup hot cinnamon tea
- 1 cup room temperature water
- 2 teaspoons gelatin
- 1/3 cup sweetener

DIRECTIONS:
1. Combine your gelatin and room temperature water, stirring until fully dissolved.
2. Stir in hot tea then leave to rest for about 2 minutes.
3. Add in the sweetener and stir until combined.
4. Transfer to serving size containers then place on a tray in the refrigerator to set for about 4 hours.
5. Enjoy!

NUTRITION FACTS:
calories: 35 |carbs: 17 g | protein: 0 g | fat: 1 g | fiber 0 g

104. HOMEY CLEAR CHICKEN BROTH

 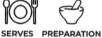

SERVES 6 | PREPARATION TIME 10 MINS | COOKING TIME 2-12 HRS | TOTAL TIME 2-12 HRS

INGREDIENTS:
- 2 pounds chicken neck
- 2 celery ribs with leaves, cut into chunks
- 2 medium carrots, cut into chunks
- 2 medium onions, quartered
- 2 bay leaves
- 2 quarts cold water
- Salt

DIRECTIONS:
1. Transfer the bones and vegetables to your stockpot. Top with enough water to cover then allow to slowly come to a boil on high heat.
2. Switch to low heat and simmer for at least 2 hours and up to 12 hours.
3. Set and pour the mixture through a fine-mesh strainer into a large bowl.
4. Taste and season with salt.
5. Serve hot.

NUTRITION FACTS:
calories: 245 |carbs: 8 g | protein: 21 g | fat: 14 g | Sodium: 58 mg | fiber 2 g

105. OXTAIL BONE BROTH

SERVES 8 | PREPARATION TIME 10 MINS | COOKING TIME 12 HRS | TOTAL TIME 12 HRS

INGREDIENTS:
- 2 pounds Oxtail
- 1 Onion, chopped in quarters
- 2 celery stalks, chopped in half
- 2 carrots, chopped in half
- 3 whole garlic cloves
- 2 bay leaves
- 1 tablespoon salt
- Filtered water (enough to cover bones)

DIRECTIONS:
1. Transfer the bones and vegetables to your stockpot. Top with enough water to cover then allow to slowly come to a boil on high heat.
2. Switch to low heat and simmer for at least 2 hours and up to 12 hours.
3. Set and pour the mixture through a fine-mesh strainer into a large bowl.
4. Taste and season with salt.
5. Serve hot.

NUTRITION FACTS:
calories: 576 |carbs: 48 g | protein: 24 g | fat: 48 g | fiber 2 g

106. CHICKEN BONE BROTH WITH GINGER AND LEMON

SERVES 8 | PREPARATION TIME 10 MINS | COOKING TIME 90 MINS | TOTAL TIME 100 MINS

INGREDIENTS:
- 3-4 pounds bones (from 1 chicken)
- 8 cups water
- 2 large carrots, cut into chunks
- 2 large stalks celery
- 1 large onion
- 3 fresh rosemary sprigs
- 3 fresh thyme sprigs
- 2 tablespoons apple cider vinegar
- 1 teaspoon kosher salt
- 1 (1/2 inches) piece fresh ginger, sliced (peeling not necessary)
- 1 large lemon, cut into quarters

DIRECTIONS:
1. Put all the ingredients in your pot and allow to sit for 30 minutes.
2. Pressure cook and adjust the time to 90 minutes.
3. Set the broth using a fine-mesh

strainer and transfer it into a storage container.
4. Can be refrigerated for 5 days or frozen for 6 months.

NUTRITION FACTS:

calories: 44 |carbs: 0 g | protein: 7 g | fat: 1 g | Sodium: 312 mg | fiber 2 g

107. VEGETABLE STOCK

SERVES 8 | PREPARATION TIME 10 MINS | COOKING TIME 40 MINS | TOTAL TIME 50 MINS

INGREDIENTS:

- 2 large carrots
- 1 large onion
- 2 large stalks celery
- 8 ounces white mushrooms
- 5 whole garlic cloves
- 2 cups parsley leaves
- 2 bay leaves
- 2 teaspoons whole black peppercorns
- 2 teaspoons kosher salt
- 10 cups water

DIRECTIONS:

1. Place all the ingredients in your pot. Secure the lid.
2. Pressure cook and adjust the time to 40 minutes.
3. Set the broth using a fine-mesh strainer and transfer it into a storage container.

NUTRITION FACTS:

calories: 9 |carbs: 2 g | protein: 0 g | fat: 1 g | Sodium: 585 mg | fiber 0 g

108. CHICKEN VEGETABLE SOUP

SERVES 8 | PREPARATION TIME 10 MINS | COOKING TIME 15 MINS | TOTAL TIME 25 MINS

INGREDIENTS:

- 2 tablespoons avocado oil
- 1 small yellow onion, peeled and chopped
- 2 large carrots, peeled and chopped
- 2 large stalks celery, ends removed and sliced
- 3 garlic cloves, minced
- 1 teaspoon dried thyme
- 1 teaspoon salt
- 8 cups chicken stock
- 3 boneless, skinless, frozen chicken breasts

DIRECTIONS:

1. Heat the oil for 1 minute. Add the onion, carrots, and celery and saute for 8 minutes.
2. Add the garlic, thyme, and salt then saute for another 30 seconds.
3. Add the stock and frozen chicken breasts to the pot. Secure the lid.
4. Pressure cook and adjust the time to 6 minutes.
5. Allow cooling into bowls to serve.

NUTRITION FACTS:

calories: 209 |carbs: 12 g | protein: 21 g | fat: 1 g | Sodium: 687 mg | fiber 1 g

109. CARROT GINGER SOUP

 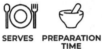

SERVES 4 | PREPARATION TIME 10 MINS | COOKING TIME 21 MINS | TOTAL TIME 31 MINS

INGREDIENTS:

- 1 tablespoon avocado oil
- 1 large yellow onion, peeled and chopped
- 1 pound carrots, peeled and chopped
- 1 tablespoon fresh ginger, peeled and minced
- 1 ½ teaspoon salt
- 3 cups vegetable broth

DIRECTIONS:

1. Add the oil to the inner pot, allowing it to heat for 1 minute.
2. Attach the onion, carrots, ginger, and salt then saute for 5 minutes.
3. Add the broth and secure the lid. Adjust the time to 15 minutes.
4. Allow the soup to cool a few minutes and then transfer it to a large blender. Merge on high until smooth and then serve.

NUTRITION FACTS:

calories: 99 |carbs: 16 g | protein: 1 g | fat: 4 g | Sodium: 1348 mg | fiber 4 g

110. TOMATO CASHEW PESTO

  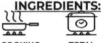

SERVES 4 | PREPARATION TIME 10 MINS | COOKING TIME 0 MINS | TOTAL TIME 10 MINS

INGREDIENTS:

- 95 g dried tomatoes
- 50 g cashew nuts
- 2 garlic cloves, minced
- 5 tablespoons extra-virgin olive oil
- 1 tablespoon oregano
- Parmesan cheese (optional)
- Salt and pepper

DIRECTIONS:

1. Puree the garlic, tomatoes, oregano, oil, and cashews with a hand blender until the mixture is even.
2. Mix with whole-wheat pasta and serve. Flavor to taste with salt and pepper then garnish with Parmesan.

NUTRITION FACTS:

calories: 29 |carbs: 2 g | protein: 1 g | fat: 4 g | fiber 1 g

111. SWEET POTATO AIOLI

SERVES 4 | PREPARATION TIME 10 MINS | COOKING TIME 35 MINS | TOTAL TIME 45 MINS

INGREDIENTS:

- 1 sweet potato
- 3 tablespoons olive oil
- 1 tablespoon mayonnaise
- 2-3 garlic cloves
- 1 tablespoon parsley, chopped

DIRECTIONS:

1. Bake the sweet potato in the oven until it is soft (about 35 minutes at 400°F - 200°C).
2. Set out of the oven, let cool down briefly, peel and mix with 1 tablespoon of mayonnaise, oil, garlic and parsley (use a hand blender).

NUTRITION FACTS:

calories: 480 |carbs: 55 g | protein: 2 g | fat:27 g | fiber 1 g

112. EGGPLANT PASTE

 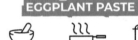

SERVES 4 | PREPARATION TIME 10 MINS | COOKING TIME 25 MINS | TOTAL TIME 35 MINS

INGREDIENTS:

- 1 eggplant
- 2 tablespoons tahini
- 2 garlic cloves
- 1 tablespoon lemon juice
- A pinch of turmeric
- 30 g black olives
- 1 tablespoon olive oil
- 1 tablespoon parsley, chopped
- Salt and pepper

DIRECTIONS:

1. Grill the eggplant in the oven at 380°F - 190°C for at least 20 minutes (until it is soft!).
2. Let cool and remove the skin. Set the eggplant in a container and use a fork to mash the meat into a paste.
3. Add the tahini, garlic, turmeric, olives, olive oil and lemon juice; mix well. Season to taste with salt and pepper.
4. Garnish with parsley.

NUTRITION FACTS:

calories: 120 |carbs: 13 g | protein: 2 g | fat: 48g | fiber 1 g

113. KULFI INDIAN ICE CREAM

SERVES	PREPARATION TIME	COOKING TIME	TOTAL TIME
16	3 HRS	0 MINS	3 HRS

INGREDIENTS:
- 2 cups heavy cream
- 14 ounces can sweeten condensed milk
- 2 teaspoon ground cardamom
- 1 teaspoon vanilla extract
- ½ cup chopped pistachios
- 1 pinch saffron + 1 tbs warm water

DIRECTIONS:
1. In a small dish, combine 1 tablespoon hot tap water. Allow a pinch of saffron to soak to absorb its color and taste.
2. Meanwhile, prepare an electric mixer fitted with a whip attachment. Pour in the heavy cream, cardamom powder, and vanilla essence. Whip the mixture at high speed until firm peaks form.
3. Using a rubber spatula, scrape the bowl. Then add the saffron and water and mix well.
4. Fold in the sweetened condensed milk using a spatula. Fold in the chopped pistachios after the mixture is smooth and uniform.
5. Insert the kulfi in an airtight container and freeze it, or spoon it into tiny cups for popsicles and place a popsicle stick in the center of each one.
6. Freeze for a minimum of 3 hours.

NUTRITION FACTS:
calories: 200 |carbs: 16 g | protein: 14 g | fat: 18 g | cholesterol: 44 mg

114. DARK CHOCOLATE WITH POMEGRANATE SEEDS

SERVES	PREPARATION TIME	COOKING TIME	TOTAL TIME
3	10 MINS	3 MINS	13 MINS

INGREDIENTS:
- 150 g dark chocolate (at least 70% cocoa)
- 120 g pomegranate seeds (from 1 pomegranate)
- 1 teaspoon sea salt

DIRECTIONS:
1. Scatter a layer of pomegranate seeds in a muffin tin (or muffin paper).
2. Melt the chocolate in the microwave.
3. Pour the chocolate into a bag, then cut a tiny hole so that it can be spread over the seeds. Add a layer of seeds and another of chocolate.
4. Sprinkle with a pinch of salt and chill in the refrigerator until the mixture is hard.
5. Enjoy cold.

NUTRITION FACTS:
calories: 82 |carbs: 19 g | protein: 2 g | fat: 1 g | fiber 4 g | sodium: 37 mg

115. COVERED BANANAS

 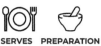

SERVES	PREPARATION TIME	COOKING TIME	TOTAL TIME
3	10 MINS	0 MINS	10 MINS

INGREDIENTS:
- 3 bananas
- 1 tablespoon oat bran
- 2 tablespoons cashew or almond butter
- 1 tablespoon honey
- 1 teaspoon chia seeds
- 1 teaspoon cinnamon

DIRECTIONS:
1. Mix the oat bran, seeds and cinnamon in a shallow bowl.
2. Mix the nut butter with honey.
3. Coat the bananas with nut butter and then add to the dry mixture so that they are coated on both sides.

NUTRITION FACTS:
calories: 11 |carbs: 3g | protein: 0 g | fat: 1 g | fiber 4 g |

116. HUMMUS WITH TAHINI AND TURMERIC

INGREDIENTS:
- 2 cans chickpeas, drained
- 50 ml lemon juice
- 60 ml tahini

 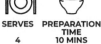

SERVES	PREPARATION TIME	COOKING TIME	TOTAL TIME
4	10 MINS	0 MINS	10 MINS

- 1 garlic clove, minced
- 2 tablespoons extra-virgin olive oil
- 1/2 tablespoon turmeric powder
- 1/2 teaspoon sea salt

DIRECTIONS:
1. Mix the tahini and lemon juice with olive oil, garlic, turmeric and salt for about 30 seconds using a hand blender or kitchen utensil.
2. Add the chickpeas and puree, making sure that no chickpeas remain unmixed on the sides. Pound until a uniform mixture is obtained.
3. Garnish with paprika powder and enjoy with any snacks, such as vegetable sticks.

NUTRITION FACTS:
calories: 33 |carbs: 9 g | protein: 2 g | fat: 1 g | fiber 1 g | sodium: 137 mg

117. PINEAPPLE ORANGE CREAMSICLE

SERVES	PREPARATION TIME	COOKING TIME	TOTAL TIME
10	4 HRS	10 MINS	4 HRS

INGREDIENTS:
- Two cups of orange-pineapple juice
- One cup heavy cream
- ½ cup granulated sugar
- 2 teaspoons vanilla extract

DIRECTIONS:
1. In a microwave-safe bowl, combine 1/2 cup juice and 1/2 sugar. Warm the juice for 1-2 minutes or until the sugar melts. Then add the remaining juice and whisk to combine.
2. Pour the heavy cream, vanilla extract, and 1 1/4 cup of the sweetened juice into a separate dish (or measuring pitcher). Stir everything together thoroughly. Then divide the mixture evenly among ten regular popsicle molds.
3. For 1 hour, place the popsicles in the freezer. Then, drizzle the remaining juice over the tops of each popsicle and insert wooden popsicle sticks. Freeze for at least 3 hours more.

NUTRITION FACTS:
calories: 145 |carbs: 15 g | protein: 17 g | fat: 8 g | cholesterol: 76 mg

118. EASY PEACH COBBLER RECIPE WITH BISQUICK

  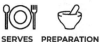

SERVES	PREPARATION TIME	COOKING TIME	TOTAL TIME
7	30 MINS	60 MINS	90 MINS

INGREDIENTS:
- 48 oz fresh or frozen sliced peaches 6 ½ cups, with or without peels
- Two cups granulated sugar
- ½ teaspoon of pumpkin pie spice or apple pie spice blend
- Cups bisquick baking mix
- 1 cup of whole milk
- 1 cup of melted butter

DIRECTIONS:
1. Preheat the oven to 350° F.. Prepare a 9-by-13-inch baking dish and a large mixing basin.
2. If you are using fresh peaches, cut them into wedges and remove the pits. Fill the baking dish halfway with fresh (or frozen)

peach slices. Then, over the peaches, add 1 cup sugar and the pumpkin pie spice. Toss the peach to coat it, then spread it out in an equal layer.
3. Combine the remaining 1 cup sugar, bisquick, and milk in a mixing basin. Whisk everything together well. Then add the melted butter and stir until combined.
4. Pour the batter over the peaches in an equal layer. Bake for 55-60 minutes, depending on the size of the baking dish.
5. After 40 minutes, check on the cobbler. If the top begins to darken, loosely cover with foil and continue baking.
6. Allow at least 15 minutes for the cobbler to cool before serving. Serve in dishes with vanilla ice cream or whipped cream.
7. Notes: you don't like peaches? Replace with an equal number of nectarines, plums, pitted cherries, or berries in this recipe.
8. How to keep leftovers: once the cobbler has completely cooled, cover it in plastic wrap or move it to a container with a lid. The fruit cobbler may be stored in the refrigerator for up to 4-5 days.
9. To put on ice: cook according to the recipe in a freezer-safe baking dish, cool, and cover the entire dish in plastic wrap. Wrap in tin foil and place in the freezer for up to 3 months. Unwrap and bake in a 350°f oven for 40-50 minutes,

NUTRITION FACTS:
calories: 420 |carbs: 59 g | protein: 11 g | fat: 20 g | cholesterol: 172 mg

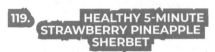
119. HEALTHY 5-MINUTE STRAWBERRY PINEAPPLE SHERBET

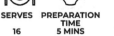

SERVES 16 | PREPARATION TIME 5 MINS | COOKING TIME 0 MINS | TOTAL TIME 5 MINS

INGREDIENTS:
- One pound frozen strawberries
- One pound has frozen pineapple chunks
- 1/2 cups plain greek yogurt
- 1/2 cup honey or palm syrup
- Two teaspoon vanilla extract
- Pinch salt

DIRECTIONS:
1. In a large food mixer, combine all of the ingredients. Pulse the frozen fruit to break it up. Then purée until completely smooth.
2. Serve immediately as soft serve, or freeze in an airtight container. Thaw for 15 minutes before scooping and serving if frozen.

Notes: this sherbet has a distinct honey taste. If you dislike the flavor of honey, use palm syrup.

NUTRITION FACTS:
calories: 70 |carbs: 16 g | protein: 2 g | fat: 1 g | cholesterol: 1 mg

120. BEST COCONUT MILK ICE CREAM (DAIRY-FREE!)

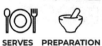

SERVES 16 | PREPARATION TIME 5 MINS | COOKING TIME 30 MINS | TOTAL TIME 35 MINS

INGREDIENTS:
- 27 ounce canned full-fat unsweetened coconut milk 2 cans
- 13.6 ounce can coconut cream
- One cup granulated sugar
- Two teaspoons of vanilla extract or vanilla bean paste
- 1/4 teaspoon salt

DIRECTIONS:
1. After making this ice cream numerous times, i learned that it does not always need to be heated/cooked before churning... This saves a huge amount of time. (this depends on the kind of coconut milk/cream and the kind of blender you use.) Put all ingredients in a blender and purée until smooth to see whether your ice cream has to be cooked. If the coconut ice cream mixture is smooth and free of clumps, you may churn it without heating.
2. Heat and stir: if there are any pieces of coconut cream in the recipe, they will freeze as hard waxy clumps in the ice cream. In this scenario, cook the mixture over medium heat until smooth, stirring often. Before churning, chill and cool to at least room temperature. *if you don't want to "test" the no-heat approach, simply combine all ingredients in a saucepot and cook over medium heat until smooth, allowing the coconut clumps and sugar to dissolve. Then take a break.
3. Set out a 1.5-2 quart ice cream machine after the ice cream mixture has cooled. Turn on the machine and place the frozen bowl inside. Fill the machine halfway with the extremely smooth ice cream mixture. Cook for 20-25 minutes, or until the mixture is thick, hard, and smooth.
4. Serve right away, or transfer to an airtight container and freeze until ready to use.

NUTRITION FACTS:
calories: 224 |carbs: 16 g | protein: 2 g | fat: 19 g | cholesterol: 27 mg

121. LEMON CRINKLE COOKIES RECIPE

SERVES 4 | PREPARATION TIME 40 MINS | COOKING TIME 10 MINS | TOTAL TIME 50 MINS

INGREDIENTS:
- 1 cup unsalted butter, softened (2 sticks)
- 3/4 cups granulated sugar
- 4 large eggs
- 2 tablespoons fresh lemon juice
- 2 tablespoon lemon zest
- 1 teaspoon vanilla extract
- 1 cup all-purpose flour (stir, spoon into the cup, and level)
- 2 teaspoon baking powder
- 1/2 teaspoon salt
- 1/4 teaspoon baking soda
- 2-5 drops yellow food coloring (optional)
- 2 cup powdered sugar

DIRECTIONS:
1. In the bowl of an electric stand mixer, combine the butter and granulated sugar. Cream the butter and sugar together on high for 3-5 minutes, or until light and creamy. Using a rubber spatula, scrape the bowl.
2. Mix in the eggs, lemon juice, lemon zest, and vanilla extract at low speed. Scrape the bowl once more. Mix in 1 cup of flour, baking powder, salt, baking soda, and food coloring on low. Once mixed, gently fold in the remaining 2 cups of flour until smooth. (be careful not to overwork the dough!)
3. Refrigerate the dough for at least 30 minutes, covered. (the longer the dough is chilled, the puffier the cookies.) Preheat the oven to 375°F. Set aside several baking sheets lined with parchment paper.
4. Set out a small dish of powdered sugar once the dough has cooled. To separate the dough into balls, use a 1 tablespoon cookie scoop. Roll each ball in powdered sugar, then place 2 inches apart on baking pans. (be careful to cover the cookies with powdered sugar generously.) You should not shrug them off.)
5. 9-10 minutes, or until the sides are golden brown and the middle appears slightly underbaked. Allow them to cool on the baking pans so that the centers continue to bake as they cool.

Note: storage suggestions: store the cookies in an airtight jar at room temperature. Consume within 7-10 days.

Citrus substitutions: in place of the lemon, you can use lime or orange juice and zest. You may also combine lemon and lime for a unique taste combination!

122. THE BEST NO-BAKE CHOCOLATE LASAGNA

SERVES: 12 | **PREPARATION TIME:** 4.5 HRS | **COOKING TIME:** 0 MINS | **TOTAL TIME:** 4.5 HRS

INGREDIENTS:

Oreo layer
- 40 oreo cookies
- 7 tablespoons melted butter
- Cream cheese layer –
- 8 oz cream cheese softened
- 3 tablespoons granulated sugar
- Two tablespoons of milk
- 16 oz of cool whip reserve half for later

Chocolate pudding layer
- 7.8 oz instant chocolate pudding mix two small boxes
- 2 ¾ cups of milk
- Two teaspoons instant coffee granules
- Whipped topping layer –
- Remaining cool whip
- 2 cup mini chocolate chips or ½ cup chocolate shavings

DIRECTIONS:

1. Set up a big food processor to make the oreo crust. In a mixing dish, combine the oreo cookies. Cover and pulse until tiny crumbs form. Then, pulse in the melted butter to coat. *if you don't have a food processor, you may smash the cookies with a rolling pin in a zip bag. Then, for the remaining processes, use a mixer.
2. Fill a 9 x 13 inch baking dish halfway with oreo crumbs. Chill after pressing into a uniform layer.
3. A layer of cream cheese: next, rinse off the food processor bowl. Combine the cream cheese, sugar, and milk in a mixing bowl. Blend until smooth. Then, using a knife, spoon half (8 oz) of the cool whip into the cream cheese. Fold the mixture with a spatula until it is smooth. Spread the mixture evenly over the crust in the baking dish. Chill.
4. Rinse the food processor bowl once more for the chocolate pudding layer. Combine the chocolate pudding powder, milk, and instant coffee in a mixing bowl. Puree till smooth, covered. In the baking dish, evenly distribute the ingredients.
5. Toppings: top the chocolate pudding with the remaining 8 oz of cool whip. Then, over the top, sprinkle with tiny chocolate chips or chocolate shavings.

6. Place in the refrigerator for at least 4 hours, covered. Freeze for 2-3 hours for optimum cutting results, then cut and serve. Allow 10-15 minutes for the frozen plated pieces to come to room temperature before serving.

Note: this is a fantastic make-ahead dessert that can be made 4-5 days ahead of time and stored in the freezer for up to 3 months.

NUTRITION FACTS:
calories: 533 | carbs: 72 g | protein: 16 g | fat: 8 g | cholesterol: 42 mg

123. EASIEST HEALTHY WATERMELON SMOOTHIE RECIPE

SERVES: 4 | **PREPARATION TIME:** 5 MINS | **COOKING TIME:** 0 MINS | **TOTAL TIME:** 5 MINS

INGREDIENTS:
- 4 cups fresh ripe watermelon cubes from a less melon
- 2 cup strawberry yogurt regular or a dairy-free variety
- 4 cups ice
- 1-2 tablespoons granulated sugar optional (only needed if the watermelon isn't very sweet.)

DIRECTIONS:
1. In a blender, combine the watermelon cubes and yogurt. Puree till smooth, covered. Taste to see if more sugar is required.
2. Pour in the ice cubes (and sugar if desired). After that, cover and purée until smooth.
3. Serve right away.

Note: garnish with cubes or slices of watermelon or cut strawberries.

NUTRITION FACTS:
calories: 120 | carbs: 27 g | protein: 27 g | fat: 19 g | cholesterol: 47 mg

124. WATERMELON

SERVES: 6 | **PREPARATION TIME:** 5 MINS | **COOKING TIME:** 0 MINS | **TOTAL TIME:** 5 MINS

INGREDIENTS:
- Whole watermelon

DIRECTIONS:
1. Stripes are well defined, with noticeable color differences between the green and yellow lines.
2. A huge yellow patch on the bottom indicates that the watermelon has been ripening on the vine in the field for some time and was not harvested too early.

NUTRITION FACTS:
calories: 111 | carbs: 16 g | protein: 29 g | fat: 18 g | cholesterol: 63 mg

3. Round versus oblong - round melons are sweeter than oblong melons. Although most watermelons fall somewhere in the middle, choose a round melon if you have the chance.
4. Weighty is ideal - choose a watermelon that appears to be heavy for its size. This indicates it's jam-packed with juice. Select a few alternatives to compare.
5. Thump the watermelon with a deep tone. The sound should be deep, showing that it is full, rather than dried out and airy on the interior.
6. Check the stem - if a stem is connected, it should be dried out and not green. A green stem indicates that the watermelon is in the process of ripening but is not quite ready.
7. Scars and blemishes are desirable - don't judge a book by its cover. Weathering on the melon's exterior is another sign that it has had plenty of time to sweeten.

Note:
How to cut a watermelon:
1. Remove the melon's short (stem) ends. Then, from stem end to stem end, cut the watermelon into quarters.
2. Start at the top of the fruit and cut straight down to the rind in 12 to 1-inch portions for slices.
3. Then, on each side, cut along the rind's edge, deep into the watermelon to remove the slices from the rind.
4. To make cubes, cut 1 inch deep into each flat side of the watermelon. Make sure to do this on both sides.
5. Then, starting at the top, cut down in 1-inch chunks.
6. Finally, cut along the rind's edge on both sides to release the rind cubes.

NUTRITION FACTS:
calories: 55 | carbs: 10 g | protein: 13 g | fat: 1 g | cholesterol: 10 mg

125. BEST ORANGE JULIUS

SERVES: 6 | **PREPARATION TIME:** 5 MINS | **COOKING TIME:** 0 MINS | **TOTAL TIME:** 5 MINS

INGREDIENTS:
- Six oz orange juice concentrate half a can
- One cup of milk 2% or whole
- ½ cup of water
- 1/3 cup granulated sugar
- Egg white about 3 tablespoons
- 2 teaspoons of vanilla extract
- ¾ cups ice cubes

DIRECTIONS:
1. Place all ingredients in the blender.

2. Puree until smooth.

Note:
This orange julius copy recipe yields 2 big (20 oz. Each) or 4 mini (10 oz.) Beverages. Do you want to make a strawberry or pineapple orange julius? Substitute 8 oz frozen strawberries or frozen pineapple pieces for the orange juice concentrate.

NUTRITION FACTS:

calories: 179 |carbs: 36 g | protein: 4 g | fat: 1 g | cholesterol: 6 mg

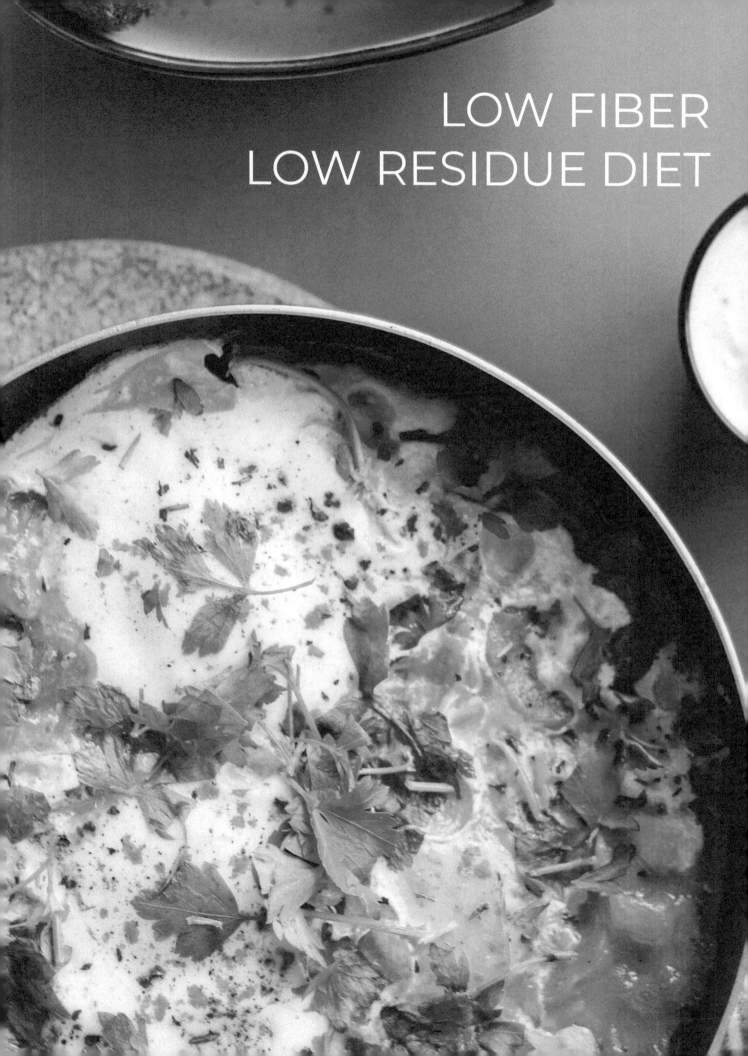

LOW FIBER
LOW RESIDUE DIET

LOW FIBER LOW RESIDUE DIET

BREAKFAST

126. LEMON BAKED EGGS

SERVES: 1 | PREPARATION TIME: 5 MINS | COOKING TIME: 10 MINS | TOTAL TIME: 15 MINS

INGREDIENTS:
- Eggs – 2g
- Cheddar cheese – 2 slices, low-fat
- Salt – to taste
- Lemon – 1 tsp, julienned
- Parsley – 2 tbsp, chopped
- Crusty white roll – one

DIRECTIONS:
1. Preheat the oven to 360°F - 180°C.
2. Spray the dish with olive oil.
3. Slice the cheddar cheese into three strips.
4. Line the edges of the dish with cheese. Break the eggs in the middle.
5. Place julienned lemon over the egg and sprinkle with fresh parsley.
6. Place dish into the oven and cook for 8 to 10 minutes.
7. Serve with crusty white bread rolls.

NUTRITION FACTS:
Calories; 233kcal, carbs; 0.6g, Fats; 16.8g Proteins; 21.3g; Fiber; 2g

127. BANANA PANCAKES

SERVES: 4 | PREPARATION TIME: 10 MINS | COOKING TIME: 10 MINS | TOTAL TIME: 20 MINS

INGREDIENTS:
- Firm silken tofu – 349g
- Dairy-free milk – 400ml
- Grapeseed oil – 4 tbsp
- Vanilla extract – 1 tbsp
- Flour – 250g, gluten-free
- Cinnamon powder – 2 tsp
- Baking powder – 1 tbsp
- Sugar – 4 tbsp
- Peanut butter – 4 tbsp. smooth
- Banana – 2, peeled, sliced
- Maple syrup, to serve

DIRECTIONS:
1. Add tofu, vanilla, cinnamon, and half of the dairy-free milk into the blender and blend until smooth.
2. Add remaining dairy-free milk to the mixture.
3. Pour baking powder and flour into another bowl. Make a hole in the centre of the dry mixture and pour the wet mixture in it and blend until smooth.
4. Add 2 tsp of oil into the pan and place it over medium flame.
5. Pour batter into the pan and cook for two minutes.
6. Flip and cook for two minutes more.
7. Spread peanut butter onto the pancakes.
8. Garnish with sliced banana.
9. Drizzle with maple syrup.

NUTRITION FACTS:
Calories; 193kcal, carbs; 29.2g, Fats; 6.6g Proteins; 5g; Fiber; 2g

128. DEVILED EGG

SERVES: 12 | PREPARATION TIME: 5 MINS | COOKING TIME: 10 MINS | TOTAL TIME: 15 MINS

INGREDIENTS:
- Whole egg mayonnaise – 3 tbsp
- Eggs – six
- Turmeric powder – one pinch
- Mustard powder – one pinch
- Salt and pepper, to taste
- Paprika – one pinch
- Water cracker – one packet

DIRECTIONS:
1. Add eggs into the saucepan and cover with water. Place it over medium flame. Bring to a boil. When boiled, cook the eggs for four and a half minutes.
2. Remove from the flame. Add eggs into the cold water for one minute.
3. Then, peel and slice them in half, lengthwise.
4. Scoop out the yolks and add them into the bowl. Let mash with pepper, salt, mustard, mayonnaise, and turmeric.
5. Slice a little piece of the rounded bottom of the egg white halves. Place onto the cracker or plate. Place yolk mixture into the white egg halves.
6. Sprinkle with paprika.

NUTRITION FACTS:
Calories; 125.3kcal, carbs; 0.7g, Fats; 10.5g Proteins; 6.4g; Fiber; 2g

129. BASIL ZOODLE FRITTATA

SERVES: 4 | PREPARATION TIME: 10 MINS | COOKING TIME: 40 MINS | TOTAL TIME: 50 MINS

INGREDIENTS:
- Bread crumbs – ½ cup
- Chives – ¼ cup, chopped
- Zucchini – two spiralized
- Eggs – six
- Cottage cheese – ½ cup
- Salt – one pinch
- Olive oil – 1 tbsp

- Basil leaves – ¼ cup

DIRECTIONS:
1. Preheat the oven to 360°F - 180° C.
2. Press breadcrumbs down onto the dish.
3. Put it into the oven and bake for ten minutes until golden.
4. Press it again. Blanch zucchini in boiled water and sprinkle with salt, and drain it onto the paper towel.
5. Add bay leaves, garlic powder, cottage cheese, chives, olive oil, and zucchini into the bowl and combine it well. Place onto the dish and press it down.
6. Beat the eggs and pour over the mixture.
7. Place it into the oven and bake for 20 to 30 minutes until golden.

NUTRITION FACTS:
Calories; 152kcal, carbs; 3.7g, Fats; 11.2g Proteins; 9.2g; Fiber; 3g

130. PEAR AND MUESLI MUFFINS

SERVES 10 | PREPARATION TIME 10 MINS | COOKING TIME 20 MINS | TOTAL TIME 30 MINS

INGREDIENTS:
- Wholemeal self-rising flour – 200g
- Muesli – 150g
- Brown sugar – ½ cup
- Pears – two, thinly sliced
- Walnuts – 75g
- Milk – one cup
- Butter – 50g, melted
- Egg – one

DIRECTIONS:
1. Preheat the oven to 360°F - 180° C.
2. Combine the walnuts, pears, sugar, flour, and muesli into the bowl.
3. Make a well in the middle of the mixture.
4. Pour butter, egg, and milk into the well and combine it well.
5. Divide the mixture into the greased muffin tray.
6. Sprinkle with muesli and bake for 18 to 20 minutes.

NUTRITION FACTS:
Calories; 372kcal, carbs; 47g, Fats; 18g Proteins; 6g, fibre; 5g

131. GREEN OMELET WITH PORTOBELLO FRIES

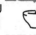
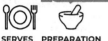

SERVES 2 | PREPARATION TIME 10 MINS | COOKING TIME 20 MINS | TOTAL TIME 30 MINS

INGREDIENTS:
Omelet:
- Zucchini – ½ cup, grated
- Fresh spinach – one cup
- Green onion – 1 tsp, green part only
- Chives – one tbsp, chopped
- Extra-virgin olive oil – 20ml
- Eggs – four
- Avocado – ½
- Lemon rind – 1 tsp
- Feta cheese – optional
- Pepper and salt – to taste

Portobello Fries:
- Portobello mushrooms – four, thickly sliced
- White breadcrumbs – 1 ½ cups
- Lemon rind – one tsp
- Parmesan cheese – one tbsp
- Eggs – two, beaten

DIRECTIONS:
Portobello fries:
1. Add parmesan cheese, lemon rind, and breadcrumbs into the bowl.
2. Let coat the mushroom slices in the beaten egg and then immerse in the breadcrumb mixture.
3. Spray the olive oil onto the baking paper. Place mushrooms onto the baking paper. Place it into the oven and bake for ten to fifteen minutes.

Omelet:
1. Add lemon rind and avocado into the bowl and keep it aside.
2. Add olive oil into the pan and heat it. Add green onion (green part only) and fry for two to three minutes. Then, add spinach and zucchini and cook for one minute until wilted.
3. Add eggs and sprinkle with chives.
4. Cook until firm.
5. Add feta cheese and turn the heat off.
6. Cut omelet in two and top with Portobello fries and sliced avocado.

NUTRITION FACTS:
Calories; 259kcal, carbs; 12g, Fats; 12g Proteins; 28g; Fiber; 3g

132. SHAKSHUKA

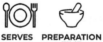

SERVES 2 | PREPARATION TIME 10 MINS | COOKING TIME 20 MINS | TOTAL TIME 30 MINS

INGREDIENTS:
- Red pepper 100g, drained, chopped
- Tomatoes – 800g, diced and cooked
- Tomato paste – 2 tbsp
- Green onion ½, minced, green part only
- Paprika – 1 ½ tsp
- Cumin – 1 tsp
- Stevia powder – ¼ tsp
- Salt and pepper to taste
- Olive oil spray
- Eggs – six
- Parsley – 1 tbsp, chopped

DIRECTIONS:
1. Place a pot over medium flame. Sprinkle with olive oil.
2. Add green onion and cook until translucent.
3. Then, add tomato paste, red pepper, and tomatoes and combine them well. Then, add stevia and spices and add them into the sauce.
4. Sprinkle with pepper. Lower the heat. Break eggs over the sauce.
5. Cover the pot with a lid and simmer for 10 to 15 minutes.
6. Garnish with fresh parsley leaves.

NUTRITION FACTS:
Calories; 146kcal, carbs; 10g, Fats; 9g Proteins; 7g; Fiber; 3g

133. SALMON FRITTER

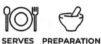

SERVES 4 | PREPARATION TIME 10 MINS | COOKING TIME 10 MINS | TOTAL TIME 20 MINS

INGREDIENTS:
- Tuna or salmon – 350g, drained
- Olive oil – 2 tbsp
- Tomato paste – 50g
- Cooked white rice – 400g
- Paprika – ½ tsp
- Oats – ½ cup
- Wholemeal flour – ¼ cup
- Egg – one

DIRECTIONS:
1. Preheat the oven to 210°F - 100° C.
2. Add rice, paprika, salmon, and oats into the bowl. Make a well and pour beaten egg and tomato paste, and blend until smooth.
3. Add white flour and shape the mixture into eight patties.
4. Place onto the baking dish and cook for five minutes.
5. Flip and cook for five minutes more.
6. Serve with tomato sauce.

NUTRITION FACTS:
Calories; 304kcal, carbs; 23.8g, Fats; 10g Proteins; 30g; Fiber; 3g

134. VANILLA ALMOND HOT CHOCOLATE

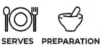

SERVES 2 | PREPARATION TIME 10 MINS | COOKING TIME 0 MINS | TOTAL TIME 10 MINS

INGREDIENTS:
- Vanilla almond milk – 600ml
- Full fat coconut cream – 30g
- Dark chocolate – 60g
- Cocoa – 1 tsp
- Stevia – to taste

DIRECTIONS:
1. Add vanilla almond milk into the pan and place it over medium flame.
2. Add stevia, cocoa powder, and chopped chocolate and heat it.
3. Top with coconut cream and chocolate shavings.

NUTRITION FACTS:
Calories; 195kcal, carbs; 33g, Fats; 4g Proteins; 8g; Fiber; 1g

135. BANANA AND PEAR PITA POCKETS

SERVES 1 | PREPARATION TIME 10 MINS | COOKING TIME 0 MINS | TOTAL TIME 10 MINS

INGREDIENTS:
- 1/2 small banana, peeled and sliced
- 1 round pita bread, made with refined white flour
- 1/2 small pear, peeled, seedless, cored, cooked and sliced
- 1/4 cup low-fat Cottage cheese

DIRECTIONS:
1. Combine the banana, pear, and Cottage cheese in a small bowl. Slice the pita bread to make a pocket.
2. Fill it with the mixture.
3. Serve.

NUTRITION FACTS:
Calories; 402kcal, carbs; 87g, Fats; 2g Proteins; 14g; Fiber; 11g

136. RIPE PLANTAIN BRAN MUFFINS

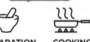

SERVES 12 | PREPARATION TIME 10 MINS | COOKING TIME 20 MINS | TOTAL TIME 30 MINS

INGREDIENTS:
- 1 ½ cup refined cereal
- 2/3 cup low-fat milk
- 4 large eggs, lightly beaten
- 1/4 cup canola oil
- 2 medium ripe plantains, mashed
- 1/2 cup brown sugar
- 1 cup refined white flour
- 2 teaspoons baking powder
- 1/2 teaspoon salt

DIRECTIONS:
1. Preheat the oven to 400°F - 200°C. In a bowl, combine the bran cereal and milk; set aside.
2. Add eggs and oil; stir in brown sugar and mashed ripe plantain. In another bowl, combine salt, flour, and baking powder.
3. Dissolve the dry ingredients into the ripe plantain mixture, stir until combined.
4. Pour the batter evenly into paper-lined muffin tins; bake for 18 minutes or until golden brown and firm. Allow cooling before serving.

NUTRITION FACTS:
Calories; 325kcal, carbs; 37g, Fats; 19g Proteins; 3g; Fiber; 2g

137. EASY BREAKFAST BRAN MUFFINS

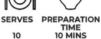

SERVES 10 | PREPARATION TIME 10 MINS | COOKING TIME 20 MINS | TOTAL TIME 30 MINS

INGREDIENTS:
- 2 cups refined cereal
- 1 cup boiling water
- 1/2 cup brown sugar
- 1/2 cup butter
- 2 eggs
- 1/2 quart buttermilk
- 2 ½ cups refined white flour
- 2 ½ teaspoons baking soda
- 1/2 teaspoon salt

DIRECTIONS:
1. Preheat the oven to 400°F - 200°C. Soak 1 cup of cereal in 1 cup of boiling water and set aside.
2. In a mixer, merge the brown sugar and butter until it is fully mixed. Add each egg separately and beat until fluffy. Then, stir in the buttermilk and the soaked cereal mixture.
3. In another bowl, combine salt, flour and baking soda. Add the flour mixture into the batter and ensure not to over mix.
4. Add in the remaining cup of cereal. Set the batter evenly into 10 greased or paper-lined muffin tins. Bake for 15-20 minutes. Allow cooling before serving.

NUTRITION FACTS:
Calories; 440kcal, carbs; 57g, Fats; 20g Proteins; 9g; Fiber; 3g

138. APPLE OATMEAL

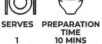

SERVES 1 | PREPARATION TIME 10 MINS | COOKING TIME 2 MINS | TOTAL TIME 12 MINS

INGREDIENTS:
- 1/2 cup instant oatmeal
- 3/4 cup milk or water
- 1/2 cup apples, peeled and cooked pureed
- 1 teaspoon brown sugar

DIRECTIONS:
1. In a microwave-safe bowl, mix oats, milk or water and apples. Cook in a microwave on high.
2. Stir and cook for another 30 seconds. Sprinkle with brown sugar and add a splash of milk.

NUTRITION FACTS:
Calories; 295kcal, carbs; 47g, Fats; 7g Proteins; 13g; Fiber; 5g

139. BREAKFAST BURRITO WRAP

SERVES 1 | PREPARATION TIME 10 MINS | COOKING TIME 15 MINS | TOTAL TIME 25 MINS

INGREDIENTS:
- 1 tablespoon extra-virgin olive oil
- 2 slices turkey bacon
- 1/4 cup green bell peppers, seeded and chopped
- 2 eggs, beaten
- 2 tablespoons milk
- 1/4 teaspoon salt
- 2 tablespoons low-fat Monterrey Jack cheese, grated
- 1 white tortilla

DIRECTIONS:
1. In a small non-stick pan, warm olive oil on medium heat and cook the turkey for about 2 minutes until slightly crispy.
2. Attach bell peppers and continue to cook until warmed through. In a small bowl beat the eggs with milk and salt.
3. Gently, stir in your eggs until almost cooked through. Turn the heat down then add the cheese.
4. Cover and continue cooking until cheese has completely melted. Place the mixture on the tortilla and roll it into a burrito.

NUTRITION FACTS:
Calories; 355kcal, carbs; 14g, Fats; 2g Proteins; 24g; Fiber; 4g

140. ZUCCHINI OMELET

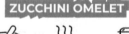

SERVES 4 | PREPARATION TIME 10 MINS | COOKING TIME 15 MINS | TOTAL TIME 25 MINS

INGREDIENTS:
- 2 tablespoons extra-virgin olive oil
- 1 medium zucchini, seeded and cubed
- 1/2 medium tomato, seeded and chopped

- 4 large eggs
- 1/4 cup milk
- 1 teaspoon salt
- 4 whole-wheat English muffins

DIRECTIONS:

1. In a large non-stick pan, warm olive oil over moderate heat. Add the zucchini and tomato.
2. Cook vegetables for 5-10 minutes or until they are soft.
3. In a separate bowl, merge the eggs, milk and salt.
4. Attach the egg mixture to the pan and stir to cook through. Set with white English muffins.

NUTRITION FACTS:

Calories; 160kcal, carbs; 14g, Fats; 10g Proteins; 6g; Fiber; 2g

141. SPICED OATMEAL

 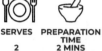 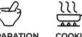

SERVES 2 | PREPARATION TIME 2 MINS | COOKING TIME 2 MINS | TOTAL TIME 4 MINS

INGREDIENTS:

- 1/3 cup quick oats
- 1/4 teaspoon ground ginger
- 1/8 teaspoon ground cinnamon
- A dash of ground nutmeg
- A dash of ground clove
- 1 tablespoon almond butter
- 1 cup Water

DIRECTIONS:

1. Combine the oats and water. Microwave for 45 seconds, then stir and cook for another 30-45 seconds.
2. Add in the spices and drizzle on the almond butter before serving.

NUTRITION FACTS:

Calories; 467kcal, carbs; 33g, Fats; 10g Proteins; 6g; Fiber; 4g

142. BREAKFAST CEREAL

SERVES 4 | PREPARATION TIME 5 MINS | COOKING TIME 0 MINS | TOTAL TIME 5 MINS

INGREDIENTS:

- 3 cups cooked old fashioned oatmeal
- 3 cups cooked quinoa
- 4 cups bananas, peeled and chopped

DIRECTIONS:

1. Combine the oatmeal and quinoa; mix well.
2. Evenly, divide into 4 bowls and top with the bananas before serving.

NUTRITION FACTS:

Calories; 228kcal, carbs; 43g, Fats; 3g Proteins; 12g; Fiber; 6g

143. SWEET POTATO HASH WITH SAUSAGE AND SPINACH

 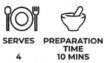

SERVES 4 | PREPARATION TIME 10 MINS | COOKING TIME 15 MINS | TOTAL TIME 25 MINS

INGREDIENTS:

- 4 small chopped sweet potatoes
- 2 apples, cored and chopped
- 1 garlic clove, minced
- 1 pound ground sausage
- 10 ounces chopped spinach
- Salt and pepper

DIRECTIONS:

1. Brown the sausage until no pink remains. Add the remaining ingredients.
2. Cook until the spinach and apples are tender. Season to taste and serve hot.

NUTRITION FACTS:

Calories; 544kcal, carbs; 65g, Fats; 2g Proteins; 12g; Fiber; 2g

144. CAJUN OMELET

  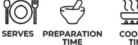

SERVES 2 | PREPARATION TIME 10 MINS | COOKING TIME 10 MINS | TOTAL TIME 20 MINS

INGREDIENTS:

- 1/4 pound spicy sausage
- 1/3 cup sliced mushrooms
- 1/2 diced onion
- 4 large eggs
- 1/2 medium bell pepper, chopped
- 2 tablespoons water
- A pinch of cayenne pepper (optional)
- Sea salt and fresh pepper to taste
- 1 tbsp. Mustard

DIRECTIONS:

1. Brown the sausage in a saucepan until cooked through. Add the mushrooms, onion and bell pepper. Cook for another 3-5 minutes, or until tender.
2. Meanwhile, whisk together the eggs, water, mustard and spices. Season with salt and pepper.
3. Top with your eggs over then reduce to low heat. Cook until the top is nearly set and then fold the omelet in half and cover.
4. Cook for another minute before serving hot.

NUTRITION FACTS:

Calories; 467kcal, carbs; 11g, Fats; 14g Proteins; 12g; Fiber; 2g

145. PEANUT BUTTER BANANA OATMEAL

SERVES 1 | PREPARATION TIME 5 MINS | COOKING TIME 0 MINS | TOTAL TIME 5 MINS

INGREDIENTS:

- 1/3 cup quick oats
- 1/4 teaspoon cinnamon (optional)
- 1/2 sliced banana
- 1 tablespoon peanut butter, unsweetened

DIRECTIONS:

1. Merge all ingredients in a bowl with a lid. Refrigerate.

NUTRITION FACTS:

Calories; 645kcal, carbs; 65g, Fats; 32g Proteins; 26g; Fiber; 5g

146. OVERNIGHT PEACH OATMEAL

SERVES 2 | PREPARATION TIME 12 HRS | COOKING TIME 0 MINS | TOTAL TIME 12 HRS

INGREDIENTS:

- 1/2 cup old fashioned oats
- 2/3 cup skim milk
- 1/2 cup plain Greek yogurt
- 1/2 teaspoon Vanilla
- 1/2 cup peach, peeled and diced
- 1 medium banana, peeled and chopped

DIRECTIONS:

1. Combine the oats, milk, yogurt, and vanilla in a bowl with a lid.
2. Refrigerate for 12 hours.
3. Top with the fruits before serving.

NUTRITION FACTS:

Calories; 282kcal, carbs; 48g, Fats; 6g Proteins; 10g; Fiber; 2g

147. MEDITERRANEAN SALMON AND POTATO SALAD

  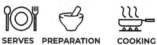

SERVES 4 | PREPARATION TIME 15 MINS | COOKING TIME 40 MINS | TOTAL TIME 55 MINS

INGREDIENTS:

- 1 pound red potatoes, peeled and cut into wedges
- 1/2 cup plus 2 tablespoons more extra-virgin olive oil
- 2 tablespoons balsamic vinegar
- 1 tablespoon fresh rosemary, minced

- 2 cups peas, cooked and drained
- 4 (4 ounces each) salmon fillets
- 2 tablespoons lemon juice
- 1/4 teaspoon salt
- 2 cups English cucumber, sliced and seedless

DIRECTIONS:

1. In a saucepan, set water to a boil and cook potatoes until tender, about 20 minutes.
2. Drain and set potatoes back into the pan. To make the dressing, in a bowl, set together 1/2 cup of olive oil, vinegar and rosemary.
3. Combine potatoes and peas with the dressing. Set aside. In a separate medium pan, warm the remaining 2 tablespoons of olive oil over medium heat.
4. Attach salmon fillets and set with lemon juice and salt.
5. Cook on both sides or until fish flakes easily. To serve, place cucumber slices on a serving plate top with potato salad and fish fillets.

NUTRITION FACTS:

Calories; 463kcal,carbs; 75g, Fats; 20g Proteins; 34g; Fiber; 3g

148. CELERY SOUP

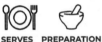

SERVES 2 | PREPARATION TIME 10 MINS | COOKING TIME 10 MINS | TOTAL TIME 20 MINS

INGREDIENTS:

- 1 tablespoon olive oil
- 3 garlic cloves, minced
- 2 pounds fresh celery, chopped into 1-inch pieces
- 6 cups vegetable stock
- 1 teaspoon salt

DIRECTIONS:

1. Reserve celery tops for later use. Warmth up the oil over medium heat in a soup pot.
2. Cook the garlic until softened, about 3-5 minutes. Add celery stalks, salt and vegetable stock then bring to a boil.
3. Cover and reduce the heat to low and simmer until the celery softens. Let the soup cool for a bit then puree with a hand blender.
4. Add and cook the celery tops on medium heat for 5 minutes.

NUTRITION FACTS:

Calories; 51 kcal,carbs; 4g, Fats; 3g Proteins; 2g; Fiber; 2g

149. PEA TUNA SALAD

SERVES 4 | PREPARATION TIME 60 MINS | COOKING TIME 0 MINS | TOTAL TIME 60 MINS

INGREDIENTS:

- 3 pounds cooked peas
- 1/2 cup low-fat mayonnaise
- 1/3 cup tarragon vinegar
- 1 teaspoon honey Dijon mustard
- 2 small shallots, thinly sliced
- 2 (6 ounces) cans tuna fish, drained
- 2 small sprigs fresh tarragon, finely chopped

DIRECTIONS:

1. In a large bowl, merge mayonnaise, vinegar and mustard. Add tuna fish, shallots and peas; toss to coat with dressing.
2. Secure and refrigerate for 1 hour before serving. Set with fresh tarragon and serve.

NUTRITION FACTS:

Calories; 246 kcal,carbs; 11g, Fats; 13g Proteins; 22g; Fiber; 1g

150. VEGETABLE SOUP

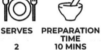

SERVES 2 | PREPARATION TIME 10 MINS | COOKING TIME 80 MINS | TOTAL TIME 90 MINS

INGREDIENTS:

- 2 tablespoons extra-virgin olive oil
- 4 garlic cloves, finely chopped
- 2 celery stalks, finely sliced
- 2 carrots, finely sliced
- 6 cups water or chicken broth
- 1/4 teaspoon thyme
- 1/4 teaspoon rosemary
- 1 bay leaf
- 1 can (14 ounces) peas
- 1/2 teaspoon salt

DIRECTIONS:

1. Warmth up the oil over medium heat in a soup pot. Add garlic, celery, and carrots and continue to cook for 5 minutes, stirring occasionally.
2. Add water or chicken broth, thyme, rosemary and bay leaf. Cook until it comes to a boil.
3. Set the heat and simmer gently for about 45-60 minutes. Add peas and season with salt.
4. Let soup cool slightly, remove the bay leaf and puree with a hand blender, until creamy.
5. Serve in warmed soup bowls.

NUTRITION FACTS:

Calories; 242 kcal,carbs; 34g, Fats; 8g Proteins; 12g; Fiber; 13g

151. CARROT AND TURKEY SOUP

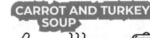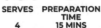

SERVES 4 | PREPARATION TIME 15 MINS | COOKING TIME 40 MINS | TOTAL TIME 55 MINS

INGREDIENTS:

- 1/2 pound lean ground turkey
- 1/2 bag frozen carrot
- 1/4 cup green peas
- 1 can (32 ounces) chicken broth
- 2 medium tomatoes, seeded and roughly chopped
- 1 teaspoon garlic powder
- 1 teaspoon paprika
- 1 teaspoon oregano
- 1 bay leaf

DIRECTIONS:

1. Over medium heat, set the ground turkey in a soup pot. Add peas, frozen carrot, paprika, tomatoes, garlic powder, bay leaf, oregano, and broth.
2. Set the pot to a boil, lower heat, cover, and simmer for 30 minutes.

NUTRITION FACTS:

Calories; 436 kcal,carbs; 20g, Fats; 12g Proteins; 59g; Fiber; 6g

152. CREAMY PUMPKIN SOUP

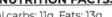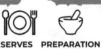

SERVES 4 | PREPARATION TIME 15 MINS | COOKING TIME 70 MINS | TOTAL TIME 85 MINS

INGREDIENTS:

- 1 pumpkin, cut lengthwise, seeds removed and peeled
- 1 sweet potato, cut lengthwise and peeled
- 2 tablespoons olive oil
- 4 garlic cloves, unpeeled
- 4 cups vegetable stock
- 1/4 cup light cream
- Salt
- 1 tbsp. chopped Shallots

DIRECTIONS:

1. Preheat the oven to 375°F - 190°C. Cut all the sides of the pumpkin, shallots and sweet potato with oil.
2. Transfer your vegetables with the garlic to a roasting pan. Set to roast for about 40 minutes or until tender.
3. Let the vegetables cool for a time and scoop out the flesh of the sweet potato and pumpkin.
4. In a soup pot, place the flesh of roasted vegetables, shallots and peeled garlic. Add the broth and set to a boil.
5. Set the heat, and let it simmer, covered for 30 minutes, stirring occasionally. Let the soup cool.
6. Set the soup with a hand blender, until smooth. Add the cream.
7. Season to taste and simmer until warmed through, about 5 minutes. Serve in warm soup bowls.

NUTRITION FACTS:

Calories; 332kcal, carbs; 32g, Fats; 18g Proteins; 12g; Fiber; 9g

153. CHICKEN PEA SOUP

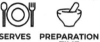

SERVES 4 | PREPARATION TIME 15 MINS | COOKING TIME 55 MINS | TOTAL TIME 70 MINS

INGREDIENTS:

- 1 pound chicken breast, skinless, boneless and cubed
- 2 tablespoons olive oil
- 3 garlic cloves, minced
- 3 carrots, grated
- 1 bay leaf
- 1 teaspoon salt
- 1 teaspoon poultry seasoning
- 8 cups chicken broth
- 1/2 cup dried split peas, washed and drained
- 1 cup green peas

DIRECTIONS:

1. Warmth up the olive oil over medium heat in a soup pot. Add the chicken and cook for 5 minutes, until lightly browned.
2. Attach the garlic, bay leaf, carrots, salt and seasoning. Cook until vegetables soften, stirring occasionally.
3. Pour the broth and split peas into the pot; bring to a boil. Set the heat, cover and simmer on low heat for 30-45 minutes.
4. Stir in green peas to the soup and heat for 5 minutes, stirring to combine all ingredients.

NUTRITION FACTS:

Calories; 176 kcal, carbs; 18g, Fats; 5g Proteins; 15g; Fiber; 6g

154. SPINACH FRITTATA

SERVES 4 | PREPARATION TIME 10 MINS | COOKING TIME 30 MINS | TOTAL TIME 40 MINS

INGREDIENTS:

- 2 teaspoons olive oil
- 1 cup red pepper, seeded and chopped
- 1 garlic clove, minced
- 3 cups spinach leaves, chopped
- 4 large eggs, beaten
- 1/2 teaspoon salt
- 1/4 cup Parmesan cheese, freshly grated

DIRECTIONS:

1. In a non-stick oven pan, heat 1 teaspoon of olive oil over medium heat.
2. Cook red peppers and garlic until vegetables are soft (about 10 minutes). In a medium bowl, combine the eggs, spinach and salt; set aside.
3. Add remaining 1 teaspoon of olive oil into the pan with vegetables and add in the egg mixture.
4. Set the heat and cook for 15 minutes. Sprinkle Parmesan cheese over the mixture and broil for an additional 4 minutes.

NUTRITION FACTS:

Calories; 106 kcal, carbs; 7g, Fats; 8g Proteins; 3g; Fiber; 2g

155. ALMOND PEANUT BUTTER FUDGE

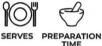

SERVES 2 | PREPARATION TIME 130 MINS | COOKING TIME 10 MINS | TOTAL TIME 140 MINS

INGREDIENTS:

- peanut butter (1 cup, unsweetened)
- vanilla almond milk (1/4 cup, unsweetened)
- coconut oil (1 cup)
- vanilla liquid stevia (2 tsps., optional)
- Salt - pinch
- For the Chocolate Sauce (topping):
- melted coconut oil (2 tbsps.)
- cocoa powder (1/4 cup, unsweetened)
- maple syrup (2 tbsps.)

DIRECTIONS:

For Chocolate Sauce:
1. Take a bowl and add the coconut oil, maple syrup and cocoa powder
2. Whisk together completely and keep it aside.

For Peanut Butter Fudge:
1. Slightly melt the coconut oil and peanut butter together over low heat on the stove (you can also use the microwave).
2. Add this melted mixture, vanilla almond milk, stevia and salt to the blender. Blend well until thoroughly combined.
3. Pour this blended mixture to a loaf pan lined with a parchment. Refrigerate for 2 hours until set.
4. Drizzle the chocolate sauce over the fudge after it has been set.
5. Refrigerate it for some more time and then serve.

NUTRITION FACTS:

Calories; 287 kcal, carbs; 4g, Fats; 30g Proteins; 15g; Fiber; 2g

156. QUICK COCOA MOUSSE

SERVES 4 | PREPARATION TIME 40 MINS | COOKING TIME 0 MINS | TOTAL TIME 40 MINS

INGREDIENTS:

- heavy whipping cream (6 tbsps., whip it and keep ready)
- butter (4 tbsps., unsalted)
- cocoa powder (1 tbsp)
- cream cheese (4 tbsps.)
- coconut oil (1 tsp)
- Stevia (as per taste)

DIRECTIONS:

1. Soften the butter in a microwave and then combine it with stevia. Stir well until it blends completely.
2. Add the cream cheese and cocoa powder to the butter mixture. Blend thoroughly until it becomes smooth.
3. Slowly add the whipped heavy cream to the mixture and keep stirring. Add 1 tsp of MCT oil or coconut oil to the mixture and blend again.
4. Spoon the smooth mixture into small glasses and refrigerate for 30 minutes.
5. Serve chilled.

NUTRITION FACTS:

227 calories, 2 g fat, 3 g carbs, 1 g fiber, 4 g protein

157. CINNAMON PEAR CHIPS

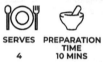

SERVES 4 | PREPARATION TIME 10 MINS | COOKING TIME 3 HRS | TOTAL TIME 3 HRS

INGREDIENTS:

- Pears (4)
- ground cinnamon (1 teaspoon)

DIRECTIONS:

1. Preheat the oven to 200°F - 100°C. Line a baking sheet with parchment paper.
2. Core the pears and cut into 1/8-inch slices. Toss pears with cinnamon.
3. Spread the pears in a single layer on the prepared baking sheet. Cook for 2 to 3 hours, until the pears are dry.
4. They will still be soft while hot but will crisp once completely cooled. Store in an airtight container for up to four days.

NUTRITION FACTS:

96 calories, 0 g fat, 26 g carbs, 1 g fiber, 1 g protein

158. CHOCOLATE YOGURT CREAM & ROASTED BANANAS

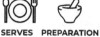

SERVES 4 | PREPARATION TIME 10 MINS | COOKING TIME 5 MINS | TOTAL TIME 15 MINS

INGREDIENTS:

- whipping cream (½ cup)
- ground cinnamon (½ tsp)
- low fat vanilla yogurt (1 ½ cups, chilled and drained)
- cold butter (1 tbsp)
- confectioner's sugar (1 tbsp)
- dark rum (1 tbsp)
- unsweetened cocoa powder (2 tbsp)
- dark brown sugar (3 tbsp)
- bananas (4, cut in strips)

DIRECTIONS:

1. Place bananas cut side up on a baking sheet coated with cooking spray.
2. Sprinkle with brown sugar, rum and cinnamon. Dot with butter.
3. Roast in a 425°F - 220°C preheated oven for five minutes.
4. Turn the broiler off until the bananas are golden.
5. Meanwhile, beat the cocoa, cream and confectioner's sugar in a large bowl using an electric mixer.
6. Add the drained yogurt and fold the cream until well combined. Plate the roasted bananas and add a dollop of chocolate cream on top.

NUTRITION FACTS:

236 calories, 0 g fat, 42g carbs, 3 g fiber, 7 g protein

159. COCONUT CELERY SMOOTHIE

 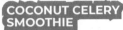

SERVES 2 | PREPARATION TIME 10 MINS | COOKING TIME 0 MINS | TOTAL TIME 10 MINS

INGREDIENTS:

- celery stalks (3, shredded)
- ground cinnamon (1 tsp)
- banana (½)
- protein powder (1 scoop)
- coconut butter (1 tbsp)
- unsweetened coconut milk (1 cup)

DIRECTIONS:

1. Toss your ingredients into a blender then process until creamy and smooth. Serve immediately and enjoy.

NUTRITION FACTS:

391 calories, 15 g fat, 42 g carbs, 1 g fiber, 29 g protein

160. APPLE SPINACH SMOOTHIE

   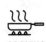

SERVES 2 | PREPARATION TIME 10 MINS | COOKING TIME 0 MINS | TOTAL TIME 10 MINS

INGREDIENTS:

- vanilla extract (¼ tsp)
- ginger (1 tsp, grated)
- maple syrup (1 tsp)
- coconut butter (1 ½ tbsp)
- yogurt (½ cup)
- apple (1, chopped)
- baby spinach (1 cup)
- unsweetened coconut milk (1 cup)

DIRECTIONS:

1. Toss your ingredients into a blender then process until creamy and smooth. Serve immediately and enjoy.

NUTRITION FACTS:

388 calories, 19 g fat, 43 g carbs, 3 g fiber, 15 g protein

LOW FIBER LOW RESIDUE DIET

LUNCH

161. BARBECUE BEEF STIR-FRY

SERVES: 4
PREPARATION TIME: 5 MINS
COOKING TIME: 10 MINS
TOTAL TIME: 15 MINS

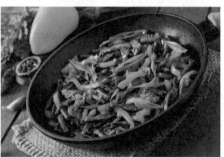

INGREDIENTS:
- Barbecue Sauce – ¼ cup
- Beef broth – three tbsp, low-sodium
- Beef sirloin steak – one lb, boneless, cut into strips
- Onion – one, sliced
- Carrot – one, thinly sliced
- Oil – one tablespoon
- Hot cooked long-grain white rice – two cups

DIRECTIONS:
1. Combine the broth and BBQ sauce into the bowl.
2. Rub one tbsp of meat and let stand for five minutes.
3. Add vegetable, meat, and oil into the skillet and cook over medium-high flame for four minutes.
4. Add remaining BBQ sauce mixture and combine well. Let simmer over medium-low flame for two minutes.
5. Serve and enjoy!

162. CHICKEN SAFFRON RICE PILAF

NUTRITION FACTS:
Calories; 310kcal, carbs; 34g, protein; 23g, fat; 9g

SERVES: 6
PREPARATION TIME: 10 MINS
COOKING TIME: 30 MINS
TOTAL TIME: 40 MINS

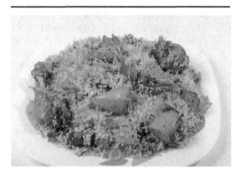

INGREDIENTS:
- Saffron – one pinch
- Ghee or olive oil – one tbsp
- Carrot – one, peeled, chopped
- Celery – one stalk, outside parts peeled, chopped
- Basmati rice or jasmine rice – 1 ½ cups
- Chicken broth – three cups, low-sodium
- Chicken breast – 1 ¼ cups, roasted, shredded
- Lemon – one
- Fresh parsley – chopped, to garnish

DIRECTIONS:
1. Add saffron and water into the bowl and soak it.
2. Add ghee into the skillet and heat it. Then, add celery and carrots and sauté for three to four minutes until softened. Add rice and sauté until toasted.
3. Add saffron and chicken broth to the skillet, bring to a boil, lower the heat, and cook for twenty-five to thirty minutes.
4. Add shredded chicken to the rice and toss to combine.
5. Let sit for five minutes.
6. When ready to serve, add lemon juice over the rice.
7. Garnish with chopped parsley leaves.

NUTRITION FACTS:
Calories; 269kcal, carbs; 41g, Fats; 5g Proteins; 13g

163. STIR-FRY GROUND CHICKEN AND GREEN BEANS

SERVES: 2
PREPARATION TIME: 5 MINS
COOKING TIME: 10 MINS
TOTAL TIME: 15 MINS

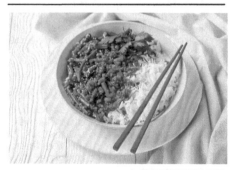

INGREDIENTS:
- Green bean – 2 cups
- Oil – one tbsp
- Ginger – one slice
- Ground chicken – ½ lb
- Soy sauce – 1 tbsp
- Rice wine – 1 tsp

- Sesame oil – 1 tsp
- Sugar – 1 tsp

DIRECTIONS:

1. Add green beans into the boiled water and cook until tender.
2. Drain it and put it into the bowl of ice water.
3. Add oil into the skillet and heat it. Then, add a ginger slice and fry for one to two minutes.
4. Add ground chicken and cook until no longer pink.
5. Add sugar, sesame oil, rice wine, and soy sauce and toss to combine.
6. Add drained green beans and cook them.
7. Serve and enjoy!

NUTRITION FACTS:

Calories; 162kcal, carbs; 10g, Fats; 18g Proteins; 22g, fiber; 2g

164. STEWED LAMB

  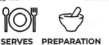   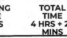

SERVES 6 | PREPARATION TIME 20 MINS | COOKING TIME 4 HRS | TOTAL TIME 4 HRS + 20 MINS

INGREDIENTS:

- Lamb leg – 1 1/2kg, boneless
- Extra-virgin olive oil – 2 tbsp
- Beef or vegetable broth – 400ml
- Red wine – 300ml
- Wholemeal flour – 80g
- Button mushrooms – 400g, sliced in half
- Fresh rosemary leaves – 1 tsp
- Potatoes – 1kg, cut into quarters, red-skinned
- Celery sticks – two chopped
- Carrots – two, cut into large chunks
- Parsley – 1 cup, chopped

DIRECTIONS:

1. Add olive oil into the saucepan and place it over medium flame.
2. Cook until browned. Add stock to the slow cooker, place the lamb with all ingredients into the slow cooker, and cook on low flame for eight hours.
3. After eight hours, turn off the slow cooker and add cooled stock to the bowl to make a paste with wholemeal flour. Stir well.
4. Add flour paste and sprinkle with pepper and salt.
5. Sprinkle with fresh parsley leaves.

NUTRITION FACTS:

Calories; 481kcal, carbs; 22g, Fats; 27g Proteins; 28g, fiber; 4g

165. PULLED CHICKEN SALAD

SERVES 4 | PREPARATION TIME 5 MINS | COOKING TIME 5 MINS | TOTAL TIME 10 MINS

INGREDIENTS:

- Pulled BBQ chicken – 200g, cooked
- Apricots – 1/3 cup, drained, thinly sliced
- Orzo pasta – 100g
- Spinach – 150g, stalks removed
- Cheddar cheese, 70g, cut into small cubes
- Parmesan cheese – 30g
- Parsley – ¼ cup, chopped
- Noodles – 1/3 cup
- Olive oil – five tbsp
- Red wine vinegar – three tbsp
- Salt and pepper, to taste

DIRECTIONS:

- Shred cooked and cooled chicken with a fork.
- Add cooked and cooled orzo pasta into the microwave dish. Top with parmesan cheese and microwave for one to two minutes.
- Add apricots, chicken, parsley, and spinach into the bowl and mix it well. Then, add red wine vinegar and olive oil, sprinkle with pepper and salt, and pour over the salad. Combine it well.
- Add crispy noodles before serving.

NUTRITION FACTS:

Calories; 352kcal, carbs; 14g, Fats; 19g Proteins; 29g, fiber; 3g

166. LEMONGRASS BEEF

SERVES 4 | PREPARATION TIME 5 MINS | COOKING TIME 10 MINS | TOTAL TIME 15 MINS

INGREDIENTS:

- Sesame oil – 2 tbsp
- Fish sauce – 1 tbsp
- Sweet chili sauce – 2 tbsp
- Basmati rice – 2 packets, microwave
- Coconut – 2 tsp, shredded
- Lemongrass paste – 1 tbsp
- Beef – 500g, minced, grass-fed
- Thai seasoning – 1 tbsp
- Cucumber – 100g, peeled and cut into chunks
- Carrots – two, peeled and julienned
- Basil – ¼ cup, chopped
- Lime – one, cut into four wedges

DIRECTIONS:

1. Add sesame oil, lemongrass paste, fish sauce, and Thai seasoning into the wok and heat it. Add the minced beef and stir well and cook for three to four minutes until browned.
2. Cook the rice according to the instructions.
3. Add one tsp shredded coconut and stir well.
4. Add carrots, cucumber, rice, and minced beef into the bowl.
5. Sprinkle with Thai basil.
6. Pour sweet chili sauce and lime wedges over it.

NUTRITION FACTS:

Calories; 450kcal, carbs; 50g, Fats; 19g Proteins; 21g, fiber; 3g

167. BEETROOT CARROT SALAD

 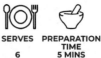

SERVES 6 | PREPARATION TIME 5 MINS | COOKING TIME 40 MINS | TOTAL TIME 45 MINS

INGREDIENTS:

- Beetroot – three, peeled
- Carrots – three, peeled
- Halloumi, 500g, thickly sliced
- Fresh oregano leaves – one tsp
- Maple syrup – 100ml
- Fresh lemon juice – 50ml
- Spinach leaves – 50g
- Tahini – 200g, hulled
- Noodles – 100g
- Extra virgin olive oil – 2 tbsp

DIRECTIONS:

1. Preheat the oven to 360°F - 180°C.
2. Wrap the beetroot and carrots into the foil and put it into the oven for forty minutes.
3. Let cool it and then cut into the wedges.
4. Add olive oil into the saucepan and place it over medium flame.
5. Turn off the flame and add oregano, lemon juice, and maple syrup and stir well.
6. Add one tbsp of hulled tahini onto the plate.
7. Top with beetroot and carrot wedges, halloumi and spinach leaves.
8. Sprinkle with crispy noodles.

NUTRITION FACTS:

Calories; 206kcal, carbs; 34.9g, Fats; 6.6g Proteins; 4.5g, fiber; 4g

168. CRUNCHY MAPLE SWEET POTATOES

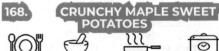 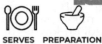 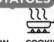

SERVES 6 | PREPARATION TIME 10 MINS | COOKING TIME 50 MINS | TOTAL TIME 60 MINS

INGREDIENTS:

- Allspice – one pinch
- Pure maple syrup – 2 tbsp
- Cashew nuts – ¼ cup, crushed
- Potatoes:
- Extra-virgin olive oil spray
- White potatoes – 500g, peeled
- Sweet potato – one, peeled
- Plain white flour – ¼ cup
- Apple juice – ½ cup
- Butter – one tbsp
- Sweet soy sauce – 1 tsp
- Maple syrup – one tbsp
- Cinnamon – one pinch
- Salt and pepper – to taste

DIRECTIONS:

1. Preheat the oven to 360°F - 180°C.
2. Mix all ingredients into the dish, place it into the oven, and bake for ten to fifteen minutes until golden and crunchy.
3. Keep it aside.

Potatoes:

1. Let boil the potatoes for fifteen to twenty minutes.
2. Spray the baking dish with extra virgin olive oil.
3. Slice potatoes into chunks and place them onto the dish.
4. Add all other ingredients into the bowl and combine them well.
5. Pour mixture over the potatoes and cover with a lid and bake for ten minutes.
6. Sprinkle with nuts.

NUTRITION FACTS:

Calories; 92kcal, carbs; 18g, Fats; 2g Proteins; 1.2g, fiber; 1g

169. VEGGIE BOWL

SERVES 2 | PREPARATION TIME 10 MINS | COOKING TIME 0 MINS | TOTAL TIME 10 MINS

INGREDIENTS:

- White basmati rice – 100g
- Green beans – six
- Red pepper, peeled, diced, and roasted
- Ripe avocado – ¼, sliced lengthways
- Cucumber – half cup, sliced
- Asparagus – six stems
- Tuna – one slice
- Pumpkin chunks – ½ cup, peeled and roasted
- Lemon – half, cut into quarters
- Ginger – 2 tsp, pickled

Dressing:

- Orange juice – ½ cup, freshly squeezed
- Sesame oil – four tbsp
- Salt and pepper, one pinch

DIRECTIONS:

1. Cook the rice and drain it well.
2. Blanche green beans.
3. Grill red pepper and remove skin and then dice it.
4. Thinly slice the avocado lengthways.
5. Cut the cucumber thinly.
6. Drain six stems of asparagus.
7. Drain tuna slices of oil.
8. Boil the pumpkin chunks.
9. Place the red pepper in a mound in the middle of the plates.
10. Arrange all ingredients on the plates.
11. Pour sesame oil over it. Sprinkle with pepper and salt.
12. Pour dressing over the bowl.

NUTRITION FACTS:

Calories; 519kcal, carbs; 59.2g, Fats; 28.4g Proteins; 13.2g, fiber; 5g

170. POMEGRANATE SALAD

SERVES 4 | PREPARATION TIME 5 MINS | COOKING TIME 10 MINS | TOTAL TIME 15 MINS

INGREDIENTS:

- Chives – one tsp, chopped
- Zucchini – 300g
- Baby spinach – 100g
- Red pepper – one, skinned
- Extra-virgin olive oil spray

Dressing:

- Walnut oil – three tbsp
- Pomegranate juice – ¼ cup
- Dijon mustard – 2 tsp
- Salt – to taste

DIRECTIONS:

1. Add all ingredients into the bowl and beat until combined for dressing.
2. Slice zucchini into chunks. Let chop the chives.
3. Spray the zucchini and chives with olive oil.
4. Place a frypan over medium flame.
5. Add chives and zucchini and fry until golden brown.
6. Then, add baby spinach leaves and stir well.
7. Turn off the flame. Pour dressing over the salad.

NUTRITION FACTS:

Calories; 273kcal, carbs; 14.9g, Fats; 21.4g Proteins; 9.5g, fiber; 2g

171. DIJON ORANGE SUMMER SALAD

SERVES 2 | PREPARATION TIME 10 MINS | COOKING TIME 0 MINS | TOTAL TIME 10 MINS

INGREDIENTS:

- Baby spinach leaves – 150g
- Oranges – two, peeled, deseeded and sliced thinly
- Crushed macadamia nuts – 60g
- Feta cheese – 100g

Dressing:

- Thyme leaves – 1 tbsp
- Extra-virgin olive oil – 4 tbsp
- Dijon mustard – 1 tbsp
- Lemon juice – 4 tbsp
- Sourdough white bread rolls – 2 crusty

DIRECTIONS:

1. Add salad ingredients into the bowl.
2. Add dressing ingredients into the jar and shake it well.
3. Pour dressing over the salad. Combine it well.
4. Serve with a sourdough white bread roll.

NUTRITION FACTS:

Calories; 27kcal, carbs; 6.7g, Proteins; 0.2g, fiber; 3g

172. PULAO RICE PRAWNS

SERVES 4 | PREPARATION TIME 5 MINS | COOKING TIME 10 MINS | TOTAL TIME 15 MINS

INGREDIENTS:

- Prawns – 20, deveined, shelled
- Extra virgin olive oil – three tbsp
- Water – 500ml
- Coconut milk – 200ml
- Cardamoms – three
- Bay leaves – two
- Red chili powder – one pinch
- Turmeric powder – ½ tsp
- Fresh coriander – ¼ cup, chopped
- Black pepper and pepper – to taste
- Garam masala powder – one pinch
- Asafoetida powder – one pinch

DIRECTIONS:

1. Add olive oil into the pan. Heat it. Then, add black pepper, cardamoms, bay leaves, and spices clove and cook for one to two minutes until fragrant, about one to two minutes.
2. Add cardamom, bay leaves, and cloves into the tea leaf ball.
3. Add asafoetida powder, turmeric, garam masala, chili powder, salt, and prawns and combine well. Drain and add rice to the pan and cover with 500ml water and 200ml coconut milk.
4. Lower the heat and simmer until cooked thoroughly.
5. Garnish with fresh coriander leaves.

NUTRITION FACTS:

Calories; 424kcal, carbs; 62g, Fats; 11g Proteins; 19g, fiber; 2g

173. WHITE RADISH CRUNCH SALAD

SERVES 2 | PREPARATION TIME 10 MINS | COOKING TIME 0 MINS | TOTAL TIME 10 MINS

INGREDIENTS:

- Radish – 200g, julienned
- Cucumber – 200g, shredded
- Noodles – 50g
- Ginger – 1 tsp, grated, steamed
- Nori – ¼ sheet, thinly sliced
- Dressing:
- Soy sauce – 1 tsp
- Rice vinegar – 1 tsp
- Maple syrup – 1 tsp
- Orange juice – 1 tbsp
- Sesame oil – 1 tbsp

DIRECTIONS:

1. Combine cucumber, ginger, and radish into the bowl. Pour dressing ingredients over it. Top with nori and noodles. Stir well.
2. Serve!

NUTRITION FACTS:

Calories; 82kcal, carbs; 5g, Fats; 7g Proteins; 1g, fiber; 2g

174. APPLE AND MUSHROOM SOUP

  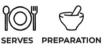

SERVES 2 | PREPARATION TIME 5 MINS | COOKING TIME 5 MINS | TOTAL TIME 10 MINS

INGREDIENTS:

- Water – 400ml
- Green apple – half, peeled, cored and grated
- Precooked rice noodles – 100g
- Green chives – ¼ cup, chopped
- Mushrooms – 2, sliced
- Silken tofu – 100g, crumbed
- Roasted seaweed – 1 slice

DIRECTIONS:

1. Rinse the rice noodles in hot water and then strain them.
2. Add all ingredients and stir for one to two minutes.
3. Then, add crushed seaweed flakes.
4. Serve!

NUTRITION FACTS:

Calories; 366kcal, carbs; 41.1g, Fats; 19g Proteins; 11g, Fibers; 3g

175. SPRING WATERCRESS SOUP

SERVES 4 | PREPARATION TIME 10 MINS | COOKING TIME 30 MINS | TOTAL TIME 40 MINS

INGREDIENTS:

- Watercress – one bunch, rinsed
- Olive oil – 1 tbsp
- Green onion – 1, diced, green part only
- Chicken stock – four cups
- Baby arugula – four cups
- Sea salt – to taste
- Chives – 1 tbsp, snipped
- Greek yogurt – 2 tbsp

DIRECTIONS:

1. Separate the thick and tough stems from the watercress leaves.
2. Dice the stems. Reserve the leaves.
3. Add oil to the pot or Dutch oven and place it over medium-high flame.
4. Then, add the green onion (green part only) and diced watercress stems into the pot, lower the heat to medium, and sprinkle with salt.
5. Cook for five minutes.
6. Add stock and bring to a boil over medium-high flame.
7. When boiled, lower the heat to medium-low and simmer for fifteen minutes.
8. Add reserved watercress leaves and arugula and cook until wilted.
9. Turn off the flame.
10. Add soup into the immersion blender and blend until smooth.
11. Place soup back in the pan/pot and warm through.
12. Garnish with chopped chives.

NUTRITION FACTS:

Calories; 174kcal, carbs; 19g, Fats; 7g Proteins; 10g

176. OYSTER SAUCE TOFU

 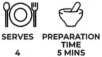

SERVES 4 | PREPARATION TIME 5 MINS | COOKING TIME 10 MINS | TOTAL TIME 15 MINS

INGREDIENTS:

- Tofu – 700g
- Oil – 2 tsp
- Ginger – one slice, peeled, minced
- Scallion – one, trimmed, chopped
- Chicken broth or vegetable broth – 1 ½ cups, low sodium
- Oyster sauce – three tbsp
- Rice wine – 2 tsp
- Cornstarch – 2 tsp
- Water – 1 tsp
- Sesame oil – 1 tsp

DIRECTIONS:

1. Slice tofu into bite-sized squares and keep it aside.
2. Add oil into the skillet and heat it.
3. Then, add ginger and green part of chopped scallions and cook for one to two minutes.
4. Add tofu, rice wine, broth, and oyster sauce and bring to a boil.
5. Lower the heat and to medium-low and simmer for five minutes.
6. Add water and cornstarch into the bowl and stir to make a slurry.
7. Add tofu into the gravy and drizzle with sesame oil, and sprinkle with green parts of scallions.

NUTRITION FACTS:

Calories; 58kcal, carbs; 4g, Fats; 3g Proteins; 2g

177. POTATO AND ROSEMARY RISOTTO

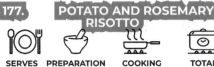

SERVES 3 | PREPARATION TIME 10 MINS | COOKING TIME 30 MINS | TOTAL TIME 40 MINS

INGREDIENTS:

- Olive oil – 2 tbsp
- Rosemary – 1 sprig, chopped
- Green onion – 1, diced, green part only
- Arborio rice – 2/3 cup
- Yukon gold potato – 1, rinsed, peeled scrubbed, diced
- Chicken stock – 3 ½ cups, low-sodium
- Parmesan cheese – 1 tbsp, grated
- Butter – 1 tsp
- Salt and pepper, to taste

DIRECTIONS:

1. Add olive oil into the Dutch oven and heat it over medium-high flame.
2. Add rosemary and cook for one minute. Then, add green onion and cook for two minutes until translucent.
3. Turn the heat down to medium and sprinkle with salt. Let sweat for eight minutes.
4. Remove the lid and elevate the heat to medium-high and then add rice to it. Combine it well.
5. Add potato and cook for one minute more.
6. Add chicken stock and bring to a boil.
7. Lower the heat to low and simmer for twenty minutes until al dente.
8. Add butter and parmesan cheese and turn off the flame.
9. Let sit for five minutes.
10. Add more stock if needed.
11. Sprinkle with black pepper.

NUTRITION FACTS:

Calories; 377kcal, carbs; 55g, Fats; 13g Proteins; 12g

178. CHEESY BAKED TORTILLAS

SERVES 4 | PREPARATION TIME 10 MINS | COOKING TIME 30 MINS | TOTAL TIME 40 MINS

INGREDIENTS:

- Pizza sauce – 255g

- Extra-virgin olive oil – 20ml
- Extra-virgin olive oil spray
- Plain Greek yoghurt – as needed
- Juice of whole lime – one
- Onion powder – 1 tsp
- Sweet paprika – ½ tsp
- Cheddar cheese – 250g, low-fat
- Chicken – 250g, cooked, shredded
- White potato – 400g, peeled
- Basmati rice – 400g, cooked and drained
- Salt and pepper – to taste
- Flour tortillas – six

DIRECTIONS:

1. Preheat the oven to 410°F - 210°C.
2. Spray the potatoes with olive oil spray.
3. Sprinkle with paprika powder and place it into the oven and bake for 20 minutes.
4. Add onion powder and olive oil into the pan and heat it for one minute.
5. Add tofu or chicken, 180g of pizza sauce, pepper, salt, and lemon juice, and combine well.
6. Layout tortillas onto the clean surface and top with chicken or tofu mixture, rice, and baked potatoes and top with cheese.
7. Roll the burritos and place them onto the dish.
8. Top with remaining cheese and bake for 15 to 20 minutes.

NUTRITION FACTS:

Calories; 389kcal,carbs; 31g, Fats; 20g Proteins; 22g, fiber; 4g

179. SMOKY RICE

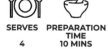

SERVES 4 | PREPARATION TIME 10 MINS | COOKING TIME 30 MINS | TOTAL TIME 40 MINS

INGREDIENTS:

- White basmati rice – 400g
- Pasta – 200ml
- Green onion – half, peeled and chopped, green part only
- Red capsicum – ¼, chopped
- Extra-virgin olive oil – 4 tbsp
- Tomato puree – 70g
- Bay leaves – three
- Paprika – one tsp
- Cumin – one tsp
- Black pepper – one pinch
- Chili – one pinch
- Coconut oil – four tbsp
- Banana – peeled and chopped
- Salt – to taste

DIRECTIONS:

Rice:
1. Rinse rice and soak for twenty minutes.
2. Let boil it for five minutes. Then, drain it.
3. Add black pepper, paprika, cumin, chili, half green onion (green part only), pasta, and red capsicum into the blender and blend until smooth.
4. Add oil into the saucepan and place it over medium flame.
5. Add capsicum mixture to the pan and sprinkle with salt and cook for few minutes until fragrant. Then, add tomato puree and bay leaves and cook for five minutes.
6. Add drained rice and one cup of water and simmer for eight minutes until the rice is soft. Discard bay leaves. Keep it aside.

Banana:
1. Add coconut oil and banana into the pan and cook until golden.
2. Add banana over the rice.
3. Serve!

NUTRITION FACTS:

Calories; 447kcal,carbs; 69g, Fats; 11g Proteins; 11g, fiber; 3g

180. ZUCCHINI LASAGNA

SERVES 4 | PREPARATION TIME 10 MINS | COOKING TIME 40 MINS | TOTAL TIME 50 MINS

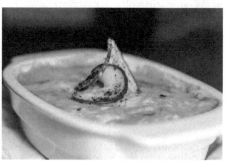

INGREDIENTS:

- Zucchini – 800g, grated
- Green onion – 1 tsp, green part only
- Chives – 1 tbsp, chopped
- Dried oregano – 1 tbsp
- Ricotta – 250g, low-fat
- Cheddar cheese – 50g, low-fat, shredded
- Passata – 350ml
- Dried lasagna sheets – nine, gluten-free
- Extra virgin oil – as needed
- Salt and pepper – to taste

DIRECTIONS:

1. Preheat the oven to 410°F - 210°C.
2. Add olive oil into the frying pan and heat it.
3. Add green onion and zucchini and cook for three minutes.
4. Lower the heat, add 25g of low-fat cheddar cheese and ricotta, and sprinkle with pepper and salt. Keep it aside.
5. Let boil the lasagna sheet in the salted water for five to six minutes.
6. Then, drain it. Add some olive oil to the pasta.
7. Place lasagna sheet onto the baking dish, add ricotta and zucchini mixture, and sprinkle with fresh chives and oregano. Then, add tomato pasata.
8. Lower the heat of the oven to 360°F - 180°C.
9. Bake the lasagna for thirty minutes.
10. Serve with salad.

NUTRITION FACTS:

Calories; 362kcal,carbs; 7g, Fats; 26g Proteins; 25g, fiber; 3g

181. GREEK CHICKEN SKEWERS

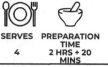

SERVES 4 | PREPARATION TIME 2 HRS + 20 MINS | COOKING TIME 20 MINS | TOTAL TIME 2 HRS + 40 MINS

INGREDIENTS:

- Lemon juice – ¼ cup
- Wok oil – ¼ cup
- Red wine vinegar – 1/8 cup
- Onion flakes – one tbsp
- Garlic – one tbsp, minced
- Lemon – one, zested
- Greek seasoning – one tsp
- Poultry seasoning – one tsp
- Dried oregano – one tsp
- Ground black pepper – one tsp
- Dried thyme – half tsp
- Chicken breasts – three, cut into 1-inch pieces, skinless and boneless

DIRECTIONS:

1. Whisk the thyme, pepper, oregano, poultry seasoning, Greek seasoning, lemon zest, garlic, onion flakes, vinegar, oil, and lemon juice into the bowl. Place it into the re-sealable plastic bag.
2. Add chicken and coat with marinade and seal the bag. Place it into the refrigerator for two hours.
3. Preheat the oven to 360°F - 180°C.
4. Discard marinade and thread chicken onto the skewers.
5. Place skewers onto the baking sheet.
6. Cook for twenty minutes until golden brown.

NUTRITION FACTS:

Calories; 248kcal,carbs; 4.1g, protein; 18.1g, fat; 17g

182. ROAST BEEF

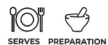

SERVES 6 | PREPARATION TIME 10 MINS | COOKING TIME 60 MINS | TOTAL TIME 70 MINS

INGREDIENTS:

- Beef eye of round roast – three pounds
- Kosher salt – half tsp

- Garlic powder – half tsp
- Freshly ground black pepper – ¼ tsp

DIRECTIONS:
1. Preheat the oven to 375°F-190°C.
2. Place roast into the pan and sprinkle with pepper, garlic powder, and salt. Cook it into the oven for one hour.
3. Let cool it for fifteen to twenty minutes.
4. Serve and enjoy!

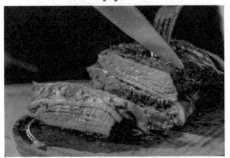

NUTRITION FACTS:
Calories; 480kcal, carbs; 0.2g, protein; 44.8g, fat; 32.4g

183. BANANA CAKE

SERVES 15 | PREPARATION TIME 20 MINS | COOKING TIME 75 MINS | TOTAL TIME 95 MINS

INGREDIENTS:
- Bananas – 1 1/3 cup, mashed
- Lemon juice – 2 ½ tbsp
- Milk – 1 ½ cups
- Flour – three cups
- Baking soda – 1 ½ tsp
- Salt – ¼ tsp
- Butter – 2/3 cup, softened
- White sugar – one cup
- Brown sugar – half cup
- Eggs – three
- Vanilla – one tsp

Frosting:
- Cream cheese – eight ounces
- Butter – 1/3 cup, softened
- Powdered sugar – 3 ½ cups
- Lemon juice – one tsp
- 1 ½ tsp lemon zest from one lemon

DIRECTIONS:
1. Preheat the oven to 360°F - 180°C. Grease and flour the pan.
2. Add 1 ½ tbsp lemon juice into the cup. Then, add one and a half cups milk and keep it aside.
3. Combine one tbsp lemon juice and mashed banana and keep it aside.
4. Add white sugar, brown sugar, and butter into the bowl and beat it well.
5. Add eggs and vanilla and combine at high speed until fluffy.
6. Mix the salt, baking soda, and flour into the bowl.
7. Add flour mixture and milk to the egg mixture and stir well.
8. Then, fold it into the bananas. Place mixture into the pan.
9. Bake it for one hour and ten minutes.
10. When done, place it into the freezer for forty-five minutes.
11. To prepare the frosting:
12. Cream the cream cheese and butter into the bowl. Add lemon juice and lemon zest and combine well.
13. Add powdered sugar and stir well. Top frosting over the cake.

NUTRITION FACTS:
Calories; 470kcal, carbs; 70g, protein; 5g, fat; 19g

184. GRILLED FISH STEAKS

SERVES 2 | PREPARATION TIME 10 MINS | COOKING TIME 70 MINS | TOTAL TIME 80 MINS

INGREDIENTS:
- Garlic, one clove, minced
- Olive oil – six tbsp
- Dried basil – one tsp
- Salt – one tsp
- Ground black pepper – one tsp
- Lemon juice – one tbsp
- Fresh parsley – one tbsp, chopped
- Halibut fillets – six ounce

DIRECTIONS:
1. Mix the parsley, lemon juice, pepper, salt, basil, olive oil, and garlic into the bowl.
2. Add halibut fillets into the glass dish and place marinade over it.
3. Place it into the refrigerator for one hour.
4. Oil the grate and preheat the grill on high heat.
5. Discard marinade and place halibut fillets onto the grill, and cook for five minutes per side.
6. When done, serve and enjoy!

NUTRITION FACTS:
Calories; 554kcal, carbs; 2.2g, protein; 36.3g, fat; 43.7g

185. APPLE PUDDING

SERVES 6 | PREPARATION TIME 10 MINS | COOKING TIME 70 MINS | TOTAL TIME 80 MINS

INGREDIENTS:
- Butter – half cup, melted
- White sugar – one cup
- All-purpose flour – one cup
- Baking powder – two tsp
- Salt – ¼ tsp
- Milk – one cup
- Apple – two cups, chopped and peeled
- Ground cinnamon – one tsp

DIRECTIONS:
1. Preheat the oven to 375°F - 190°C.
2. Mix the milk, salt, baking powder, flour, sugar, and butter into the baking dish.
3. Mix the cinnamon and apples into the bowl and microwave it for two to five minutes. Place apple into the middle of the batter.
4. Place it into the oven and bake for a half-hour.
5. Serve and enjoy!

NUTRITION FACTS:
Calories; 384kcal, carbs; 57.5g, protein; 3.8g, fat; 16g

186. LAMB CHOPS

SERVES 2 | PREPARATION TIME 40 MINS | COOKING TIME 10 MINS | TOTAL TIME 50 MINS

INGREDIENTS:
- Lamb chops – 2lb, cut ¾" thick, 4 pieces
- Kosher salt and Black pepper – for seasoning
- Garlic – one tbsp, minced
- Rosemary – two tsp, chopped
- Thyme – two tsp, chopped
- Parsley – half tsp, chopped
- Extra-virgin olive oil – ¼ cup

DIRECTIONS:
1. Rub the lamb chops with pepper and salt.
2. Mix the two tbsp olive oil, parsley, thyme, rosemary, and garlic into the bowl.
3. Rub this paste on each side of the lamb chops and let marinate it for a half-hour.
4. Place two tbsp olive oil into the frying pan over medium-high flame.
5. Add lamb chops and cook for two to three minutes.
6. Flip and cook for three to four minutes more.
7. Let cool it for ten minutes.
8. Serve and enjoy!

NUTRITION FACTS:
Calories; 465kcal, carbs; 12g, protein; 14g, fat; 38g

187. EGGPLANT CROQUETTES

SERVES 6 | PREPARATION TIME 15 MINS | COOKING TIME 20 MINS | TOTAL TIME 35 MINS

INGREDIENTS:
- Eggplants – two, peeled and cubed
- Cheddar cheese – one cup,

- shredded
- Italian seasoned bread crumbs – one cup
- Eggs – two, beaten
- Dried parsley – two tbsp
- Onion – two tbsp, chopped
- Garlic – one clove, minced
- Vegetable oil – one cup, for frying
- Salt – one tsp
- Ground black pepper – half tsp

DIRECTIONS:
1. Microwave the eggplant over medium-high heat for three minutes.
2. Flip and cook for two minutes more.
3. If eggplant did not tender, cook for two minutes more.
4. Then, drain it and mash the eggplants.
5. Mix the salt, garlic, onion, parsley, eggs, cheese, breadcrumbs, and mashed eggplant.
6. Make the patties from the eggplant mixture.
7. Add oil into the skillet and heat it. Place eggplant patties into the skillet and fry until golden brown for five minutes.
8. Serve and enjoy!

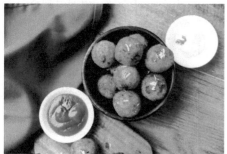

NUTRITION FACTS:
Calories; 266kcal, carbs; 23.6g, protein; 12g, fat; 14.4g

188. CUCUMBER EGG SALAD

SERVES 4 | PREPARATION TIME 15 MINS | COOKING TIME 20 MINS | TOTAL TIME 35 MINS

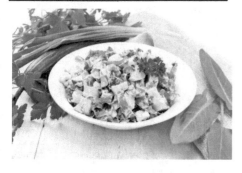

INGREDIENTS:
- Eggs – four
- Cucumbers – four, seedless
- Dill pickles – four
- Mayonnaise – three tbsp

DIRECTIONS:
1. Add eggs into the saucepan and cover it with cold water. Let boil it.
2. Remove from the flame. Let stand eggs in hot water for ten to twelve minutes.
3. Remove from the hot water and cool it.
4. Peel eggs and chop them. Add it into the salad bowl.
5. Cube and pickled the cucumber and add to the eggs.
6. Add mayonnaise and combine it well.
7. Place it into the fridge until chill.

NUTRITION FACTS:
Calories; 176kcal, carbs; 8g, protein; 7.6g, fat; 13.4g

189. SHRIMP AND MANGO SALSA LETTUCE WRAPS

 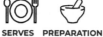

SERVES 6 | PREPARATION TIME 15 MINS | COOKING TIME 3 MINS | TOTAL TIME 18 MINS

INGREDIENTS:
For the Salsa:
- 1 mango, peeled, pitted and chopped
- 1/4 cup red onion, finely chopped
- 1/2 cup red bell pepper
- 1/4 cup fresh cilantro, chopped
- 1 jalapeño pepper, seeded and finely chopped
- 2 tablespoons fresh lime juice
- Salt and freshly ground black pepper

For the Shrimp Wraps:
- 1 teaspoon organic olive oil
- 2 pounds large shrimp, peeled, deveined and chopped
- 1/2 teaspoon ground cumin
- 1 tablespoon red chili powder
- Salt and freshly ground black pepper
- 2 heads butter lettuce, leaves separated

DIRECTIONS:
For the salsa:
1. In a large bowl, mix all ingredients. Keep aside.

For the Shrimp Wraps:
1. In a skillet, heat oil on medium heat.
2. Add the shrimp and seasoning. Cook for approximately 2-3 minutes.
3. Remove from the heat and cool slightly.
4. Divide the shrimp mixture over lettuce leaves lightly.
5. Top with mango salsa evenly and serve.

NUTRITION FACTS:
Calories; 463kcal, carbs; 75g, protein; 34g, fat; 4.g fiber 18g

190. BACON-WRAPPED ASPARAGUS

SERVES 6 | PREPARATION TIME 25 MINS | COOKING TIME 30 MINS | TOTAL TIME 55 MINS

INGREDIENTS:
- 10 bacon slices cut in half
- 1 pound fresh asparagus, trimmed
- 1 tablespoon extra-virgin olive oil
- 1 tablespoon balsamic vinegar
- Freshly ground black pepper, to taste
- 1 lemon, sliced

DIRECTIONS:
1. Heat the oven to 400°F - 200°C.
2. Line a substantial baking dish with foil paper.
3. Wrap 1 bacon slice around each asparagus piece.
4. Arrange asparagus in the prepared baking dish.
5. 4. Set with oil and vinegar. Sprinkle with black pepper.
6. Bake for approximately 15 minutes. Change the inside and bake for 10-15 minutes more.
7. Serve immediately with lemon slices.

NUTRITION FACTS:
Calories; 645kcal, carbs; 65g, protein; 26g, fat; 32.g fiber 5g

191. ZUCCHINI PASTA WITH SHRIMP

 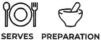

SERVES 4 | PREPARATION TIME 15 MINS | COOKING TIME 6 MINS | TOTAL TIME 21 MINS

INGREDIENTS:
- 2 tablespoons ghee or coconut oil
- 1 tablespoon extra-virgin olive oil
- 3 garlic cloves, minced
- 1 pound shrimp, peeled and deveined
- 4 large zucchini, spiralized with blade C
- Salt and freshly ground black pepper
- 4-6 fresh basil leaves, chopped

Directions:
1. In a big skillet, heat the ghee and essential olive oil on medium heat.
2. Add garlic and saute for approximately 1 minute.
3. Set the shrimp and cook for approximately 2-3 minutes.
4. Add the zucchini, tossing occasionally and cook for approximately 2-3 minutes.
5. Stir in salt and black pepper and take off from the heat.

6. Serve while using the garnishing of basil leaves.

NUTRITION FACTS:

Calories; 59kcal, carbs; 14g, protein; 1g, fat; 1.g fiber 1 g Sodium: 304 mg

192. SWEET POTATO BUNS SANDWICH

SERVES 1 | PREPARATION TIME 25 MINS | COOKING TIME 25 MINS | TOTAL TIME 50 MINS

INGREDIENTS:

For Sweet Potato Buns:
- 1 ½ tablespoon extra-virgin olive oil, divided
- 1 large sweet potato, peeled and spiralized with blade C
- 2 teaspoons garlic powder
- Salt and freshly ground black pepper
- 1 large organic egg
- 1 organic egg white

For the Sandwich:
- 1 (1/2 ounce) salmon piece
- Salt and freshly ground black pepper
- 1 teaspoon fresh lime juice
- 1 tomato, sliced
- 1 onion, sliced
- 1/2 avocado, peeled, pitted and chopped
- 2 teaspoons fresh cilantro, chopped
- 1 large bit fresh kale
- 1 bacon piece

DIRECTIONS:

For the buns:
1. In a sizable skillet, heat 1/2 tablespoon of oil on medium heat.
2. Add the sweet potato and sprinkle with garlic powder, salt and black pepper.
3. Cook for 5-7 minutes. Transfer the sweet potato mixture to a bowl.
4. Add the egg and egg white; mix well. Now, transfer a combination into 2 (6 ounces) ramekins, midway full.
5. Cover the ramekins with wax paper. Now, place them over noodles to press firmly down. Refrigerate for about 15-20 minutes.

For the Sandwich:
1. Preheat the grill to medium heat. Grease it.
2. In another bowl, add salmon, salt, black pepper and lime juice. Toss to coat well.
3. In a substantial skillet, heat the remaining oil on medium-low heat.
4. Carefully, transfer the sweet potato patties to the skillet.
5. Cook for 3-4 minutes. Change the medial side and cook for 2-3 minutes more.

6. Place the salmon, onion and tomato slices over the grill.
7. Grill the tomato slice for 1 minute. Grate the onion slice for approximately 2 minutes.
8. Cook the salmon for approximately 4-5 minutes or till the desired doneness.
9. In a bowl, add the avocado and cilantro; mash well.
10. On a plate, place the onion slice, salmon, tomato, bacon and kale over the bun.
11. Spread the avocado mash around the bottom side of another bun. Place the bun, avocado mash side downwards over the kale.
12. Secure having a toothpick and serve.

NUTRITION FACTS:

Calories; 76kcal, carbs; 8g, protein; 14, fat; 2g

193. SHRIMP, SAUSAGE AND VEGGIE SKILLET

 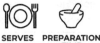

SERVES 3 | PREPARATION TIME 15 MINS | COOKING TIME 13 MINS | TOTAL TIME 28 MINS

INGREDIENTS:

- 3 tablespoons organic olive oil, divided
- 1 pound shrimp, peeled and deveined
- 1/2 medium yellow onion, chopped
- 3/4 cup green peppers, seeded and chopped
- 3/4 cup green peppers, seeded and chopped
- 1 zucchini, chopped
- 6 ounces cooked sausage, chopped
- 2 garlic cloves, minced
- 1/4 cup chicken broth
- A pinch of red pepper flakes, crushed
- Salt and freshly ground black pepper

DIRECTIONS:

1. In a sizable skillet, heat 1 tablespoon of oil on medium-high heat.
2. Attach the shrimp and cook for around 3-4 minutes. Transfer it to a bowl.
3. In the same skillet, heat the remaining oil on medium heat.
4. Add the onion and sweet peppers. Saute for about 4-5 minutes.
5. Stir in the zucchini and sausage. Cook for approximately 2 minutes.
6. Add the garlic and cooled shrimp. Cook for approximately 1 minute.
7. Pour the broth and mix to combine well. Stir in red pepper

flakes, salt and black pepper. Cook for approximately 1 minute.
8. Serve hot.

NUTRITION FACTS:

Calories: 332 Fat: 18 g Carbs: 32 g Fiber: 9 g Protein: 12 g

194. SEA SCALLOPS WITH SPINACH AND BACON

  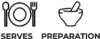

SERVES 4 | PREPARATION TIME 10 MINS | COOKING TIME 25 MINS | TOTAL TIME 35 MINS

INGREDIENTS:

- 3 bacon slices
- 1 ½ pound jumbo sea scallops
- Salt and freshly ground black pepper
- 1 cup onion, chopped
- 6 garlic cloves, minced
- 12 ounces fresh baby spinach

DIRECTIONS:

1. Heat a sizable non-stick skillet on medium-high heat.
2. Add the bacon and cook for approximately 8-10 minutes.
3. Transfer the bacon into a bowl, reserving 1 tablespoon of bacon fat within the skillet.
4. Chop the bacon and keep it aside.
5. Attach the scallops and sprinkle with salt and black pepper.
6. Immediately, boost the heat to high heat.
7. Cook for about 5 minutes, turning once after 2 ½ minutes.
8. Transfer the scallops into another bowl. Cover having foil paper to ensure that they're warm.
9. In the same skillet, add the onion and garlic minimizing the temperature to medium-high.
10. Saute them for around 3 minutes.
11. Add the spinach and cook for approximately 2-3 minutes. Season with salt and black pepper. Remove from the heat.
12. Divide the spinach among serving plates. Top with scallops and bacon evenly. Serve immediately.

NUTRITION FACTS:

Calories: 246 Fat: 13 g Carbs: 11 g Fiber: 1 g Protein: 22 g

195. LIVER WITH ONION AND PARSLEY ONE

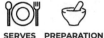

SERVES 4 | PREPARATION TIME 10 MINS | COOKING TIME 25 MINS | TOTAL TIME 35 MINS

INGREDIENTS:

- 3 tablespoons coconut oil, divided
- 2 large onions, sliced
- Salt to taste

- 1 pound grass-fed beef liver, cut into 1/2-inch thick slices
- Freshly ground black pepper, to taste
- 1/2 cup fresh parsley
- 2 tablespoons freshly squeezed lemon juice

DIRECTIONS:

1. In a sizable skillet, heat 1 tablespoon of oil on high heat.
2. Attach the onions plus some salt and saute for about 5 minutes.
3. Set the heat to medium. Saute them for 10-15 minutes more.
4. Place the onion right into a plate.
5. In the same skillet, heat another 1 tablespoon of oil on medium-high heat.
6. Add the liver and sprinkle with salt and black pepper.
7. Cook for approximately 1-2 minutes or till browned.
8. Flip alongside it and cook for approximately 1-2 minutes till browned. Set the liver right into a plate.
9. In the skillet, heat the remaining oil on medium heat.
10. Attach the cooked onion, parsley and lemon juice; stir well. Cook for about 2-3 minutes.
11. Set the onion mixture over the liver and serve immediately.

NUTRITION FACTS:
Calories: 228 Fat: 3 g Carbs: 43 g Fiber: 6 g Protein: 12 g

196. EGG AND AVOCADO WRAPS

SERVES 5 | PREPARATION TIME 10 MINS | COOKING TIME 0 MINS | TOTAL TIME 10 MINS

INGREDIENTS:

- 1 ripe avocado, peeled, pitted and chopped
- 1 tablespoon freshly squeezed lemon juice
- 1 tablespoon fresh parsley, chopped
- 2 tablespoons celery stalk, chopped
- 4 organic hard-boiled eggs, peeled and finely chopped
- Salt and freshly ground black pepper
- 4-5 endive bulbs
- 2 cooked bacon slices, chopped

DIRECTIONS:

1. In a bowl, add the avocado and freshly squeezed lemon juice and mash till smooth and creamy.
2. Add parsley, celery, eggs, salt and black pepper. Stir to mix well.
3. Separate the endive leaves. Divide the avocado mixture over endive leaves evenly.
4. Top with bacon and serve immediately.

NUTRITION FACTS:
Calories: 404 Fat: 7 g Carbs: 47 g Fiber: 6 g Protein: 15 g

197. CREAMY SWEET POTATO PASTA WITH PANCETTA

SERVES 4 | PREPARATION TIME 10 MINS | COOKING TIME 25 MINS | TOTAL TIME 35 MINS

INGREDIENTS:

For the Creamy Sauce:
- 4-5 cups cauliflower florets
- 1 small shallot, minced
- 1 large garlic herb, chopped
- A pinch of red pepper flakes, crushed
- 1 cup chicken broth
- 1 tablespoon nutritional yeast
- Salt to taste
- For the Pancetta:
- 8 pancetta slices, cubed

For the Sweet Potato Pasta:
- 1 tablespoon extra-virgin olive oil
- 3 medium sweet potatoes, peeled and spiralized with blade C
- 3 cups leeks
- Salt and freshly ground black pepper
- 1 tablespoon fresh parsley, chopped

DIRECTIONS:

1. In a pan of salted boiling water, attach cauliflower florets and cook for around 7-8 minutes. Drain well.
2. Meanwhile, heat a large non-stick skillet on medium heat.
3. Add pancetta slices and cook for approximately 5-7 minutes.
4. Transfer the pancetta into a bowl.
5. In the same skillet, add shallot, garlic and red pepper flakes. Saute for around 2 minutes.
6. Transfer the shallot mixture into a higher speed blender.
7. Add the cauliflower and the remaining sauce ingredients. Pulse till smooth and creamy.
8. In the identical skillet, heat extra-virgin olive oil on medium heat.
9. Add sweet potatoes and leeks. Cook, tossing occasionally for approximately 8-10 minutes.
10. Stir in the sauce and cook for about 1 minute.
11. Serve this creamy pasta with all the topping of the pancetta and parsley.

NUTRITION FACTS:
Calories; 465kcal, carbs; 12g, protein; 14g, fat; 38g

198. ROASTED BEET PASTA WITH KALE AND PESTO

INGREDIENTS:

For the Pesto:
- 3 cups fresh basil leaves
- 1 large garlic oil
- 1/4 cup organic olive oil
- 1/4 cup pine nuts
- Salt and freshly ground black pepper

For the Beet Pasta:
- 2 medium beets, trimmed, peeled and spiralized with blade C
- Olive oil cooking spray, as required
- Salt and freshly ground black pepper

For the Kale:
- 2 cups fresh baby kale

SERVES 3 | PREPARATION TIME 10 MINS | COOKING TIME 25 MINS | TOTAL TIME 35 MINS

DIRECTIONS:

1. Heat the oven to 425°F - 220°C. Lightly, grease a large baking sheet.
2. In a mixer, add all pesto ingredients and pulse till smooth. Keep aside.
3. Place the beet pasta in the prepared baking sheet.
4. Drizzle with cooking spray and sprinkle with salt and black pepper. Gently, toss to coat well.
5. Roast for around 5-10 minutes or till the desired doneness.
6. Transfer the pasta to a sizable bowl.
7. Add the kale and pesto. Gently, toss to coat well.

NUTRITION FACTS:
Calories: 37 Fat: 1 g Carbs: 3 g Fiber: 0 g Protein: 4 g Sodium: 58 mg

199. VEGGIES AND APPLE WITH ORANGE SAUCE

SERVES 4 | PREPARATION TIME 30 MINS | COOKING TIME 16 MINS | TOTAL TIME 46 MINS

INGREDIENTS:

For the Sauce:
- 1 (1 inch) fresh ginger, minced
- 2 garlic cloves, minced
- 1 tablespoon fresh orange zest, grated finely
- 1/2 cup fresh orange juice
- 2 tablespoons white wine vinegar
- 2 tablespoons coconut aminos
- 1 tablespoon red boat fish sauce

For the Veggies and Apple:
- 1 tablespoon extra-virgin olive oil
- 1 cup carrot, peeled and julienned
- 1 cup celery, chopped
- 1 cup onion, chopped
- 2 apples, cored and sliced

DIRECTIONS:

1. In a sizable bowl, mix all sauce ingredients. Keep aside.
2. In a big skillet, set the oil on medium-high heat.
3. Add the carrot and stir fry for about 4-5 minutes.
4. Attach celery and onion. Stir fry for approximately 4-5 minutes.
5. Pour the sauce and stir to combine. Cook approximately 2-3 minutes.
6. Stir in apple slices and cook for about 2-3 minutes more.
7. Serve hot.

NUTRITION FACTS:
Calories: 29 Fat: 1 g Carbs: 2 g Fiber: 1 g Protein: 1 g

200. CAULIFLOWER RICE WITH PRAWNS AND VEGGIES

Preparation Time: 15 minutes

Cooking Time: 21 minutes

Servings: 4

INGREDIENTS:
- 2 tablespoons coconut oil, divided
- 14 prawns, peeled and deveined
- 2 organic eggs, beaten
- 1 brown onion, chopped
- 1 garlic clove, minced
- 1 small fresh red chili, chopped
- 1/2 pound grass-fed ground chicken
- 1 cauliflower head, cut into florets, processed like rice consistency
- 1/4 red cabbage, chopped
- 1/2 cup green peas, shelled
- 1 head small broccoli
- 1 large carrot, peeled and finely chopped
- 1 small red bell pepper
- 2 bok choy, sliced thinly
- 3 tablespoons coconut aminos
- Salt and freshly ground black pepper

DIRECTIONS:
1. In a substantial skillet, heat 1/2 tablespoon of oil on medium-high heat.
2. Add the prawns and cook for approximately 3-4 minutes. Transfer to a large bowl.
3. In the same skillet, heat 1/2 tablespoon of oil on medium heat.
4. Add the beaten eggs and with the back of a spoon, spread the eggs. Cook for around 2 minutes.
5. Remove the eggs from the skillet and cut them into strips.
6. In the identical skillet, heat the remaining oil on high heat. Add the onion, garlic and red chili. Saute for about 4-5 minutes.
7. Add the chicken and cook for about 4-5 minutes.
8. Add the cauliflower rice and remaining veggies except for the bok choy and coconut aminos and cook for around 2-3 minutes.
9. Add the bok choy, coconut aminos, cooked eggs, prawns, salt and black pepper. Cook for 2 minutes more.

NUTRITION FACTS:
Calories: 75 Carbs: 0.1 g Protein: 13.4 g Fat: 1.7 g Sugar: 0 g Sodium: 253 mg

201. LENTILS WITH TOMATOES AND TURMERIC

Preparation Time: 15 minutes

Cooking Time: 10 minutes

Servings: 2

INGREDIENTS:
- 1/2 onion, finely chopped
- 1/2 teaspoon garlic powder
- 1/2 (14 ounces) can chopped tomatoes, drained
- 1/8 teaspoon ground black pepper
- 1 tablespoon extra-virgin olive oil, plus extra for garnishing
- 1/2 tablespoon ground turmeric
- 1/2 (14 ounces) can lentils, drained
- 1/4 teaspoon sea salt

DIRECTIONS:
1. Heat the olive oil in a pot over medium-high heat until it starts shimmering.
2. Cook, stirring regularly, for around 5 minutes until the onion and turmeric are tender.
3. Add the garlic powder, salt, tomatoes, lentils, and pepper.
4. Cook, stirring regularly, for 5 minutes

NUTRITION FACTS:
Calories: 248 Fat: 8 g Carbs: 34 g Sugar: 5 g Fiber: 15 g Protein: 12 g Sodium: 243 mg

202. FRIED RICE WITH KALE

Preparation Time: 10 minutes

Cooking Time: 12 minutes

Servings: 2

INGREDIENTS:
- 4 ounces tofu chopped
- 1 cup kale, stemmed and chopped
- 2 tablespoons stir-fry sauce
- 1 tablespoon extra-virgin olive oil
- 3 sliced scallions
- 1 ½ cup cooked brown rice

DIRECTIONS:
1. Heat the olive oil in a big skillet or pan over medium-high heat until it starts shimmering.
2. Add the scallions, tofu, and kale. Cook until the vegetables are tender.
3. Combine the stir-fry sauce and brown rice in a mixing bowl. Cook, stirring regularly until thoroughly heated.

NUTRITION FACTS:
Calories: 301 Fat: 11 g Carbs: 36 g Sugar: 1 g Fiber: 3 g Protein: 16 g Sodium: 2,535 mg

203. TOFU AND RED PEPPER STIR-FRY

Preparation Time: 10 minutes

Cooking Time: 12 minutes

Servings: 2

INGREDIENTS:
- 1 chopped red bell peppers
- 1 tablespoon extra-virgin olive oil
- 1/2 chopped onion
- 1/4 cup ginger teriyaki sauce
- 4 ounces chopped tofu

DIRECTIONS:
1. Heat the olive oil in a skillet or pan over medium-high heat until it starts shimmering.
2. Add the onion, red bell peppers, and tofu. Cook, stirring regularly.
3. Apply the teriyaki sauce to the skillet or pan after whisking it together. Cook, stirring occasionally for 3-4 minutes, or until it thickens.

NUTRITION FACTS:
Calories: 166 Fat: 10 g Carbs: 17 g Sugar: 12 g Fiber: 2 g Protein: 7 g Sodium: 892 mg

204. SWEET POTATO AND BELL PEPPER HASH WITH A FRIED EGG

Preparation Time: 10 minutes

Cooking Time: 25 minutes

Servings: 2

INGREDIENTS:
- 1/2 chopped onion
- 2 cups peeled and cubed potatoes
- 2 tablespoons extra-virgin olive oil
- 1/2 chopped red bell pepper
- 1/2 teaspoon sea salt
- 2 eggs
- A pinch of freshly ground black pepper

DIRECTIONS:
1. Heat olive oil in a big non-stick pan over medium-high heat until it starts shimmering.
2. Add the red bell pepper, onion, and sweet potato. Season with salt and a pinch of black pepper. Cook, stirring regularly until the potatoes are soft and browned.
3. Serve the potatoes in 4 bowls.
4. Return the skillet or pan to heat,

turn the heat down to medium-low, and swirl to secure the bottom of the pan with the remaining olive oil.
5. Scatter some salt over the eggs and carefully smash them into the tray. Cook until the whites are set, around 3-4 minutes.
6. Flip the eggs gently and remove them from the heat. Allow to rest for 1 minute in the hot skillet or pan. 1 egg should be placed on top of each serving of hash.

NUTRITION FACTS:

Calories: 384 Fat: 19 g Carbs: 47 g Sugar: 16 g Fiber: 8 g Protein: 10 g Sodium: 603 mg

205. QUINOA FLORENTINE

Preparation Time: 5 minutes

Cooking Time: 25 minutes

Servings: 2

INGREDIENTS:
- 1/2 chopped onion
- 2 minced garlic cloves
- 2 cups no-salt-added vegetable broth
- A pinch of freshly ground black pepper
- 1 tablespoon extra-virgin olive oil
- 1 ½ cup fresh baby spinach
- 1 cup quinoa, rinsed well
- 1/4 teaspoon sea salt

DIRECTIONS:
1. Heat the olive oil over medium-high heat until it starts shimmering.
2. Add the spinach and onion. Cook, stirring regularly, for 3 minutes.
3. Cook, stirring continuously, for 30 seconds after adding the garlic.
4. Combine the vegetable broth, salt, quinoa, and pepper in a mixing bowl. Set to a simmer, then reduce to low heat. Cook, covered, for 15-20 minutes, or until the liquid has been absorbed. Using a fork, fluff the mixture.

NUTRITION FACTS:
Calories: 403 Fat: 12 g Carbs: 62 g Sugar: 4 g Fiber: 7 g Protein: 13 g Sodium: 278 mg

206. TOMATO ASPARAGUS FRITTATA

Preparation Time: 5 minutes

Cooking Time: 20 minutes

Servings: 2

INGREDIENTS:
- 5 trimmed asparagus spears
- 3 eggs
- 1 tablespoon extra-virgin olive oil
- 5 cherry tomatoes
- 1/2 tablespoon chopped fresh thyme
- A pinch of freshly ground black pepper
- 1/4 teaspoon sea salt

DIRECTIONS:
1. Preheat the broiler to the highest setting.
2. Heat the olive oil in a big ovenproof skillet or pan over medium-high heat until it starts shimmering.
3. Toss in the asparagus. Cook, stirring regularly, for 5 minutes.
4. Add in the tomatoes. Cook for 3 minutes, stirring once in a while.
5. Whisk together the thyme, salt, eggs, and pepper in a medium mixing cup. Carefully, spill over the tomatoes and asparagus, turning them about in the pan to ensure that they are equally distributed.
6. Turn the heat down to medium. Cook for 3 minutes, or until the eggs are hardened around the outside
7. Place the pan under the broiler and cook for 3-5 minutes, or until puffed and brown. To eat, cut into wedges.

NUTRITION FACTS:
Calories: 224 Fat: 14 g Carbs: 15 g Sugar: 10 g Fiber: 5 g Protein: 12 g Sodium: 343 mg

207. TOFU SLOPPY JOES

Preparation Time: 5 minutes

Cooking Time: 15 minutes

Servings: 2

INGREDIENTS:
- 1/2 chopped onion
- 1 (14 ounces) can crushed tomatoes
- 1/2 tablespoon chili powder
- 1 tablespoon extra-virgin olive oil
- 5 ounces chopped tofu
- 2 tablespoons apple cider vinegar
- 1/2 teaspoon garlic powder
- a pinch of freshly ground black pepper
- 1/4 teaspoon sea salt

DIRECTIONS:
1. Heat the olive oil in a big pot over medium-high heat until it starts shimmering.
2. Combine the tofu and onion in a mixing bowl. Cook, stirring regularly until the onion is tender.
3. Add the tomatoes, apple cider vinegar, salt, garlic powder, chili powder, and pepper in a large mixing bowl. Simmer for 10 minutes, stirring regularly, to enable the flavors to meld.

NUTRITION FACTS:
Calories: 209 Fat: 10 g Carbs: 21 g Sugar: 13 g Fiber: 8 g Protein: 11 g Sodium: 644 mg

208. BROCCOLI AND EGG "MUFFINS"

Preparation Time: 5 minutes

Cooking Time: 20 minutes

Servings: 2

INGREDIENTS:
- 1 tablespoon extra-virgin olive oil
- 1/2 cup chopped broccoli florets
- 1/2 teaspoon garlic powder
- 2 tablespoons freshly ground black pepper
- Non-stick cooking spray
- 1/2 chopped onion
- 4 beaten eggs
- 1/4 teaspoon sea salt

DIRECTIONS:
1. Preheat the oven to 350°F.
2. Using non-stick cooking oil, coat a muffin pan.
3. Add the broccoli and onion. Let it be for 3 minutes in the oven. Divide the vegetables equally among the four muffin cups.
4. Add the eggs, salt, garlic powder, and pepper. They can be poured over the vegetables in the muffin tins.
5. Bake for 15-17 minutes, or until the eggs are cooked through.

NUTRITION FACTS:
Calories: 207 Fat: 16 Carbs: 5 g Sugar: 2 g Fiber: 1 g Protein: 12 g Sodium: 366 mg

209. SHRIMP SCAMPI

Preparation Time: 10 minutes

Cooking Time: 15 minutes

Servings: 2

INGREDIENTS:
- 1/2 finely chopped onion
- 1 pound shrimp, peeled and tails removed
- 1 lemon juice
- 2 tablespoons extra-virgin olive oil
- 1/2 chopped red bell pepper
- 3 minced garlic cloves
- 1 lemon zest
- A pinch of freshly ground black pepper
- 1/4 teaspoon sea salt

DIRECTIONS:
1. Heat the olive oil in a big non-stick pan over medium-high heat until it starts shimmering.
2. Add the red bell pepper and onion. Cook, stirring regularly, for around 6 minutes, or until tender.

3. Cook for around 5 minutes, or until the shrimp are yellow.
4. Add the garlic. Cook for 30 seconds while continuously stirring.
5. Stir in the zest and lemon juice, as well as the pepper and salt. Cook for 3 minutes on low heat.

NUTRITION FACTS:

Calories: 345 Fat: 16 Carbs: 10 g Sugar: 3 g Fiber: 1 g Protein: 40 g Sodium: 424 mg

 210. SHRIMP WITH CINNAMON SAUCE

Preparation Time: 5 minutes

Cooking Time: 10 minutes

Servings: 2

INGREDIENTS:
- 1 pound shrimp, peeled
- 1/2 cup no-salt-added chicken broth
- 1/2 teaspoon onion powder
- 1/8 teaspoon ground black pepper
- 1 tablespoon extra-virgin olive oil
- 1 tablespoon Dijon Mustard
- 1/2 teaspoon ground cinnamon
- 1/4 teaspoon sea salt

DIRECTIONS:
1. Heat the olive oil in a big non-stick skillet or pan over medium-high heat until it starts shimmering.
2. Toss in the shrimp. Cook, stirring regularly, for around 4 minutes, or until it is opaque.
3. Whisk together the chicken broth, mustard, onion powder, salt, cinnamon, and pepper in a shallow cup. Pour this into the skillet or pan and fry, stirring regularly, for another 3 minutes.

NUTRITION FACTS:

Calories: 270 Fat: 11g Carbs: 4 g Sugar: 1 g Fiber: 1 g Protein: 39 g Sodium: 664 mg

 211. SUPER-FOOD SCRAMBLE

Preparation Time: 10 minutes

Cooking Time: 7 minutes

Servings: 3

INGREDIENTS:
- 2 C. fresh spinach, chopped finely
- 1 tbsp. olive oil
- Salt and freshly ground black pepper, to taste
- ½ C. cooked salmon, chopped finely
- 4 eggs, beaten

DIRECTIONS:

1. In a skillet, heat the oil over high heat and cook the spinach with black pepper for about 2 minutes.
2. Stir in the salmon and reduce the heat to medium.
3. Add the eggs and cook for about 3-4 minutes, stirring frequently.
4. Serve immediately.

NUTRITION FACTS:

calories: 179;carbs: 1.2g; Protein: 15.3g; Fat: 12.9g; Sugar: 0.5g; Sodium: 165mg; Fiber: 0.4g

 212. FAMILY FAVORITE SCRAMBLE

Preparation Time: 10 minutes

Cooking Time: 5 minutes

Servings: 2

INGREDIENTS:
- 4 eggs
- ¼ tsp. red pepper flakes, crushed
- Salt and freshly ground black pepper, to taste
- ¼ C. fresh basil, chopped
- ½ C. tomatoes, peeled, seeded and chopped
- 1 tbsp. olive oil

DIRECTIONS:
1. In a large bowl, add eggs, red pepper flakes, salt and black pepper and beat well.
2. Add the basil and tomatoes and stir to combine.
3. In a large non-stick skillet, heat the oil over medium-high heat.
4. Add the egg mixture and cook for about 3-5 minutes, stirring continuously.
5. Serve immediately.

NUTRITION FACTS:

calories: 195;carbs: 2.6g; Protein: 11.6g; Fat: 15.9g; Sugar: 1.9g; Sodium: 203mg; Fiber: 0.7g

213. TASTY VEGGIE OMELET

Preparation Time: 15 minutes

Cooking Time: 25 minutes

Servings: 4

INGREDIENTS:
- 6 large eggs
- Sea salt and freshly ground black pepper, to taste
- ½ C. low-fat milk
- 1/3 C. fresh mushrooms, cut into slices
- 1/3 C. red bell pepper, seeded and chopped
- 1 tbsp. chives, minced

DIRECTIONS:
1. Preheat the oven to 350°F - 180°C. Lightly, grease a pie dish.
2. In a bowl, add the eggs, salt, black pepper and coconut oil and beat until well combined.
3. In another bowl, mix together the onion, bell pepper and mushrooms.
4. Transfer the egg mixture into the prepared pie dish evenly.
5. Top with vegetable mixture evenly and sprinkle with chives evenly.
6. Bake for about 20-25 minutes.
7. Remove from the oven and set aside for about 5 minutes.
8. With a knife, cut into equal sized wedges and serve.

NUTRITION FACTS:

calories: 125;carbs: 3.1g; Protein: 10.8g; Fat: 7.8g; Sugar: 2.8g; Sodium: 158mg; Fiber: 0.2g

 214. GARDEN VEGGIES QUICHE

Preparation Time: 15 minutes

Cooking Time: 20 minutes

Servings: 4

INGREDIENTS:
- 6 eggs
- ½ C. low-fat milk
- Salt and freshly ground black pepper, to taste
- 2 C. fresh baby spinach, chopped
- ½ C. green bell pepper, seeded and chopped
- 1 scallion, chopped
- ¼ C. fresh parsley, chopped
- 1 tbsp. fresh chives, minced

DIRECTIONS:
1. Preheat the oven to 400°F- 200°C. Lightly grease a pie dish.
2. In a bowl, add eggs, almond milk, salt and black pepper and beat until well combined. Set aside.
3. In another bowl, add the vegetables and herbs and mix well.
4. In the bottom of prepared pie dish, place the veggie mixture evenly and top with the egg mixture.
5. Bake for about 20 minutes or until a wooden skewer inserted in the center comes out clean.
6. Remove pie dish from the oven and set aside for about 5 minutes before slicing.
7. Cut into desired sized wedges and serve warm.

NUTRITION FACTS:

calories: 118;carbs: 4.3g; Protein: 10.1g; Fat: 7g; Sugar: 3g; Sodium: 160mg; Fiber: 0.8g

 215. FLUFFY PUMPKIN PANCAKES

Preparation Time: 10 minutes

Cooking Time: 40 minutes

Servings: 10

INGREDIENTS:
- 2 eggs
- 1 C. buckwheat flour
- 1 tbsp. baking powder
- 1 tsp. pumpkin pie spice
- ½ tsp. salt
- 1 C. pumpkin puree
- ¾ C. plus 2 tbsp. low-fat milk
- 3 tbsp. pure maple syrup
- 2 tbsp. olive oil
- 1 tsp. vanilla extract

DIRECTIONS:
1. In a blender, add all ingredients and pulse until well combined.
2. Transfer the mixture into a bowl and set aside for about 10 minutes.
3. Heat a greased non-stick skillet over medium heat.
4. Place about ¼ C. of the mixture and spread in an even circle.
5. Cook for about 2 minutes per side.
6. Repeat with the remaining mixture.
7. Serve warm.

NUTRITION FACTS:
calories: 113;carbs: 16.5g; Protein: 3.6g; Fat: 4.4g; Sugar: 5.9g; Sodium: 143mg; Fiber: 2g

 216. SPER-TASTY CHICKEN MUFFINS

Preparation Time: 15 minutes

Cooking Time: 45 minutes

Servings: 8

INGREDIENTS:
- 8 eggs
- Salt and freshly ground black pepper, as required
- 2 tbsp. filtered water
- 7 oz. cooked chicken, chopped finely
- 1½ C. fresh spinach, chopped
- 1 C. green bell pepper, seeded and chopped finely
- 2 tbsp. fresh parsley, chopped finely

DIRECTIONS:
1. Preheat the oven to 350°F - 180°C. Grease 8 C. of a muffin tin.
2. In a bowl, add eggs, salt, black pepper and water and beat until well combined.
3. Add the chicken, spinach, bell pepper and parsley and stir to combine.
4. Transfer the mixture into the prepared muffin C. evenly.
5. Bake for about 18-20 minutes or until golden brown.
6. Remove the muffin tin from oven and place onto a wire rack to cool for about 10 minutes.
7. Carefully invert the muffins onto a platter and serve warm.

NUTRITION FACTS:
calories: 107;carbs: 1.7g; Protein: 13.1g; Fat: 5.2g; Sugar: 1.1g; Sodium: 102mg; Fiber: 0.4g

217. CLASSIC ZUCCHINI BREAD

Preparation Time: 15 minutes

Cooking Time: 45 minutes

Servings: 24

INGREDIENTS:
- 3 C. all-purpose flour
- 2 tsp. baking soda
- 1 tsp. ground cinnamon
- 1 tsp. ground nutmeg
- 2 C. Splenda
- 1 C. olive oil
- 3 eggs, beaten
- 2 tsp. vanilla extract
- 2 C. zucchini, peeled, seeded and grated

DIRECTIONS:
1. Preheat the oven to 325°F - 160°C. Arrange a rack in the center of oven. Grease 2 loaf pans.
2. In a medium bowl, mix together the flour, baking soda and spices.
3. In another large bowl, add the Splenda and oil and beat until well combined.
4. Add the eggs and vanilla extract and beat until well combined.
5. Add the flour mixture and mix until just combined.
6. Gently, fold in the zucchini.
7. Place the mixture into the bread loaf pans evenly.
8. Bake for about 45-50 minutes or until a toothpick inserted in the center of bread comes out clean.
9. Remove the bread pans from oven and place onto a wire rack to cool for about 15 minutes.
10. Carefully, invert the breads onto the wire rack to cool completely before slicing.
11. With a sharp knife, cut each bread loaf into desired-sized slices and serve.

NUTRITION FACTS:
calories: 219;carbs: 28.4g; Protein: 16.3g; Fat: 9.2g; Sugar: 16.3g; Sodium: 113mg; Fiber: 0.6g

 218. GREEK INSPIRED CUCUMBER SALAD

Preparation Time: 10 minutes

Cooking Time: 0 minutes

Servings: 4

INGREDIENTS:
- 4 medium cucumbers, peeled, seeded and chopped
- ½ C. low-fat Greek yogurt
- 1½ tbsp. fresh dill, chopped
- 1 tbsp. fresh lemon juice
- Salt and freshly ground black pepper, as required

DIRECTIONS:
1. In a large bowl, add all the ingredients and mix well.
2. Serve immediately.

NUTRITION FACTS:
calories: 71;carbs: 13.8g; Protein:4g; Fat: 0.8g; Sugar: 7.3g; Sodium: 69mg; Fiber: 1.7g

219. LIGHT VEGGIE SALAD

Preparation Time: 10 minutes

Cooking Time: 0 minutes

Servings: 5

INGREDIENTS:
- 2 C. cucumbers, peeled, seeded and chopped
- 2 C. red tomatoes, peeled, seeded and chopped
- 2 tbsp. extra-virgin olive oil
- 2 tbsp. fresh lime juice
- Salt, to taste

DIRECTIONS:
1. In a large serving bowl, add all the ingredients and toss to coat well.
2. Serve immediately.

NUTRITION FACTS:
calories: 68;carbs: 04.4g; Protein: 0.9g; Fat: 5.8g; Sugar: 2.6g; Sodium: 35mg; Fiber: 1.1g

220. EASTERN EUROPEAN SOUP

Cooking Time: 5 minutes

Preparation Time: 10 minutes

Servings: 3

INGREDIENTS:
- 2 C. fat-free yogurt
- 4 tsp. fresh lemon juice
- 2 C. beets, trimmed, peeled and chopped
- 2 tbsp. fresh dill
- Salt, as required
- 1 tbsp. fresh chives, minced

DIRECTIONS:
1. In a high-speed blender, add all ingredients except for chives and pulse until smooth.
2. Transfer the soup into a pan over medium heat and cook for about 3-5 minutes or until heated through.
3. Serve immediately with the garnishing of chives.

NUTRITION FACTS:
calories: 149;carbs: 25.2g; Protein: 11.8g; Fat: 0.6g; Sugar: 21.7g; Sodium:

269mg; Fiber: 2.5g

221. CITRUS GLAZED CARROTS

Preparation Time: 15 minutes

Cooking Time: 15 minutes

Servings: 6

INGREDIENTS:
- 1½ lb. carrots, peeled and sliced into ½-inch pieces diagonally
- ½ C. water
- 2 tbsp. olive oil
- Salt, to taste
- 3 tbsp. fresh orange juice

DIRECTIONS:
1. In a large skillet, add the carrots, water, boil and salt over medium heat and bring to a boil.
2. Reduce heat to low and simmer; covered for about 6 minutes.
3. Add the orange juice and stir to combine.
4. Increase the heat to high and cook, uncovered for about 5-8 minutes, tossing frequently.
5. Serve immediately.

NUTRITION FACTS:
calories: 90;carbs: 12g; Protein: 1g; Fat: 4.7g; Sugar: 6.2g; Sodium: 106mg; Fiber: 2.8g

222. BRAISED ASPARAGUS

Preparation Time: 10 minutes

Cooking Time: 8 minutes

Servings: 2

INGREDIENTS:
- ½ C. chicken bone broth
- 1 tbsp. olive oil
- 1 (½-inch) lemon peel
- 1 C. asparagus, trimmed

DIRECTIONS:
1. In a small pan add the broth, oil and lemon peel over medium heat and bring to a boil.
2. Add the asparagus and cook, covered for about 3-4 minutes.
3. Discard the lemon peel and serve.

NUTRITION FACTS:
calories: 82;carbs: 2.6g; Protein: 3.7g; Fat: 7.1g; Sugar: 1.3g; Sodium: 25mg; Fiber: 1.4g

223. SPRING FLAVORED PASTA

Preparation Time: 10 minutes

Cooking Time: 10 minutes

Servings: 4

INGREDIENTS:
- 2 tbsp. olive oil
- 1 lb. asparagus, trimmed and cut into 1½-inch pieces
- Salt and freshly ground black pepper, to taste
- ½ lb. cooked hot pasta, drained

DIRECTIONS:
1. In a large cast-iron skillet, heat the oil over medium heat and cook the asparagus, salt and black pepper for about 8-10 minutes, stirring occasionally.
2. Place the hot pasta and toss to coat well.
3. Serve immediately.

NUTRITION FACTS:
calories: 246carbs: 35.2g; Protein: 8.9g; Fat: 8.4g; Sugar: 2.1g; Sodium: 17mg; Fiber: 2.4g

224. VERSATILE MAC 'N CHEESE

Preparation Time: 15 minutes

Cooking Time: 12 minutes

Servings: 1

INGREDIENTS:
- 2 C. elbow macaroni
- 1½ s butternut squash, peeled and cubed
- 1 C. low-fat Swiss cheese, shredded
- 1/3 C. low-fat milk
- 1 tbsp. olive oil
- Salt and freshly ground black pepper, to taste

DIRECTIONS:
1. In a large pan of the salted boiling water, cook the macaroni for about 8-10 minutes.
2. Drain the macaroni and transfer into a bowl.
3. Meanwhile, in a pan of the boiling water, cook the squash cubes for about 6 minutes or until soft.
4. Drain the squash cubes completely and return to the same pan.
5. With a masher, mash the squash and place over low heat.
6. Add the cheese and milk and cook for about 2-3 minutes, stirring continuously.
7. Add the macaroni, oil, salt and black pepper and stir to combine.
8. Remove from the heat and serve hot.

NUTRITION FACTS:
calories: 321;carbs: 40g; Protein: 14g; Fat: 11.9g; Sugar: 3.7g; Sodium: 65mg; Fiber: 2.4g

225. GLUTEN-FREE CURRY

Preparation Time: 15 minutes

Cooking Time: 20 minutes

Servings: 6

INGREDIENTS:
- 2 C. tomatoes, peeled, seeded and chopped
- 1½ C. water
- 2 tbsp. olive oil
- 1 tsp. fresh ginger, chopped
- ¼ tsp. ground turmeric
- 2 C. fresh shiitake mushrooms, sliced
- 5 C. fresh button mushrooms, sliced
- ¼ C. fat-free yogurt, whipped
- Salt and freshly ground black pepper, to taste

DIRECTIONS:
1. In a food processor, add the tomatoes and ¼ C. of water and pulse until a smooth paste forms.
2. In a pan, heat the oil over medium heat and sauté the ginger and turmeric for about 1 minute.
3. Add the tomato paste and cook for about 5 minutes.
4. Stir in the mushrooms, yogurt and remaining water and bring to a boil.
5. Cook for about 10-12 minutes, stirring occasionally.
6. Season with the salt and black pepper and remove from the heat.
7. Serve hot.

NUTRITION FACTS:
calories: 70;carbs: 5.3g; Protein: 3g; Fat: 5g; Sugar: 3.4g; Sodium: 41mg; Fiber: 1.4g

226. NEW YEAR'S LUNCHEON MEAL

Preparation Time: 10 minutes

Cooking Time: 0 minutes

Servings: 2

INGREDIENTS:
- 1 large avocado, halved and pitted
- 1 (5-oz.) can water-packed tuna, drained and flaked
- 3 tbsp. fat-free yogurt
- 2 tbsp. fresh lemon juice
- 1 tsp. fresh parsley, chopped finely
- Salt and freshly ground black pepper, to taste

DIRECTIONS:
1. Carefully, remove abut about 2-3 tbsp. of flesh from each avocado half.
2. Arrange the avocado halves onto a platter and drizzle each with 1 tsp. of lemon juice.
3. Chop the avocado flesh and transfer into a bowl.
4. In the bowl of avocado flesh, add tuna, yogurt, parsley, remaining lemon juice, salt, and black pepper, and stir to combine.
5. Divide the tuna mixture in both

avocado halves evenly.
6. Serve immediately.

NUTRITION FACTS:
calories: 215; carbs: 7g; Protein: 20.6g; Fat: 11.8g; Sugar: 2.4g; Sodium: 137mg; Fiber: 3.2g

227. ENTERTAINING WRAPS

Preparation Time: 15 minutes

Cooking Time: 10 minutes

Servings: 5

INGREDIENTS:
For Chicken:
- 2 tbsp. olive oil
- 1 tsp. fresh ginger, minced
- 1¼ lb. ground chicken
- Salt and freshly ground black pepper, to taste

For Wraps:
- 10 romaine lettuce leaves
- 1½ C. carrot, peeled and julienned
- 2 tbsp. fresh parsley, chopped finely
- 2 tbsp. fresh lime juice

DIRECTIONS:
1. In a skillet, heat the oil over medium heat and sauté the ginger for about 1 minute.
2. Add the ground chicken, salt, and black pepper and cook for about 7-9 minutes, breaking up the meat into smaller pieces with a wooden spoon.
3. Remove from the heat and set aside to cool.
4. Arrange the lettuce leaves onto serving plates.
5. Place the cooked chicken over each lettuce leaf and top with carrot and cilantro.
6. Drizzle with lime juice and serve immediately.

NUTRITION FACTS:
calories: 280; carbs: 3.8g; Protein: 33.2g; Fat: 14g; Sugar: 1.7g; Sodium: 153mg; Fiber: 0.9g

DIVERTICULITIS COOKBOOK

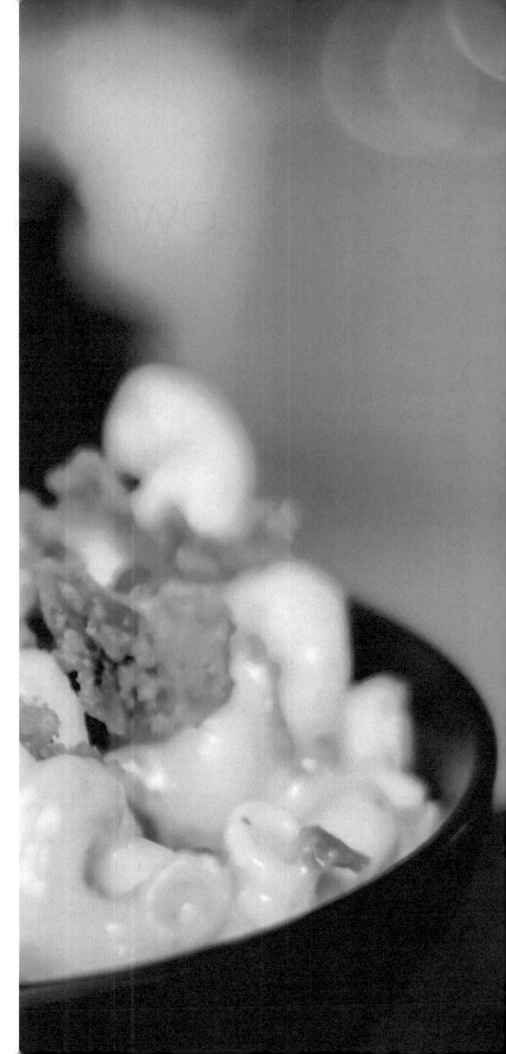

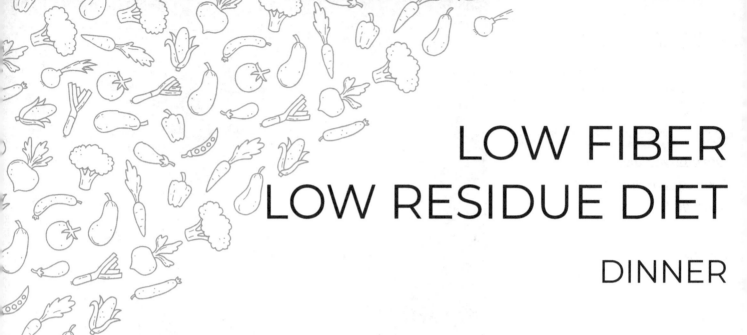

LOW FIBER LOW RESIDUE DIET
DINNER

228. ITALIAN STYLED STUFFED ZUCCHINI BOATS

Preparation Time: 10 minutes

Cooking Time: 25 minutes

Servings: 2

INGREDIENTS:
- 6 large zucchini
- 1/2 tablespoon olive oil
- Kosher salt
- Freshly ground black pepper
- 1/4 teaspoon garlic powder
- 1 small yellow onion, diced
- 2 garlic cloves, minced
- 1 pound ground turkey
- 1 (28 ounces) can crush tomatoes
- 4 ounces Mozzarella cheese, shredded
- 1 ounce Parmesan cheese, freshly grated
- Flat-leaf parsley for garnishing
- Cooking spray

DIRECTIONS:
1. Turn your oven on and allow to preheat up to 425°F - 220°C and lightly grease a 9x13-inch baking dish with cooking spray.
2. Divide the zucchini in half lengthwise and then scoop out the seeds. Brush with olive oil and season with salt, pepper and garlic powder.
3. Roast in the prepared dish for 20 minutes, or until it begins to soften.
4. Meanwhile, saute the onions and garlic in 1/2 tablespoon of olive oil over medium-high heat in a large skillet.
5. Cook for 3-4 minutes, then add the ground turkey and brown. Attach the tomatoes and bring them to a boil.
6. Reduce the heat to medium and then let simmer until the zucchini are done. Stir in 1/2 teaspoon salt and pepper to taste.
7. Set to bake for about 5 minutes or at least until the Mozzarella cheese you added has melted, about 3-5 minutes.
8. Serve hot, garnished with Parmesan cheese and parsley.

NUTRITION FACTS:
Calories: 298 Fat: 7 g Carbs: 14 g Fiber: 2 g Protein: 25 g

229. CHICKEN CUTLETS

Preparation Time: 10 minutes

Cooking Time: 15 minutes

Servings: 4

INGREDIENTS:
- 4 teaspoons red wine vinegar
- 2 teaspoons minced garlic cloves
- 2 teaspoons dried sage leaves
- 1 pound chicken breast cutlets
- Salt and pepper, to taste
- 1/4 cup refined white flour
- 2 teaspoons olive oil

DIRECTIONS:
1. Set a good amount of plastic wrap on the kitchen counter; sprinkle with half the combined sage, garlic and vinegar.
2. Put the chicken breast on the plastic wrap; sprinkle with the rest of the vinegar mixture. Season lightly with pepper and salt.
3. Secure the chicken with the second sheet of plastic wrap. Use a kitchen mallet to pound the breast until it is flattened. Let stand 5 minutes.
4. Set the chicken on both sides with flour. In a skillet, heat the oil over medium heat.
5. Add half of the chicken breast and cook for 1 ½ minute or until it is browned on the bottom.
6. Turn on the other side and let it cook for 3 minutes.
7. Remove the chicken breast and place it on an oven-proof serving plate so that you can keep warm.
8. Reduce the liquid by half. Pour the mixture over the chicken breast; serve immediately.

NUTRITION FACTS:
Calories: 549 Fat: 6 g Carbs: 7 g Fiber: 1 g Protein: 114 g

230. SLOW COOKER SALSA TURKEY

Preparation Time: 8 minutes

Cooking Time: 7 hours

Servings: 4

INGREDIENTS:
- 2 pounds turkey breasts, boneless and skinless
- 1 cup salsa
- 1 cup small tomatoes, diced, canned choose low-sodium
- 2 tablespoons taco seasoning
- 1/2 cup celery, finely diced
- 1/2 cup carrots, shredded
- 3 tablespoons low-fat sour cream

DIRECTIONS:
1. Add the turkey to your slow cooker. Season it with taco seasoning then top with salsa and vegetables.
2. Add in 1/2 cup of water. Set to cook on low for 7 hours (internal temperature should be 165°F when done).
3. Shred the turkey with 2 forks, add in sour cream and stir. Enjoy.

NUTRITION FACTS:

Calories: 178 Fat: 4 g Carbs: 7 g Fiber: 2 g Protein: 27 g

231. SRIRACHA LIME CHICKEN AND APPLE SALAD

Preparation Time: 20 minutes

Cooking Time: 15 minutes

Servings: 4

INGREDIENTS:

Sriracha Lime Chicken:
- 2 organic chicken breasts
- 3 tablespoons sriracha
- 1 lime, juiced
- 1/4 teaspoon fine sea salt
- 1/4 teaspoon freshly ground pepper

Fruit Salad:
- 4 apples, peeled, cored and diced
- 1 cup organic grape tomatoes
- 1/3 cup red onion, finely chopped

Lime Vinaigrette:
- 1/3 cup light olive oil
- 1/4 cup apple cider vinegar
- 2 limes, juiced
- A dash of fine sea salt

DIRECTIONS:

1. Use salt and pepper to season the chicken on both sides. Spread on the sriracha and lime and let sit for 20 minutes.
2. Cook the chicken per side over medium heat, or until done. Grill the apple with the chicken.
3. Meanwhile, whisk together the dressing and season to taste.
4. Arrange the salad, topping it with red onion and tomatoes.
5. Serve as a side to the chicken and apple.

NUTRITION FACTS:

Calories: 484 Fat: 28 g Carbs: 32 g Fiber: 8 g Protein: 30 g

232. PAN-SEARED SCALLOPS WITH LEMON-GINGER VINAIGRETTE

Preparation Time: 10 minutes

Cooking Time: 10 minutes

Servings: 2

INGREDIENTS:

- 1 pound sea scallops
- 1 tablespoon extra-virgin olive oil
- 1/4 teaspoon sea salt
- 2 tablespoons lemon-ginger vinaigrette
- A pinch of freshly ground black pepper

DIRECTIONS:

1. Heat the olive oil in a non-stick skillet or pan over medium-high heat until it starts shimmering.
2. Add the scallops to the skillet or pan after seasoning them with pepper and salt. Cook for 3 minutes per side or until the fish is only opaque.
3. Serve with a dollop of vinaigrette on top.

NUTRITION FACTS:

Calories: 280 Fat: 16 Carbs: 5 g Sugar: 1 g Fiber: 0 g Protein: 29 g Sodium: 508 mg

233. ROASTED SALMON AND ASPARAGUS

Preparation Time: 5 minutes

Cooking Time: 15 minutes

Servings: 2

INGREDIENTS:

- 1 tablespoon extra-virgin olive oil
- 1 pound salmon, cut into two fillets
- 1/2 lemon zest and slices
- 1/2 pound asparagus spears, trimmed
- 1 teaspoon sea salt, divided
- 1/8 teaspoon freshly cracked black pepper

DIRECTIONS:

1. Preheat the oven to 425°F - 220°C.
2. Stir the asparagus with half of salt and olive oil. At the base of a roasting tray, spread in a continuous sheet.
3. Season the salmon with salt and pepper. Place the asparagus on top of the skin-side down.
4. Lemon zest should be sprinkled over the asparagus, salmon, and lemon slices. Set them over the top.
5. Roast for around 15 minutes until the flesh of the fish is opaque, in the preheated oven.

NUTRITION FACTS:

Calories: 308 Fat: 18 g Carbs: 5 g Sugar: 2 g Fiber: 2 g Protein: 36 g Sodium: 542 mg

234. ORANGE AND MAPLE-GLAZED SALMON

Preparation Time: 15 minutes

Cooking Time: 15 minutes

Servings: 2

INGREDIENTS:

- 1 orange zest
- 1 tablespoon low-sodium soy sauce
- 2 (4-6 ounces) salmon fillets, pin bones removed
- 1 orange juice
- 2 tablespoons pure maple syrup
- 1 teaspoon garlic powder

DIRECTIONS:

1. Preheat the oven to 400°F- 200°C.
2. Set the orange juice and zest, soy sauce, maple syrup, and garlic powder in a little shallow bowl.
3. Place the salmon parts in the dish flesh-side down. Allow resting 10 minutes for marinating.
4. Put the salmon on a rimmed baking dish, skin-side up, and bake for 15 minutes, or until the flesh is opaque.

NUTRITION FACTS:

Calories: 297 Fat: 11 Carbs: 18 g Sugar: 15 g Fiber: 1 g Protein: 34 g Sodium: 528 mg

235. COD WITH GINGER AND BLACK BEANS

Preparation Time: 10 minutes

Cooking Time: 15 minutes

Servings: 2

INGREDIENTS:

- 2 (6 ounces) cod fillets
- 1/2 teaspoon sea salt, divided
- 3 minced garlic cloves
- 2 tablespoons chopped fresh cilantro leaves
- 1 tablespoon extra-virgin olive oil
- 1/2 tablespoon grated fresh ginger
- 2 tablespoons freshly ground black pepper
- 1/2 (14 ounces) can black beans, drained

DIRECTIONS:

1. Heat the olive oil in a big non-stick skillet or pan over medium-high heat until it starts shimmering.
2. Half of the salt, ginger, and pepper are used to season the fish. Cook for around 4 minutes per side in the hot oil until the fish is opaque. Detach the cod from the pan and place it on a plate with aluminum foil tented over it.
3. Add the garlic to the skillet or pan and return it to the heat. Cook for 30 seconds while continuously stirring.
4. Mix the black beans and the remaining salt. Cook, stirring regularly, for 5 minutes.
5. Add the cilantro and serve the black beans on top of the cod.

NUTRITION FACTS:

Calories: 419 Fat: 2 g Carbs: 33 g Sugar: 1 g Fiber: 8 g Protein: 50 g Sodium: 605 mg

236. HALIBUT CURRY

Preparation Time: 10 minutes

Cooking Time: 10 minutes

Servings: 2

INGREDIENTS:

- 1 teaspoon ground turmeric
- 1 pound halibut, skin, and bones removed, cut into 1-inch pieces
- 1/2 (14 ounces) can coconut milk
- 1/8 teaspoon ground black pepper
- 1 tablespoon extra-virgin olive oil
- 1 teaspoon curry powder
- 2 cups no-salt-added chicken broth
- 1/4 teaspoon sea salt

DIRECTIONS:

1. Heat the olive oil in a non-stick skillet or pan over medium-high heat until it starts shimmering.
2. Add the curry powder and turmeric to a bowl. To bloom the spices, cook for 2 minutes, stirring continuously.
3. Stir in the halibut, coconut milk, chicken broth, pepper, and salt. Lower the heat to medium-low and bring to a simmer. Cook, stirring regularly, for 6-7 minutes, or until the fish is opaque.

NUTRITION FACTS:

Calories: 429 Fat: 47 g Carbs: 5 g Sugar: 1 g Fiber: 1 g Protein: 27 g Sodium: 507 mg

 ## 237. CHICKEN CACCIATORE

Preparation Time: 10 minutes

Cooking Time: 20 minutes

Servings: 2

INGREDIENTS:

- 1 pound skinless chicken, cut into bite-size pieces
- 1/4 cup black olives, chopped
- 1/2 teaspoon onion powder
- A pinch of freshly ground black pepper
- 1 tablespoon extra-virgin olive oil
- 1 (28 ounces) can crushed tomatoes, drained
- 1/2 teaspoon garlic powder
- 1/4 teaspoon sea salt

DIRECTIONS:

1. Heat the olive oil in a non-stick skillet or pan over medium-high heat until it starts shimmering.
2. Cook until the chicken is browned.
3. Add the tomatoes, garlic powder, olives, salt, onion powder, and pepper, then stir to combine. Cook, stirring regularly, for 10 minutes.

NUTRITION FACTS:

Calories: 305 Fat: 11 g Carbs: 34 g Sugar: 23 g Fiber: 13 g Protein: 19 g Sodium: 1,171 mg

 ## 238. CHICKEN AND BELL PEPPER SAUTE

Preparation Time: 5 minutes

Cooking Time: 15 minutes

Servings: 2

INGREDIENTS:

- 1 chopped bell pepper
- 1 pound skinless chicken breasts, cut into bite-size pieces
- 1 ½ tablespoon extra-virgin olive oil
- 1/2 chopped onion
- 3 minced garlic cloves
- 1/8 teaspoon ground black pepper
- 1/4 teaspoon sea salt

DIRECTIONS:

1. Heat the olive oil in a non-stick skillet or pan over medium-high heat until it starts shimmering.
2. Add the onion, red bell pepper, and chicken. Cook, stirring regularly, for 10 minutes.
3. Stir in the salt, garlic, and pepper in a mixing bowl. Cook for 30 seconds while continuously stirring.

NUTRITION FACTS:

Calories: 179 Fat: 13 g Carbs: 6 g Sugar: 3 g Fiber: 1 g Protein: 10 g Sodium: 265 mg

 ## 239. CHICKEN SALAD SANDWICHES

Preparation Time: 15 minutes

Cooking Time: 0 minutes

Servings: 2

INGREDIENTS:

- 2 tablespoons anti-inflammatory mayonnaise
- 1 tablespoon chopped fresh tarragon leaves
- 1 cup chicken, chopped, cooked and skinless (from 1 rotisserie chicken)
- 1/2 minced red bell pepper
- 1 teaspoon Dijon mustard
- 4 slices whole-wheat bread
- 1/4 teaspoon sea salt

DIRECTIONS:

1. Combine the chicken, red bell pepper, mayonnaise, mustard, tarragon, and salt in a medium mixing bowl.
2. Spread on 2 pieces of bread and top it with the remaining bread.

NUTRITION FACTS:

Calories: 315 Fat: 9 g Carbs: 30 g Sugar: 6 g Fiber: 4 g Protein: 28 g Sodium: 677 mg

240. ROSEMARY CHICKEN

Preparation Time: 15 minutes

Cooking Time: 20 minutes

Servings: 2

INGREDIENTS:

- 1 tablespoon extra-virgin olive oil
- 1 pound chicken breast tenders
- 1 tablespoon chopped fresh rosemary leaves
- 1/8 teaspoon ground black pepper
- 1/4 teaspoon sea salt

DIRECTIONS:

1. Preheat the oven to 425°F-220°C.
2. Set the chicken tenders on a baking sheet with a rim. Sprinkle with salt, rosemary, and pepper after brushing them with olive oil.
3. For 15-20 minutes, keep in the oven, just before the juices run clear.

NUTRITION FACTS:

Calories: 389 Fat: 20 g Carbs: 1 g Sugar: 0 g Fiber: 1 g Protein: 49 g Sodium: 381 mg

 ## 241. GINGERED TURKEY MEATBALLS

Preparation Time: 10 minutes

Cooking Time: 10 minutes

Servings: 2

INGREDIENTS:

- 1/2 cup shredded cabbage
- 1/2 tablespoon grated fresh ginger
- 1/2 teaspoon onion powder
- 1 pound ground turkey
- 2 tablespoons chopped fresh cilantro leaves
- 1/2 teaspoon garlic powder
- 1/4 teaspoon sea salt
- 1 tablespoon olive oil
- A pinch of freshly ground black pepper

DIRECTIONS:

1. Combine the cabbage, turkey, cilantro, ginger, onion powder, garlic powder, pepper, and salt in a big mixing bowl. Mix well. Make 10 (3/4 inch) meatballs out of the turkey mixture.
2. Heat the oil in a big non-stick skillet or pan over medium-high heat until it starts shimmering.
3. Cook for about 10 minutes, rotating the meatballs while they brown and you are done.

NUTRITION FACTS:

Calories: 408 Fat: 26 g Carbs: 4 g Sugar: 1 g Fiber: 1 g Protein: 47 g Sodium: 426 mg

 ## 242. TURKEY AND KALE SAUTE

Preparation Time: 15 minutes

Cooking Time: 35 minutes

Servings: 2

INGREDIENTS:

- 1 pound ground turkey breast
- 1/2 chopped onion
- 1/2 teaspoon sea salt
- 3 minced garlic cloves
- 1 tablespoon extra-virgin olive oil
- 1 cup stemmed and chopped kale
- 1 tablespoon fresh thyme leaves
- A pinch of freshly ground black pepper

DIRECTIONS:

1. Heat the olive oil in a big non-stick skillet or pan over medium-high heat until it starts shimmering.
2. Add the turkey, onion, kale, thyme, pepper, and salt. Cook, crumbling the turkey with a spoon until it browns, for about 5 minutes.
3. Garlic can be included now. Cook for 30 minutes while continuously stirring.

NUTRITION FACTS:

Calories: 413 Fat: 20 g Carbs: 7 g Sugar: 1 g Fiber: 1 g Protein: 50 g Sodium: 358 mg

243. TURKEY WITH BELL PEPPERS AND ROSEMARY

Preparation Time: 15 minutes

Cooking Time: 10 minutes

Servings: 2

INGREDIENTS:

- 1 chopped red bell peppers
- 1 pound boneless, skinless turkey breasts, cut into bite-size pieces
- 1/4 teaspoon sea salt
- 2 minced garlic cloves
- 2 tablespoons extra-virgin olive oil
- 1/2 chopped onion
- 1 tablespoon chopped fresh rosemary leaves
- A pinch of freshly ground black pepper

DIRECTIONS:

1. Heat the olive oil in a non-stick skillet or pan over medium-high heat until it starts shimmering.
2. Add the onion, red bell peppers, rosemary turkey, salt, and pepper. Cook until the turkey is cooked and the veggies are soft.
3. Garlic can be included now. Cook for an additional 30 seconds.

NUTRITION FACTS:

Calories: 303 Fat: 14 g Carbs: 15 g Sugar: 10 g Fiber: 2 g Protein: 30 g Sodium: 387 mg

244. MUSTARD AND ROSEMARY PORK TENDERLOIN

Preparation Time: 20 minutes

Cooking Time: 15 minutes

Servings: 2

INGREDIENTS:

- 2 tablespoons Dijon mustard
- 2 tablespoons fresh rosemary leaves
- 1/4 teaspoon sea salt
- 1/2 (1 ½ pound) pork tenderloin
- 1/4 cup fresh parsley leaves
- 3 garlic cloves
- 1 ½ tablespoon extra-virgin olive oil
- 1/8 teaspoon ground black pepper

DIRECTIONS:

1. Preheat the oven to 400°F - 200°C.
2. Combine the mustard, parsley, garlic, olive oil, rosemary, pepper, and salt in a blender or food processor. Pulse 20 times in 1-second intervals before a paste emerges. Rub the tenderloin with the paste and place it on a rimmed baking sheet.
3. Bake the pork for around 15 minutes or until an instant-read meat thermometer, reads 165°F-75°C.
4. Allow resting for 5 minutes before slicing and serving.

NUTRITION FACTS:

Calories: 362 Fat: 18 g Carbs: 5 g Sugar: 1 g Fiber: 2 g Protein: 2 g Sodium: 515 mg

245. THIN-CUT PORK CHOPS WITH MUSTARDY KALE

Preparation Time: 10 minutes

Cooking Time: 25 minutes

Servings: 2

INGREDIENTS:

1. 1 teaspoon sea salt, divided
2. 2 tablespoons Dijon mustard, divided
3. 1/2 finely chopped red onion
4. 1 tablespoon apple cider vinegar
5. 2 thin-cut pork chops
6. 1/8 teaspoon ground black pepper, divided
7. 1 ½ tablespoon extra-virgin olive oil
8. 2 cups stemmed and chopped kale

DIRECTIONS:

1. Preheat the oven to 425°F - 220°C.
2. Half of salt and pepper are used to season the pork chops. Place them on a rimmed baking sheet and spread 1 tablespoon of mustard over them. Bake for 15 minutes until an instant-read meat thermometer detects a temperature of 165°F-75°C.
3. When the pork cooks, heat the olive oil in a big non-stick skillet or pan over medium-high heat until it starts shimmering.
4. Add the red onion and kale. Cook, stirring regularly, for around 7 minutes, or until the veggies soften.
5. Whisk together the remaining tablespoon of mustard, the remaining half salt, the cider vinegar, and the remaining pepper in a wide mixing bowl. Toss with the kale. Cook for 2 minutes, stirring occasionally.

NUTRITION FACTS:

Calories: 504 Fat: 39 g Carbs: 10 g Sugar: 1 g Fiber: 2 g Protein: 28 g Sodium: 755 mg

246. BEEF TENDERLOIN WITH SAVORY BLUEBERRY SAUCE

Preparation Time: 10 minutes

Cooking Time: 15 minutes

Servings: 2

INGREDIENTS:

1. 1 teaspoon sea salt, divided
2. 2 tablespoons extra-virgin olive oil
3. 1/4 cup tawny port
4. 1 ½ tablespoon very cold butter, cut into pieces
5. 2 beef tenderloin fillets, about 3/4 inch thick
6. 1/8 teaspoon ground black pepper, divided
7. 1 finely minced shallot
8. 1 cup fresh blueberries

DIRECTIONS:

1. Half salt and pepper are to be used to season the beef.
2. Heat the olive oil in a big skillet or pan over medium-high heat until it starts shimmering.
3. Add the seasoned steaks to the pan. Cook per side until an instant-read meat thermometer detects an internal temperature of 130°F-55°C. Set aside on a plate of aluminum foil tented over it.
4. Get the skillet or pan back up to heat. Add the port, shallot, blueberries, and the remaining salt and pepper to the pan. Scrape some browned pieces off the bottom of the skillet or pan with a wooden spoon. Set the heat to medium-low and bring to a simmer. Cook, stirring from time to time, and gently crushing the blueberries for around 4 minutes or until the liquid has reduced by half.
5. Set in the butter 1 slice at a time. Toss the meat back into the skillet or pan. Mix it once with the sauce

to coat it. The rest of the sauce can be spooned over the meat before serving.

NUTRITION FACTS:

Calories: 554 Fat: 32 g Carbs: 14 g Sugar: 8 g Fiber: 2 g Protein: 50 g Sodium: 632 mg

247. GROUND BEEF CHILI WITH TOMATOES

Preparation Time: 10 minutes

Cooking Time: 15 minutes

Servings: 2

INGREDIENTS:

- 1/2 chopped onion
- 1 (14 ounces) can kidney beans, drained
- 1/2 pound extra-lean ground beef
- 1 (28 ounces) can chopped tomatoes, undrained
- 1/2 tablespoon chili powder
- 1/4 teaspoon sea salt
- 1/2 teaspoon garlic powder

DIRECTIONS:

- Cook the beef and onion in a big pot over medium-high heat for around 5 minutes.
- Add the kidney beans, tomatoes, garlic powder, chili powder, salt, and stir to combine. Bring to boil, then reduce to low heat.
- Cook for 10 minutes, stirring occasionally.

NUTRITION FACTS:

Calories: 890 Fat: 20 g Carbs: 63 g Sugar: 13 g Fiber: 17 g Protein: 116 g Sodium: 562 mg

248. FISH TACO SALAD WITH STRAWBERRY AVOCADO SALSA

Preparation Time: 20 minutes

Cooking Time: 15 minutes

Servings: 2

INGREDIENTS:

For the salsa:
- 2 hulled and diced strawberries
- 1/2 diced small shallot
- 2 tablespoons finely chopped fresh cilantro
- 2 tablespoons freshly squeezed lime juice
- 1/8 teaspoon cayenne pepper
- 1/2 diced avocado
- 2 tablespoons canned black beans, rinsed and drained
- 1 thinly sliced green onions
- 1/2 teaspoon finely chopped peeled ginger
- 1/4 teaspoon sea salt

For the fish salad:
- 1 teaspoon agave nectar
- 2 cups arugula
- 1 tablespoon extra-virgin olive or avocado oil
- 1/2 tablespoon freshly squeezed lime juice
- 1 pound light fish (halibut, cod, or red snapper), cut into 2 fillets
- 1/4 teaspoon ground black pepper
- 1/2 teaspoon sea salt

DIRECTIONS:

For the salsa:
1. Preheat the grill, whether it's gas or charcoal.
2. Add the avocado, beans, strawberries, shallot, cilantro, green onions, salt, ginger, lime juice, and cayenne pepper in a medium mixing cup. Put aside after mixing until all the components are well combined.

For the fish salad:
1. Whisk the agave, oil, and lime juice in a small bowl. Set the arugula with the vinaigrette in a big mixing bowl.
2. Season the fish fillets with pepper and salt. Grill the fish for 7-9 minutes over direct high heat, flipping once during cooking. The fish should be translucent and quickly flake.
3. Place 1 cup of arugula salad on each plate to eat. Cover each salad with a fillet and a heaping spoonful of salsa.

NUTRITION FACTS:

Calories: 878 Fat: 26 g Carbs: 53 g Sugar: 15 g Fiber: 18 g Protein: 119 g Sodium: 582 mg

249. BEEF AND BELL PEPPER STIR-FRY

Preparation Time: 5 minutes

Cooking Time: 10 minutes

Servings: 2

INGREDIENTS:

- 3 scallions, white and green parts, chopped
- 1 tablespoon grated fresh ginger
- 2 minced garlic cloves
- 1/2 pound extra-lean ground beef
- 1 chopped red bell peppers
- 1/4 teaspoon sea salt

DIRECTIONS:

1. Cook the beef for around 5 minutes in a big non-stick skillet or pan until it browns.
2. Add the scallions, ginger, red bell peppers, and salt. Cook, stirring occasionally, for around 4 minutes or until the bell peppers are tender.
3. Garlic can be included now. Cook for 30 seconds while continuously stirring. Switch off the flame, and you are done.

NUTRITION FACTS:

Calories: 599 Fat: 19 g Carbs: 9 g Sugar: 4 g Fiber: 2 g Protein: 97 g Sodium: 520 mg

250. VEGGIE PIZZA WITH CAULIFLOWER-YAM CRUST

Preparation Time: 5 minutes

Cooking Time: 1 hour 10 minutes

Servings: 2

INGREDIENTS:

- 1/2 medium peeled and chopped garnet yam
- 1 teaspoon sea salt, divided
- 1/2 tablespoon coconut oil, plus more for greasing pizza stone
- 1/4 cup sliced cremini mushrooms
- 1/4 medium head cauliflower, cut into small florets
- 1/2 tablespoon dried Italian herbs
- 1/2 cup flour brown rice
- 1/2 sliced small red onion
- 1/2 zucchini or yellow summer squash
- 2 tablespoons vegan pesto
- 1/2 cup spinach

DIRECTIONS:

1. Heat the oven to 400°F -200°C or preheat the pizza stone in case you have one.
2. Set a big pot with 1 inch of water, place a steamer basket. Put the yam and cauliflower in the steamer basket and steam for 15 minutes, or until both are quickly pricked with a fork. If you overcook the vegetables, they can get too soggy.
3. Place the vegetables in a food blender or processor and pulse until smooth. Blend in the Italian herbs and half a teaspoon of salt until smooth. Set the mixture in a big mixing bowl. Gradually whisk in the flour until it is well mixed.
4. Use coconut oil to grease the pizza stone or a pizza plate. In the middle of the pizza stone, pile the cauliflower mixture. Spread the pizza dough uniformly in a round or circular way (much like frosting) with a spatula until the crust is around 1/8 inches thick.
5. Bake for around 45 minutes. To get the top crispy, switch on the broiler and cook it for 2 minutes.
6. In a medium skillet or pan, melt the coconut oil over medium heat. Cook for 2 minutes after adding the onion. Add the squash, mushrooms, and the remaining ingredients to a large mixing bowl. Saute for 3-4 minutes with a quarter teaspoon of salt. Detach the spinach from the heat as soon as it starts to wilt.
7. Evenly, plate the pesto around the pizza crust. Over the pesto, spread the sautéed vegetables. It's time to slice the pizza and eat it.

NUTRITION FACTS:

Calories: 329 Fat: 17 g Carbs: 9 g Sugar: 3 g Fiber: 5 g Protein: 37 g Sodium: 430 mg

251. TOASTED PECAN QUINOA BURGERS

Preparation Time: 5 minutes

Cooking Time: 30 minutes

Servings: 2

INGREDIENTS:

- 2 cups vegetable broth, divided
- 1 teaspoon sea salt
- 2 tablespoons sesame seeds
- 1/2 teaspoon dried oregano
- 1/4 cup canned black beans,
- 2 tablespoons pecans
- 1/2 cup quinoa, rinsed and drained
- 1/4 cup sunflower seeds
- 1/2 teaspoon ground cumin
- 1/2 shredded carrot
- Freshly ground black pepper
- 1/2 thinly sliced avocado
- 1/2 teaspoon coconut or sunflower oil

DIRECTIONS:

1. Preheat the oven to 375°F-190°C.
2. Roast the pecans for 5-7 minutes on a baking sheet.
3. In a big saucepan, bring 1 cup of broth, quinoa, and salt to a boil over medium-high heat. Set the heat to a minimum, cover, and cook for 20 minutes, stirring occasionally.
4. In a food processor, grind the pecans, cumin, sesame seeds, sunflower seeds, and oregano to a medium-coarse texture.
5. Combine a half cup of quinoa, carrots, nut mixture, and beans in a big mixing bowl. Slowly, pour the remaining cup of broth, constantly stirring, before the paste becomes tacky. Season with pepper and salt as per taste.
6. Set the mixture into 2 (1/2-inch thick) patties and cook, refrigerate them right away.
7. In a big skillet or pan over medium-high heat, melt the coconut oil. Cook for around 2 minutes on either side. Carry on for the remaining patties in the same manner. Avocado slices can be placed on top of the burgers.

NUTRITION FACTS:

Calories: 432 Fat: 12 g Carbs: 12 g Sugar: 5 g Fiber: 3 Protein: 57 g Sodium: 566 mg

252. SIZZLING SALMON AND QUINOA

Preparation Time: 10 minutes

Cooking Time: 30 minutes

Servings: 2

INGREDIENTS:

- 1/2 teaspoon extra-virgin olive oil
- 1/2 cup quinoa, rinsed and drained
- 1/4 pound sliced chanterelle mushrooms
- 1/2 cup frozen small peas
- 1 tablespoon chopped fresh basil
- 1 head garlic
- 1 ½ cup mushroom broth, divided
- 1 tablespoon coconut oil
- 1/2 cup shredded brussels sprouts
- 1 tablespoon nutritional yeast
- 1/2 tablespoon dried oregano
- Sea salt and freshly ground black pepper
- 1/4 pound salmon, skin, and bones removed, cut into 1-inch cubes

DIRECTIONS:

1. Preheat the oven to 350°F-180°C.
2. Detach the top of the garlic head to reveal the cloves. Cover the head in foil and drizzle with olive oil. Set in the oven for 50 minutes to roast.
3. Meanwhile, in a big saucepan, mix 1 cup of broth and the quinoa. Set to a boil over high heat, then reduce to low heat, cover, and simmer without stirring for 20 minutes. To make this dish, measure 1/4 cup of quinoa, reserving any leftovers for another use.
4. Heat the coconut oil in a big skillet or pan over medium heat. Saute for 5 minutes, or before the mushrooms release liquid and become tender.
5. Cook for 3 minutes with the brussels sprouts, adding up to 1/4 cup of broth if required to keep the mushrooms and sprouts from sticking to the skillet or pan.
6. Saute for 5 minutes, stirring regularly, with the peas, basil, nutritional yeast, and oregano.
7. Toss the salmon in the pan to mix. Squeeze the garlic cloves gently into it. Cook, secured, for 4-5 minutes, stirring periodically.
8. Stir in the remaining 1/4 cup of broth and 1/4 cup of quinoa in the skillet or pan until all is well mixed. Season with pepper and salt to taste.
9. Serve.

NUTRITION FACTS:

Calories: 599 Fat: 20 g Carbs: 10 g Sugar: 4 g Fiber: 6 g Protein: 88 g Sodium: 662 mg

253. PAPAYA-MANGO SMOOTHIE

Preparation Time: 5 minutes

Cooking Time: 0 minutes

Servings: 2

INGREDIENTS:

- 1 cup mango, diced
- 1 cup papaya chunks
- 1 cup almond or lactose-free milk
- 1 tablespoon honey or maple syrup

DIRECTIONS:

1. Blend all ingredients in a blender and then pulse until smooth.
2. Pour into a large glass. Enjoy!

NUTRITION FACTS:

Calories: 554 Fat: 32 g Carbs: 14 g Sugar: 8 g Fiber: 2 g Protein: 50 g Sodium: 632 mg

254. CANTALOUPE SMOOTHIE

Preparation Time: 5 minutes

Cooking Time: 0 minutes

Servings: 2

INGREDIENTS:

- 1 cup cantaloupe, diced
- 1/2 cup vanilla yogurt or lactose-free yogurt
- 1/2 cup of orange juice
- 1 tablespoon honey or maple syrup
- 2 ice cubes

DIRECTIONS:

1. Merge all ingredients in a blender and then pulse until smooth.
2. Pour into a large glass. Enjoy!

NUTRITION FACTS:

Calories: 179 Fat: 13 g Carbs: 6 g Sugar: 3 g Fiber: 1 g Protein: 10 g Sodium: 265 mg

255. CANTALOUPE-MIX SMOOTHIE

Preparation Time: 5-10 minutes

Cooking Time: 0 minutes

Servings: 2

INGREDIENTS:

- 1 cup cantaloupe, diced
- 1/2 cup mango, diced
- 1/2 cup almond milk or lactose-free cow milk
- 1/2 cup of orange juice
- 2 tablespoons lemon
- 1 tablespoon honey or maple syrup
- 2 ice cubes

DIRECTIONS:

1. Merge all ingredients in a blender until smooth.
2. Pour into a large glass. Enjoy!

NUTRITION FACTS:
Calories: 329 Fat: 17 g Carbs: 9 g Sugar: 3 g Fiber: 5 g Protein: 37 g Sodium: 430 mg

256. APPLESAUCE-AVOCADO SMOOTHIE

Preparation Time: 5-10 minutes

Cooking Time: 0 minutes

Servings: 1

INGREDIENTS:
- 1 cup unsweetened almond or lactose-free milk
- 1/2 avocado
- 1/2 cup applesauce
- 1/4 teaspoon ground cinnamon
- 1/2 cup ice
- 1/2 teaspoon stevia or 1 tablespoon honey, for sweetness (optional)

DIRECTIONS:
1. Blend all ingredients in a blender. Pulse the mix until smooth.
2. Pour into a large glass. Enjoy!

NUTRITION FACTS:
Calories: 270 Fat: 11 g Carbs: 4 g Sugar: 1 g Fiber: 1 g Protein: 39 g Sodium: 664 mg

257. PINA COLADA SMOOTHIE

Preparation Time: 5-10 minutes

Cooking Time: 0 minutes

Servings: 1

INGREDIENTS:
- 1 cup papaya chunks
- 1/2 cup unsweetened almond milk or lactose-free milk
- 1 banana
- 1/2 teaspoon vanilla extract, to taste
- 1 tablespoon honey, maple syrup or 1 teaspoon stevia (optional)

DIRECTIONS:
1. Blend all ingredients in a blender and then pulse until smooth and creamy.
2. Pour into a large glass. Enjoy!

NUTRITION FACTS:
Calories: 329 Fat: 17g Carbs: 9g Sugar: 3g Fiber: 5g Protein: 37g Sodium: 430mg

258. DICED FRUITSDICED FRUITS

Preparation Time: 10 minutes

Cooking Time: 40 minutes

Servings: 6

INGREDIENTS:
- 4 peaches, skin removed and thinly sliced
- 1 pound apple, pitted and skin removed
- 1 teaspoon cinnamon powder
- 1 cup honey or maple syrup
- 1 teaspoon vanilla extract

DIRECTIONS:
1. In a large pot, cook the fruits in boiling water over medium heat until softened.
2. In a large bowl, mix well all ingredients (except the fruits).
3. Pour the syrup over fruits and let the compote be thickened.
4. Pour the compote into a jar. Serve hot or cold. Enjoy!

NUTRITION FACTS:
Calories: 178 Fat: 4 g Carbs: 7 g Fiber: 2 g Protein: 27 g

APPLESAUCE

Preparation Time: 10 minutes

Cooking Time: 30 minutes

Servings: 4

INGREDIENTS:
- 6 organic apples, peeled, cored and cubed
- 1/2 cup boiling water
- 1/2 teaspoon cinnamon powder
- 1/4 cup sugar or 4 tablespoons honey
- 2 tablespoons fresh lemon juice
- 1/4 teaspoon salt

DIRECTIONS:
1. In a large pot, cook apples with boiling water, lemon juice, cinnamon, sugar or honey, and salt over medium-low heat until softened. Remove from the heat.
2. You can mash all ingredients by using a fork or blend with a blender or a food processor.
3. Pour the applesauce into a suitable container or jar. Serve warm or cold. Enjoy!

NUTRITION FACTS:
Calories: 51 Fat: 3 g Carbs: 4 g Fiber: 2 g Protein: 2 g

259. AVOCADO DIP

Preparation Time: 10 minutes

Cooking Time: 0 minutes

Servings: 4

INGREDIENTS:
- 6 avocados, peeled
- 1/2 tablespoon extra-virgin olive oil
- 1/4 cup chopped fresh cilantro
- 2 tablespoons fresh lime juice
- 1 teaspoon fresh lemon juice
- 1/2 teaspoon salt

DIRECTIONS:
1. In a large bowl, set avocados with a fork.
2. Add extra-virgin olive oil and the other ingredients.
3. Enjoy!

NUTRITION FACTS:
Calories: 75 Carbs: 0.1 g Protein: 13.4 g Fat: 1.7 g Sugar: 0 g Sodium: 253 mg

260. HOMEMADE HUMMUS

Preparation Time: 10 minutes

Cooking Time: 60 minutes

Servings: 4

INGREDIENTS:
- 1/4 pound dried chickpeas (soaked in water for a night)
- 1 1/2 tablespoon tahini
- 1 tablespoon lemon juice
- 2 tablespoons extra-virgin olive oil, divided
- 1/4 teaspoon cumin powder
- 1/2 teaspoon salt
- 1 tablespoon water
- 1 teaspoon baking soda (optional)
- 1 teaspoon paprika powder (optional)

DIRECTIONS:
1. First, you need to soak the chickpeas overnight in water and optionally add baking soda to the water.
2. Cook your chickpeas in a large pot with water, over medium heat for about 1 hour. Check if they are cooked well by crushing one of them with a fork in your hand.
3. When chickpeas are cooked, drain and put them in a blender.
4. Add 1 tablespoon of extra-virgin olive oil, lemon juice, tahini, cumin powder, and salt to the blender. Blend until your hummus gets a soft, creamy texture equally.
5. Drizzle with 1 tablespoon of extra-virgin olive oil or paprika powder (optional).
6. Serve immediately or fridge it.

NUTRITION FACTS:
Calories: 207 Fat: 16 g Carbs: 5 g Sugar: 2 g Fiber: 1 g Protein: 12 g Sodium: 366 mg

261. TOFU

Preparation Time: 10 minutes

Cooking Time: 25 minutes

Servings: 4

INGREDIENTS:
- 1 ½ cup firm tofu, pressed and drained
- 1 avocado, cubed
- 1 tablespoon extra-virgin olive oil
- Salt and pepper, to taste

DIRECTIONS:
1. Preheat the oven to 400°F-200°C.
2. Choose a baking sheet, cover it with parchment paper or spray extra-virgin olive oil. Cut tofu cubes of 1/2 inch and spray extra-virgin olive oil on them.
3. Let it bake for 15 minutes until golden brown and crispy. Flip tofu and cook for another 10 minutes. Remove from the oven. Let it rest for 10 minutes.
4. Cube the avocado on a plate. Add salt and pepper.
5. Mix the tofu with avocado in a bowl. Enjoy!

NUTRITION FACTS:
Calories: 645 Fat: 32 g Carbs: 65 g Fiber: 5 g Protein: 26 g

262. ALMOND BUTTER SANDWICH

Preparation Time: 10 minutes

Cooking Time: 5 minutes

Servings: 1

INGREDIENTS:
- 2 slices white bread or white gluten-free bread
- 1 tablespoon organic smooth almond butter

DIRECTIONS:
1. Set 1 piece of bread with almond butter.
2. Toast and enjoy!

NUTRITION FACTS:
Calories: 178 Fat: 4 g Carbs: 7 g Fiber: 2 g Protein: 27 g

263. 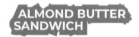 GLUTEN-FREE MUFFINS

Preparation Time: 15 minutes

Cooking Time: 30 minutes

Servings: 10-15

INGREDIENTS:
- 2 tablespoons extra-virgin olive oil
- 2 ½ cups almond flour, blanched
- 3 large organic free-range eggs
- 1/4 cup organic maple syrup
- 2 teaspoons vanilla extract
- 1/4 cup banana, mashed
- 1 teaspoon lemon juice
- 3/4 teaspoon baking soda
- 1/4 teaspoon cinnamon powder
- 1/2 teaspoon salt

DIRECTIONS:
1. Preheat your oven to 375°F-190°C.
2. In a bowl, set almond flour, cinnamon, baking soda, and salt. Mix well.
3. In another bowl, add extra-virgin olive oil, vanilla extract, eggs, ripe banana, maple syrup, and lemon juice. Whisk well.
4. Mix both bowls and stir with a wooden spoon until the flour is mixed well with the other ingredients.
5. Prepare 10 muffin cups. Pour them to the top and then bake for 15 minutes.
6. To avoid browning quickly, loosely cover muffins with aluminum foil. Cook for another 15 minutes.
7. Put a toothpick in a muffin to check if it cooks well or not. If cooked well, the toothpick should not stick to the muffin.
8. Remove from the oven. Let the muffins cool for 15 more minutes. Enjoy!

NUTRITION FACTS:
Calories: 408 Fat: 26 g Carbs: 4 g Sugar: 1 g Fiber: 1 g Protein: 47 g Sodium: 426 mg

264. OUTDOOR CHICKEN KABOBS

Preparation Time: 15 minutes

Cooking Time: 7 minutes

Servings: 4

INGREDIENTS:
- ¼ C. low-fat Parmesan cheese, grated
- 3 tbsp. olive oil
- 1 C. fresh basil leaves, chopped
- Salt and freshly ground black pepper, to taste
- 1¼ lb. boneless, skinless chicken breast, cut into 1-inch cubes

DIRECTIONS:
1. In a food processor, add the cheese, oil, garlic, basil, salt, and black pepper, and pulse until smooth.
2. Transfer the basil mixture into a large bowl.
3. Add the chicken cubes and mix well.
4. Cover the bowl and refrigerate to marinate for at least 4-5 hours.
5. Preheat the grill to medium-high heat. Generously, grease the grill grate.
6. Thread the chicken cubes onto pre-soaked wooden skewers.
7. Place the skewers onto the grill and cook for about 3-4 minutes.
8. Flip and cook for about 2-3 minutes more.
9. Remove from the grill and place onto a platter for about 5 minutes before serving.
10. Serve hot.

NUTRITION FACTS:
calories: 270; carbs: 0.3g; Protein: 31.5g; Fat: 15.3g; Sugar: 0g; Sodium: 207mg; Fiber: 0.1g

265. FLAVORFUL SHRIMP KABOBS

Preparation Time: 15 minutes

Cooking Time: 8 minutes

Servings: 4

INGREDIENTS:
- ¼ C. olive oil
- 2 tbsp. fresh lime juice
- 1 tsp. honey
- ½ tsp. paprika
- ¼ tsp. ground cumin
- Salt and freshly ground black pepper, to taste
- 1 lb. medium raw shrimp, peeled and deveined

DIRECTIONS:
1. In a large bowl, add all the ingredients except for shrimp and mix well.
2. Add the shrimp and coat with the herb mixture generously.
3. Refrigerate to marinate for at least 30 minutes.
4. Preheat the grill to medium-high heat. Grease the grill grate.
5. Thread the shrimp onto pre-soaked wooden skewers.
6. Place the skewers onto the grill and cook for about 2-4 minutes per side.
7. Remove from the grill and place onto a platter for about 5 minutes before serving.

NUTRITION FACTS:
calories: 250; carbs: 3.4g; Protein: 25.9g; Fat: 14.6g; Sugar: 01.5g; Sodium: 316mg; Fiber: 0.1g

266. PAN-SEARED SCALLOPS

Preparation Time: 15 minutes

Cooking Time: 7 minutes

Servings: 4

INGREDIENTS:
- 1¼ lb. fresh sea scallops, side muscles removed
- Salt and freshly ground black pepper, to taste
- 2 tbsp. olive oil
- 1 tbsp. fresh parsley, minced

DIRECTIONS:
1. Sprinkle the scallops with salt and black pepper.
2. In a large skillet, heat the oil over

medium-high heat and cook the scallops for about 2-3 minutes per side.
3. Stir in the parsley and remove from the heat.
4. Serve hot.

NUTRITION FACTS:

calories: 185;carbs: 3.4g; Protein: 23.8g; Fat: 8.1g; Sugar: 0g; Sodium: 268mg; Fiber: 0g

267. MEDITERANEAN SHRIMP SALAD

Preparation Time: 15 minutes

Cooking Time: 3 minutes

Servings: 5

INGREDIENTS:
- 1 lb. shrimp, peeled and deveined
- 1 lemon, quartered
- 2 tbsp. olive oil
- 2 tsp. fresh lemon juice
- Salt and freshly ground black pepper, to taste
- 3 tomatoes, peeled, seeded and sliced
- ¼ C. olives, pitted
- ¼ C. fresh cilantro, chopped finely

DIRECTIONS:
1. In a pan of the lightly salted water, add the quartered lemon and bring to a boil.
2. Add the shrimp and cook for about 2-3 minutes or until pink and opaque.
3. With a slotted spoon, transfer the shrimp into a bowl of ice water to stop the cooking process.
4. Drain the shrimp completely and then pat dry with paper towels.
5. In a small bowl, add the oil, lemon juice, salt, and black pepper, and beat until well combined.
6. Divide the shrimp, tomato, olives, and cilantro onto serving plates.
7. Drizzle with oil mixture and serve.

NUTRITION FACTS:

calories: 178;carbs: 5g; Protein: 21.4g; Fat: 8g; Sugar: 2.1g; Sodium: 315mg; Fiber: 1.2g

268. HELTH CONSCIOUS PEOPLE'S SALAD

Preparation Time: 15 minutes

Cooking Time: 0 minutes

Servings: 2

INGREDIENTS:
- ¼ C. low-fat mozzarella cheese, cubed
- ¼ C. tomato, peeled, seeded and chopped
- 1 tbsp. fresh dill, chopped
- 1 tsp. fresh lemon juice
- Salt, to taste

- 6 oz. cooked salmon, chopped

DIRECTIONS:
1. In a small bowl, add all the ingredients and stir to combine.
2. Serve immediately.

NUTRITION FACTS:

calories: 131;carbs: 1.9g; Protein: 18g; Fat: 6g; Sugar: 0.6g; Sodium: 141mg; Fiber: 0.5g

269. ITALIAN PASTA SOUP

Cooking Time: 25 minutes

Preparation Time: 15 minutes

Servings: 5

INGREDIENTS:
- 1 potato, peeled and chopped
- 1 carrot, peeled and chopped
- 5¼ C. chicken bone broth
- ½ C. tomato, peeled, seeded and chopped
- ¾ lb. asparagus tips
- ½ C. cooked small pasta
- Salt and freshly ground black pepper, to taste

DIRECTIONS:
1. In a pan, add the potato, carrot and broth over medium-high heat and bring to a boil.
2. Reduce the heat to low and cook, covered for about 15 minutes or until vegetables become tender.
3. Add the tomatoes and asparagus and cook or about 4-5 minutes.
4. Stir in the cooked pasta, salt and black pepper and cook for about 2-3 minutes.
5. Serve hot.

NUTRITION FACTS:

calories: 147;carbs: 23.2g; Protein: 13.6g; Fat: 0.5g; Sugar: 3.5g; Sodium: 108mg; Fiber: 3g

270. PURE COMFORT SOUP

Cooking Time: 20 minutes

Preparation Time: 10 minutes

Servings: 4

INGREDIENTS:
- 6 C. chicken bone broth
- 1/3 C. orzo
- 6 large egg yolks
- 1½ C. cooked chicken, shredded
- ¼ C. fresh lemon juice
- Salt and freshly ground black pepper, to taste

DIRECTIONS:
1. In a large pan, add the broth over medium-high heat and bring to a boil.
2. Add the pasta and cook for about

8-9 minutes.
3. In a slowly, add in 1 C. of the hot broth, beating continuously.
4. Add the egg mixture to the pan, stirring continuously.
5. Reduce the heat to medium and cook for about 5-7 minutes, stirring, frequently.
6. Stir in the cooked chicken, salt and black pepper and cook for about 1-2 minutes.
7. Remove from the heat and serve hot.

NUTRITION FACTS:

calories: 269;carbs: 11.9g; Protein: 34.6g; Fat: 8.7g; Sugar: 1.2g; Sodium: 230mg; Fiber: 0.6g

271. GOOF-FOR-YOU STEW

Cooking Time: 18 minutes

Preparation Time: 15 minutes

Servings: 8

INGREDIENTS:
- 2½ C. fresh tomatoes, peeled, seeded and chopped
- 4 C. fish bone broth
- 1 lb. salmon fillets, cubed
- 1 lb. shrimp, peeled and deveined
- 2 tbsp. fresh lime juice
- Salt and freshly ground black pepper, to taste
- 3 tbsp. fresh parsley, chopped

DIRECTIONS:
1. In a large soup pan, add the tomatoes and broth and bring to a boil.
2. Reduce the heat to medium and simmer for about 5 minutes.
3. Add the salmon and simmer for about 3-4 minutes.
4. Stir in the shrimp and cook for about 4-5 minutes.
5. Stir in lemon juice, salt, and black pepper, and remove from heat.
6. Serve hot with the garnishing of parsley.

NUTRITION FACTS:

calories: 173;carbs: 3.2g; Protein: 27.1g; Fat: 5.5g; Sugar: 1.5g; Sodium: 368mg; Fiber: 0.7g

272. ZERO-FIBER CHICKEN DISH

Cooking Time: 10 minutes

Preparation Time: 16 minutes

Servings: 6

INGREDIENTS:
- 4 (6-oz.) boneless, skinless chicken breast halves
- Salt and freshly ground black pepper, to taste
- 2 tbsp. olive oil

DIRECTIONS:

1. Season each chicken breast half with salt and black pepper evenly.
2. Place chicken breast halves over a rack set in a rimmed baking sheet.
3. Refrigerate for at least 30 minutes.
4. Remove from refrigerator and pat dry with paper towels.
5. In a skillet, heat the oil over medium-low heat.
6. Place the chicken breast halves, smooth-side down, and cook for about 9-10 minutes, without moving.
7. Flip the chicken breasts and cook for about 6 minutes or until cooked through.
8. Remove from the heat and let the chicken stand in the pan for about 3 minutes.
9. Now, place the chicken breasts onto a cutting board.
10. Cut each chicken breast into slices and serve.

NUTRITION FACTS:

calories: 255;carbs: 0g; Protein: 32.8g; Fat: 13.1g; Sugar: 0g; Sodium: 125mg; Fiber: 0g

273. AMAZING CHICKEN PLATTER

Cooking Time: 18 minutes

Preparation Time: 15 minutes

Servings: 6

INGREDIENTS:

- 2 tbsp. olive oil, divided
- 4 (4-oz.) boneless, skinless chicken breasts, cut into small pieces
- Salt and freshly ground black pepper, to taste
- 1 tsp. fresh ginger, grated
- 4 C. fresh mushrooms, sliced
- 1 C. chicken bone broth

DIRECTIONS:

1. In a large skillet, heat 1 tbsp. of oil over medium-high heat and stir fry the chicken pieces, salt, and black pepper for about 4-5 minutes or until golden-brown.
2. With a slotted spoon, transfer the chicken pieces onto a plate.
3. In the same skillet, heat the remaining oil over medium heat and sauté the onion, ginger for about 1 minute.
4. Add the mushrooms and cook for about 6-7 minutes, stirring frequently.
5. Add the cooked chicken and coconut milk and stir fry for about 3-4 minutes
6. Add in the salt and black pepper and remove from the heat.
7. Serve hot.

NUTRITION FACTS:

calories: 200;carbs: 1.6g; Protein: 24.8g; Fat: 10.4g; Sugar: 0.8g; Sodium: 111mg; Fiber: 0.5g

274. COLORFUL CHICKEN DINNER

Cooking Time: 20 minutes

Preparation Time: 15 minutes

Servings: 6

INGREDIENTS:

- 3 tbsp. olive oil, divided
- 1 large yellow bell pepper, seeded and sliced
- 1 large red bell pepper, seeded and sliced
- 1 large green bell pepper, seeded and sliced
- 1 lb. boneless, skinless chicken breasts, sliced thinly
- 1 tsp. dried oregano, crushed
- ¼ tsp. garlic powder
- ¼ tsp. ground cumin
- Salt and freshly ground black pepper, to taste
- ¼ C. chicken bone broth

DIRECTIONS:

1. In a skillet, heat 1 tbsp. of oil over medium-high heat and cook the bell peppers for about 4-5 minutes.
2. With a slotted spoon, transfer the peppers mixture onto a plate.
3. In the same skillet, heat the remaining over medium-high heat and cook the chicken for about 8 minutes, stirring frequently.
4. Stir in the thyme, spices, salt, black pepper, and broth, and bring to a boil.
5. Add the peppers mixture and stir to combine.
6. Reduce the heat to medium and cook for about 3-5 minutes or until all the liquid is absorbed, stirring occasionally.
7. Serve immediately.

NUTRITION FACTS:

calories: 226;carbs: 4.8g; Protein: 22.9g; Fat: 12.8g; Sugar: 3g; Sodium: 98mg; Fiber: 0.9g

275. EASIEST TUNA SALAD

Preparation Time: 15 minutes

Cooking Time: 0 minutes

Servings: 4

INGREDIENTS:

For Dressing:
- 2 tbsp. fresh dill, minced
- 2 tbsp. olive oil
- 1 tbsp. fresh lime juice
- Salt and freshly ground black pepper, to taste

For Salad:
- 2 (6-oz.) cans water-packed tuna, drained and flaked
- 6 hard-boiled eggs, peeled and sliced
- 1 C. tomato, peeled, seeded and chopped
- 1 large cucumber, peeled, seeded and sliced

DIRECTIONS:

1. For dressing: in a small bowl, add all the ingredients and beat until well combined.
2. For salad: in another large serving bowl, add all the ingredients and mix well.
3. Divide the tuna mixture onto serving plates.
4. Drizzle with dressing and serve.

NUTRITION FACTS:

calories: 277;carbs: 5.9g; Protein: 31.2g; Fat: 14.5g; Sugar: 3g; Sodium: 181mg; Fiber: 1.1g

276. LEMONY SALMON

Preparation Time: 10 minutes

Cooking Time: 14 minutes

Servings: 4

INGREDIENTS:

- 1 tbsp. fresh lemon zest, grated
- 2 tbsp. extra-virgin olive oil
- 2 tbsp. fresh lemon juice
- Salt and freshly ground black pepper, to taste
- 4 (6-oz.) boneless, skinless salmon fillets

DIRECTIONS:

1. Preheat the grill to medium-high heat. Grease the grill grate.
2. In a bowl, place all ingredients except for salmon fillets and mix well.
3. Add the salmon fillets and coat with garlic mixture generously.
4. Place the salmon fillets onto grill and cook for about 6-7 minutes per side.
5. Serve hot.

NUTRITION FACTS:

calories: 290;carbs: 1g; Protein: 33.2g; Fat: 21.5g; Sugar: 0.3g; Sodium: 116mg; Fiber: 0.2g

277. HERBED SALMON

Cooking Time: 8 minutes

Preparation Time: 10 minutes

Servings: 4

INGREDIENTS:

- 1 tsp. dried oregano, crushed
- 1 tsp. dried basil, crushed
- Salt and freshly ground black

pepper, to taste
- ¼ C. olive oil
- 2 tbsp. fresh lemon juice
- 4 (4-oz.) salmon fillets

DIRECTIONS:

1. In a large bowl, add all ingredients except for salmon and mix well.
2. Add the salmon and coat with marinade generously.
3. Cover the bowl and refrigerate to marinate for at least 1 hour.
4. Preheat the grill to medium-high heat. Grease the grill grate.
5. Place the salmon onto the grill and cook for about 4 minutes per side.
6. Serve hot.

NUTRITION FACTS:

calories: 261;carbs: 0.4g; Protein: 22.1g; Fat: 19.7g; Sugar: 0.2g; Sodium: 80mg; Fiber: 0.2g

278. DELICIOUS COMBO DINNER

Preparation Time: 15 minutes

Cooking Time: 15 minutes

Servings: 5

INGREDIENTS:

- 2 tbsp. olive oil
- 1 lb. prawns, peeled and deveined
- 1 lb. asparagus, trimmed
- Salt and freshly ground black pepper, to taste
- 1 tsp. fresh ginger, minced
- 2 tbsp. fresh lemon juice

DIRECTIONS:

1. In a skillet, heat 1 tbsp. of oil over medium-high heat and cook the prawns with salt and black pepper for about 3-4 minutes.
2. With a slotted spoon, transfer the prawns into a bowl. Set aside.
3. In the same skillet, heat the remaining oil over medium-high heat and cook the asparagus, ginger, salt and black pepper for about 6-8 minutes, stirring frequently.
4. Stir in the prawns and cook for about 1 minute.
5. Stir in the lemon juice and remove from the heat.
6. Serve hot.

NUTRITION FACTS:

calories: 176;carbs: 5.1g; Protein: 22.7g; Fat: 7.3g; Sugar: 1.9g; Sodium: 255mg; Fiber: 1.9g

 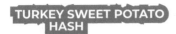

279. TURKEY SWEET POTATO HASH

Preparation Time: 10 minutes

Cooking Time: 12 minutes

Servings: 4

INGREDIENTS:

- 1 ½ tablespoon avocado oil
- 1 medium yellow onion, peeled and diced
- 2 garlic cloves, minced
- 1 medium sweet potato, cut into cubes (peeling not necessary)
- 1/2 pound lean ground turkey
- 1/2 teaspoon salt
- 1 teaspoon Italian seasoning blend

DIRECTIONS:

1. Attach the oil and allow it to heat for 1 minute. Add the onion and cook until softened, about 5 minutes. Attach the garlic and cook for an additional 30 seconds.
2. Add the sweet potato, turkey, salt, and Italian seasoning and cook for another 5 minutes.

NUTRITION FACTS:

Calories: 172 Fat: 9 g Protein: 12 g Sodium: 348 mg Fiber: 1 g Carbs: 10 g Sugar: 3 g

280. CHICKEN TENDERS WITH HONEY MUSTARD SAUCE

Preparation Time: 5 minutes

Cooking Time: 10 minutes

Servings: 4

INGREDIENTS:

- 1 pound chicken tenders
- 1 tablespoon fresh thyme leaves
- 1/2 teaspoon salt
- 1/4 teaspoon black pepper
- 1 tablespoon avocado oil
- 1 cup chicken stock
- 1/4 cup Dijon mustard
- 1/4 cup raw honey

DIRECTIONS:

1. Dry the chicken tenders with a towel and then season them with thyme, salt, and pepper.
2. Attach the oil and let it heat for 2 minutes. Add the chicken tenders and seer them until brown on both sides, about 1 minute per side. Press the Cancel button.
3. Remove the chicken tenders and set them aside. Add the stock to the pot. Use a spoon to scrape up any small bits from the bottom of the pot.
4. Set the steam rack in the inner pot and place the chicken tenders directly on the rack.
5. While the chicken is cooking, prepare the sauce.
6. In a bowl, combine the Dijon mustard and honey then stir to combine.
7. Serve the chicken tenders with the honey mustard sauce.

NUTRITION FACTS:

Calories: 223 Fat: 5 g Protein: 22 g Sodium: 778 mg Fiber: 0 g Carbs: 19 g Sugar: 18 g

281. CHICKEN BREASTS WITH CABBAGE AND MUSHROOMS

Preparation Time: 10 minutes

Cooking Time: 18 minutes

Servings: 4

INGREDIENTS:

- 2 tablespoons avocado oil
- 1 pound sliced Baby Bella mushrooms
- 1 ½ teaspoon salt, divided
- 2 garlic cloves, minced
- 8 cups chopped green cabbage
- 1 ½ teaspoon dried thyme
- 1/2 cup chicken stock
- 1 ½ pound boneless, skinless chicken breasts

DIRECTIONS:

- Add the oil. Allow it to heat for 1 minute. Attach the mushrooms and 1/4 teaspoon of salt. Saute until they have cooked down and released their liquid, about 10 minutes.
- Add the garlic and saute for another 30 seconds. Press the Cancel button.
- Attach the cabbage, 1/4 teaspoon of salt, thyme, and the stock to the inner pot. Stir to combine.
- Dry the chicken breasts and sprinkle both sides with the remaining salt. Place on top of the cabbage mixture.
- Transfer to plates and spoon the juices on top.

NUTRITION FACTS:

Calories: 337 Fat: 10 g Protein: 44 g Sodium: 1,023 mg Fiber: 4 g Carbs: 14 g Sugar: 2 g

282. DUCK WITH BOK CHOY

Preparation Time: 15 minutes

Cooking Time: 12 minutes

Servings: 6

INGREDIENTS:

- 2 tablespoons coconut oil
- 1 onion, sliced thinly
- 2 teaspoons fresh ginger, grated finely
- 2 minced garlic cloves
- 1 tablespoon fresh orange zest, grated finely
- 1/4 cup chicken broth
- 2/3 cup fresh orange juice
- 1 roasted duck, meat picked
- 3 pounds bok choy leaves
- 1 orange, peeled, seeded and segmented

DIRECTIONS:

1. In a sizable skillet, melt the coconut oil on medium heat. Attach the onion, saute for around 3 minutes. Add ginger and garlic then saute for about 1-2 minutes.
2. Stir in the orange zest, broth and orange juice.
3. Add the duck meat and cook for around 3 minutes.
4. Transfer the meat pieces to a plate. Add the bok choy and cook for about 3-4 minutes.
5. Divide the bok choy mixture into serving plates and top with duck meat.
6. Serve with the garnishing of orange segments.

NUTRITION FACTS:

Calories: 290 Fat: 4 g Fiber: 6 g Carbs: 8 g Protein: 14 g

 283. BEEF WITH MUSHROOM AND BROCCOLI

Preparation Time: 60 minutes

Cooking Time: 12 minutes

Servings: 4

INGREDIENTS:

For Beef Marinade:
- 1 garlic clove, minced
- 1 piece fresh ginger, minced
- Salt and freshly ground black pepper
- 3 tablespoons white wine vinegar
- 3/4 cup beef broth
- 1 pound flank steak, trimmed and sliced into thin strips

For Vegetables:
- 2 tablespoons coconut oil
- 2 garlic cloves
- 3 cups broccoli rabe
- 4 ounces shiitake mushrooms
- 8 ounces cremini mushrooms

DIRECTIONS:

For the marinade:
1. In a substantial bowl, mix all ingredients except the beef. Add it and coat with the marinade generously. Refrigerate to soak for around 1/4 hour.
2. In a substantial skillet, warm oil on medium-high heat.
3. Detach the beef from the bowl, reserving the marinade.

For the Vegetables:
1. Attach the beef and garlic and cook for about 3-4 minutes or till browned.
2. In the same skillet, add the reserved marinade, broccoli and mushrooms. Cook for approximately 3-4 minutes.
3. Set in the beef and cook for about 3-4 minutes.

NUTRITION FACTS:

Calories: 200 Carbs: 31 g Cholesterol: 93 mg Fat: 4 g Protein: 10 g Fiber: 2 g

 284. GROUND BEEF WITH VEGGIES

Preparation Time: 60 minutes

Cooking Time: 22 minutes

Servings: 4

INGREDIENTS:

- 1-2 tablespoons coconut oil
- 1 red onion,
- 2 red jalapeño peppers
- 2 minced garlic cloves
- 1 pound lean ground beef
- 1 small head broccoli, chopped
- 1/2 head cauliflower
- 3 carrots, peeled and sliced
- 3 celery ribs
- Chopped fresh thyme, to taste
- Dried sage, to taste
- Ground turmeric, to taste
- Salt and freshly ground black pepper

DIRECTIONS:

1. In a large skillet, dissolve the coconut oil on medium heat.
2. Stir in the onion, jalapeño peppers and garlic. Saute for about 5 minutes.
3. Attach the beef and cook for around 4-5 minutes, entering pieces using the spoon.
4. Add the remaining ingredients and cook, stirring occasionally for about 8-10 minutes.
5. Serve hot.

NUTRITION FACTS:

Calories: 141 Cholesterol: 50 mg Carbs: 6 g Fat: 1 g Sugar: 3 g Fiber: 2 g

285. GROUND BEEF WITH GREENS AND TOMATOES

Preparation Time: 15 minutes

Cooking Time: 15 minutes

Servings: 4

INGREDIENTS:

- 1 tablespoon organic olive oil
- 1/2 white onion, chopped
- 2 garlic cloves, finely chopped
- 1 jalapeño pepper, finely chopped
- 1 pound lean ground beef
- 1 teaspoon ground coriander
- 1 teaspoon ground cumin
- 1/2 teaspoon ground turmeric
- 1/2 teaspoon ground ginger
- 1/2 teaspoon ground cinnamon
- 1/2 teaspoon ground fennel seeds
- Salt and freshly ground black pepper
- 8 fresh cherry tomatoes, quartered
- 8 collard green leaves, stemmed and chopped
- 1 teaspoon fresh lemon juice

DIRECTIONS:

1. In a big skillet, warm oil on medium heat.
2. Add the onion and saute for approximately 4 minutes.
3. Stir in the garlic and jalapeño pepper. Saute for approximately 1 minute.
4. Attach the beef and spices; cook for approximately 6 minutes breaking into pieces while using a spoon.
5. Set in tomatoes and greens. Cook, stirring gently for about 4 minutes.
6. Whisk in lemon juice and take away from the heat.

NUTRITION FACTS:

Calories: 444 Fat: 15 g Carbs: 20 g Fiber: 2 g Protein: 37 g

286. ROASTED CARROT STICKS IN A HONEY GARLIC MARINADE

Preparation Time: 10 minutes

Cooking Time: 25-30 minutes

Servings: 4

INGREDIENTS:

- 1 bunch carrots, halved lengthways
- 2 garlic cloves, minced
- 1 tablespoon honey
- 1 tablespoon lemon juice (alternatively apple cider vinegar)
- 40 g butter
- 3 tablespoons parsley, chopped

DIRECTIONS:

1. Place the halved carrots on baking paper.
2. For the marinade, first, melt the butter. Add the garlic, honey and lemon/vinegar, mix well.
3. Set over the carrots so that they are all covered with the marinade.
4. Bake in the oven at 355°F-180°C for about 25-30 minutes. Turn regularly.
5. Garnish with parsley and serve with herb quark or yogurt.

NUTRITION FACTS:

Calories: 216 Fat: 1 g Carbs: 37 g Fiber: 4 g Protein: 8 g

 287. APPLE AND PISTACHIO SALAD ON SPINACH

Preparation Time: 10 minutes

Cooking Time: 5 minutes

Servings: 4

INGREDIENTS:

- 1 ½ tablespoon butter
- 1 pack baby spinach

- 1 apple, diced small
- 1 teaspoon ginger, grated
- 60 g pistachios
- 1 tablespoon mustard
- 40 g Ricotta cheese
- 1 tablespoon honey
- 1 tablespoon lemon juice
- Salt and pepper

DIRECTIONS:

1. Dissolve the butter in the pan, add the apple pieces, honey, ginger and mustard. Fry over medium heat until the apples are lightly caramelized for (about 3-5 minutes).
2. Wash the spinach and divide between 2 bowls. Place the apples on the salad, garnish with Ricotta and season with a little lemon juice, pistachios, salt and pepper as desired.

NUTRITION FACTS:

Calories: 37 Fat: 1 g Carbs: 3 g Fiber: 0 g Protein: 4 g Sodium: 58 mg

288. CATALAN STYLE SPINACH

Preparation Time: 10 minutes

Cooking Time: 5 minutes

Servings: 4

INGREDIENTS:

- 200 g fresh spinach
- 2 garlic cloves
- 2 tablespoons cashew nuts
- 3 tablespoons raisins
- 2-3 tablespoons extra-virgin olive oil

DIRECTIONS:

1. Warm the oil and fry the garlic over medium heat.
2. After 1-2 minutes add the cashews and raisins. Fry for another minute.
3. Add the spinach (do not boil!), stir well.
4. Serve with Goat cheese and wholemeal baguette.

NUTRITION FACTS:

Calories: 59 Fat: 1 g Carbs: 14 g Fiber: 1 g Protein: 1 g Sodium: 304 mg

289. ENERGY BALLS

Preparation Time: 50 minutes

Cooking Time: 0 minutes

Servings: 4

INGREDIENTS:

- 120 g oat bran
- 80 ml honey
- 120 g coconut flakes (health food store, drugstore)
- 60 g choice nuts, ground
- 40 g dark chocolate, finely chopped
- 1 teaspoon yeast flakes
- 1 teaspoon sea salt

DIRECTIONS:

1. Mix all ingredients well in a container.
2. Set small balls and put them in the fridge for about 45 minutes.

NUTRITION FACTS:

Calories: 75 Carbs: 0.1 g Protein: 13.4 g Fat: 1.7 g Sugar: 0 g Sodium: 253 mg Fiber: 0 g

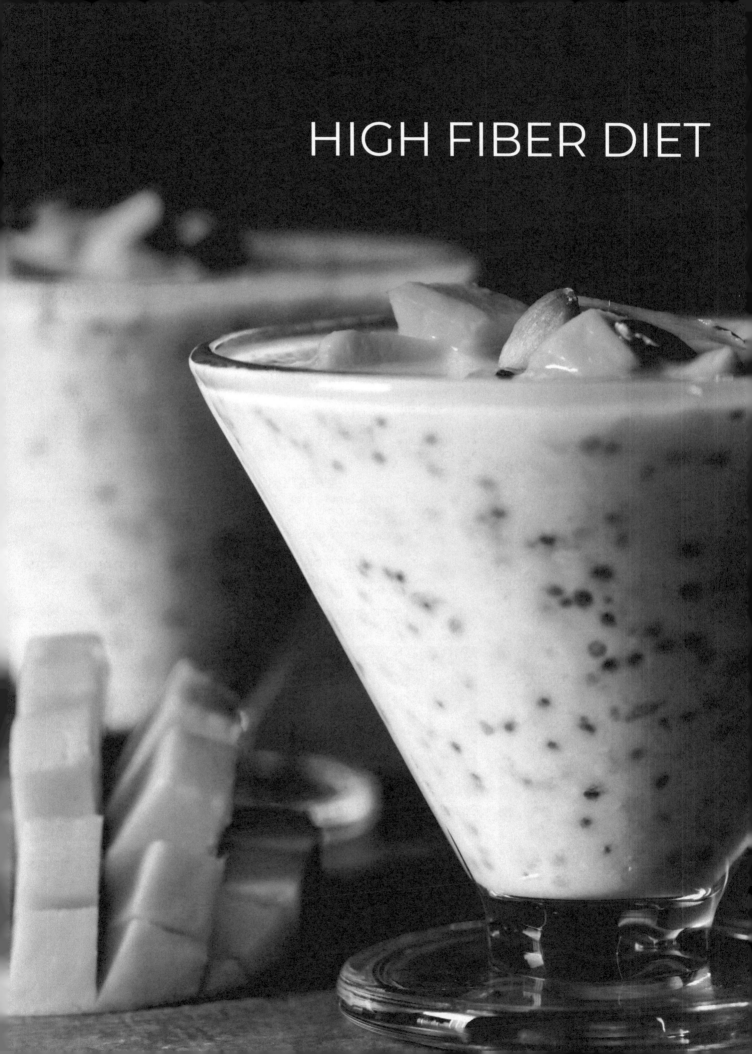
HIGH FIBER DIET

HIGH FIBER DIET

BREAKFAST

290. CHERRY SPINACH SMOOTHIE

Preparation time: 5 minutes

Serving: 1

INGREDIENTS:
- Kefir – one cup, low-fat
- Frozen cherries – one cup
- Baby spinach leaves – half cup
- Avocado – ¼ cup, mashed
- Salted almond butter – one tbsp
- Ginger – ½-inch piece, peeled
- Chia seeds – one tsp

DIRECTIONS:
1. Add all ingredients into the blender and blend on high, about two to three minutes.
2. Pour smoothie into the glass.
3. Garnish with chia seeds.

NUTRITION FACTS:
Calories; 410kcal, carbs; 46.6g, Fats; 20.1g Proteins; 17.4g, fiber; 10.1g

291. BANANA CACAO SMOOTHIE

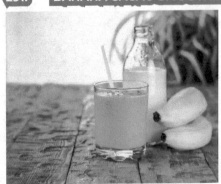

Preparation time: 5 minutes

Serving: 2

INGREDIENTS:
- Frozen banana – two, sliced
- Cacao Bliss – ¼ cup
- Almond butter – ¼ cup
- Hemp hearts – 2 tbsp
- Non-dairy milk – 2 cups
- Ice – ½ cup

DIRECTIONS:
1. Add all ingredients into the blender and blend on high, about two to three minutes.
2. Pour smoothie into the glass.

NUTRITION FACTS:
Calories; 515kcal, carbs; 48g, Fats; 31g Proteins; 22g, fiber; 11g

292. SPINACH AND EGG SCRAMBLE WITH RASPBERRIES

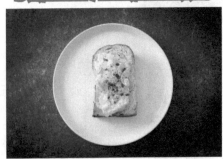

Preparation time: 10 minutes

Serving: 1

INGREDIENTS:
- Canola oil – 1 tsp
- Baby spinach – 1 ½ cups
- Eggs – 2, beaten
- Kosher salt – one pinch
- ground pepper – one pinch
- Whole-grain bread – one slice, toasted
- Fresh raspberries – half cup

DIRECTIONS:
1. Add oil into the skillet and heat it over medium-high flame.
2. Add spinach and cook for one to two minutes until wilted.
3. Transfer the spinach to the medium plate.
4. Clean the pan and place it over medium flame. Then, add eggs and cook for one to two minutes.
5. Add pepper, salt, and spinach and stir well.
6. Top with raspberries. Serve with toasted bread.

NUTRITION FACTS:
Calories; 296kcal, carbs; 20.9g, Fats; 15.7g Proteins; 17.8g, fiber; 7g

293. BLACKBERRY SMOOTHIE

Preparation time: 5 minutes

Serving: 1

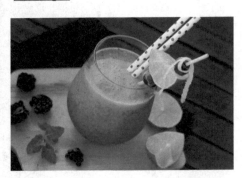

INGREDIENTS:
- Fresh blackberries – one cup
- Banana – half
- Plain whole-milk Greek yogurt – half cup
- Honey – one tbsp
- Fresh lemon juice – 1 ½ tsp
- Fresh ginger – 1 tsp, chopped

DIRECTIONS:
1. Add all ingredients into the blender and blend on high, about two to three minutes.
2. Pour smoothie into the glass.

NUTRITION FACTS:
Calories; 316kcal, carbs; 53g, Fats; 7g Proteins; 15g, fiber; 10g

VEGGIE FRITTATA

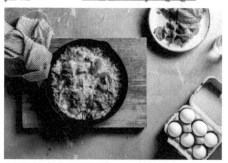

Preparation time: 5 minutes

Cooking time: 10 minutes

Serving: 1

INGREDIENTS:
- Canola oil – one tbsp
- Scallions – two green and white parts separated, thinly sliced
- Mixed veggies – one cup carrots, broccoli, and cauliflower, chopped
- Salt – 1/8 tsp
- Eggs – 2, beaten
- Cheddar cheese – 2 tbsp, shredded
- Orange – 1, cut into wedges

DIRECTIONS:
1. Add oil into a skillet and place it over medium-high flame.
2. Add salt, veggies, and whites scallions and cook for three to five minutes until browned. Add green scallions and stir well.
3. Pour eggs over the vegetables and sprinkle with cheese.
4. Cover with a foil and remove from the flame.
5. Let sit for four to five minutes.
6. Serve with orange wedges.

NUTRITION FACTS:
Calories; 491kcal, carbs; 37g, Fats; 29g Proteins; 22g, fiber; 7g

CHOCOLATE BANANA PROTEIN SMOOTHIE

Preparation time: 5 minutes

Serving: 1

INGREDIENTS:
- Banana – one, frozen
- Red lentils – half cup, cooked
- Milk – half cup, non-fat
- Unsweetened cocoa powder – 2 tsp
- Pure maple syrup – one tsp

Directions:
- Mix the syrup, cocoa, milk, lentils, and banana into the blender and blend until smooth.
- Serve!

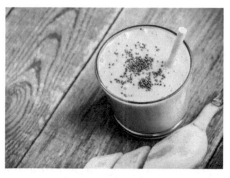

NUTRITION FACTS:
Calories; 310kcal, carbs; 63.8g, Fats; 1.8g Proteins; 15.3g, fiber; 8.5g

296. COCOA ALMOND FRENCH TOAST

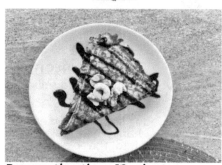

Preparation time: 10 minutes

Cooking time: 10 minutes

Serving: 2

INGREDIENTS:
- Unsweetened almond milk – ½ cup
- Egg – 1
- Ground cinnamon – ½ tsp
- Ground nutmeg – ½ tsp
- Almond – ¼ cup, chopped
- Non-stick cooking spray
- Whole wheat bread – four slices
- Chocolate syrup – 2 tbsp, sugar-free
- Raspberries – ¼ cup

DIRECTIONS:
1. Add nutmeg, cinnamon, eggs, and almond milk into the dish and keep ½ tbsp of chopped almonds to garnish.
2. Place remaining chopped almonds in another bowl.
3. Let coat the griddle with a cooking spray.
4. Heat the griddle over medium flame.
5. Meanwhile, immerse each bread slice into the egg mixture.
6. Then, dip soaked bread in the almonds and coat on both sides.
7. Place coated bread slices onto the griddle and cook for four to six minutes until golden brown.
8. Cut bread in half, lengthwise. Place onto the two serving plates.
9. Drizzle with chocolate syrup.
10. Top with raspberries and chopped almonds.

NUTRITION FACTS:
Calories; 250kcal, carbs; 28.6g, Fats; 11.7g Proteins; 15g, fiber; 7.9g

297. MUESLI WITH RASPBERRIES

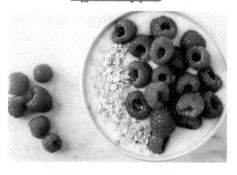

Preparation time: 5 minutes

Serving: 1

INGREDIENTS:
- Muesli – 1/3 cup
- Raspberries – one cup
- Milk – ¾ cup, low-fat

DIRECTIONS:
1. Place muesli into the bowl. Top with raspberries.
2. Serve with warm or cold water.

NUTRITION FACTS:
Calories; 288kcal, carbs; 51.8g, Fats; 6.6g Proteins; 13g, fiber; 13.3g

298. MOCHA OVERNIGHT OATS

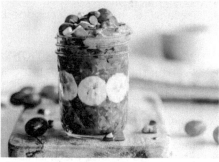

Preparation time: 10 minutes

Chill time: 8 hours

Serving: 1

INGREDIENTS:

- Rolled oats – half cup
- Milk – half cup, low fat
- Cooled coffee – ¼ cup
- Pure maple syrup – one tbsp
- Chia seeds – 1 ½ tsp
- Cocoa powder – 1 ½ tsp
- Walnuts – 1 tbsp, toasted, chopped
- Cacao nibs – one tsp

DIRECTIONS:

1. Mix the cocoa powder, chia seeds, maple syrup, coffee, milk, and oats into the bowl. Cover with a lid and put it into the fridge overnight or for eight hours.
2. Top with cacao nibs and walnuts.

NUTRITION FACTS:

Calories; 379kcal, carbs; 53g, Fats; 15.1g Proteins; 12.6g, fiber; 9.1g

299. BAKED BANANA-NUT OATMEAL CUPS

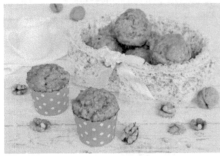

Preparation time: 10 minutes

Baking time: 25 minutes

Serving: 12

INGREDIENTS:

- Rolled oats – three cups
- Low-fat milk – 1 ½ cups
- Bananas – two, mashed
- Brown sugar – 1/3 cup
- Eggs – two, beaten
- Baking powder – one tsp
- Ground cinnamon – one tsp
- Vanilla extract – one tsp
- Salt – half tsp
- Pecans – half cup, chopped, toasted

DIRECTIONS:

1. Preheat the oven to 375°F-190°C.
2. Let coat the muffin tin with cooking spray.
3. Mix the salt, vanilla, cinnamon, baking powder, eggs, brown sugar, bananas, milk, and oats into the bowl.
4. Fold in the pecans. Place mixture into the muffin cups and bake for twenty-five minutes.
5. Let cool it for ten minutes.
6. Serve and enjoy!

NUTRITION FACTS:

Calories; 176kcal, carbs; 26.4g, protein; 5.2g, fat; 6.2g, fiber; 3.1g

300. PINEAPPLE GREEN SMOOTHIE

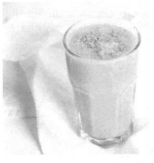

Preparation time: 5 minutes

Serving: 1

INGREDIENTS:

- Unsweetened almond milk – half cup
- Plain Greek yogurt – 1/3 cup, non-fat
- Baby spinach – one cup
- Frozen banana slices – one cup
- Frozen pineapple chunks – half cup
- Chia seeds – one tbsp
- Pure maple syrup or honey – one to two tsp

DIRECTIONS:

1. Add yogurt and almond milk into the blender and blend until smooth.
2. Then, add spinach, pineapple, bananas, honey or maple syrup, and chia into the blender and blend until smooth.
3. Serve and enjoy!

NUTRITION FACTS:

Calories; 297kcal carbs; 54.3g, protein; 12.8g, fat; 5.7g, fiber; 9.8g

301. PUMPKIN BREADPUMPKIN BREAD

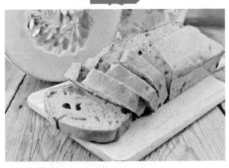

Preparation time: 10 minutes

Cooking time: 1 hour 15 minutes

Serving: 12

INGREDIENTS:

- Water – five tbsp
- Flaxseed meal – two tbsp
- Unsweetened almond milk – ¾ cup
- Sugar – ¾ cup
- Canola oil – 1/3 cup
- Vanilla extract – one tsp
- Unseasoned pumpkin puree – 1 ½ cups
- White whole-wheat flour – two cups
- Baking powder – two tsp
- Pumpkin pie spice or cinnamon – one tsp
- Salt – half tsp
- Bittersweet chocolate chips – half cup

DIRECTIONS:

1. Preheat the oven to 350°F-180°C.
2. Let coat the loaf pan with cooking spray.
3. Mix the flaxseed meal and water into the bowl. Let sit for few minutes.
4. Whisk the flaxseed mixture, vanilla, oil, sugar, and almond milk into the bowl. Then, add pumpkin puree and stir well.
5. Whisk the salt, pumpkin pie spice, flour, and baking powder into the bowl. Add wet ingredients and stir well.
6. Add chocolate chips and stir well.
7. Transfer the batter to the pan. Bake for one hour and fifteen minutes.
8. Let cool it for one hour.
9. Serve and enjoy!

NUTRITION FACTS:

Calories; 191kcal, carbs; 30.5g, protein; 3.3g, fat; 7g, fiber; 3.3g

302. BANANA-BRAN MUFFINS

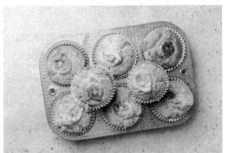

Preparation time: 10 minutes

Cooking time: 25 minutes

Serving: 12

INGREDIENTS:

- Eggs – two
- Brown sugar – 2/3 cup
- Ripe bananas – one cup, mashed
- Buttermilk – one cup
- Unprocessed wheat bran – one cup
- Canola oil – ¼ cup
- Vanilla extract – one tsp
- Whole-wheat flour – one cup
- All-purpose flour – ¾ cup
- Baking powder – 1 ½ tsp
- Baking soda – half tsp
- Ground cinnamon – half tsp

- Salt – ¼ tsp
- Chocolate chips – half cup
- Walnuts – 1/3 cup, chopped

DIRECTIONS:
1. Preheat the oven to 400°F-200°C.
2. Let coat twelve muffin cups with cooking spray.
3. Whisk the brown sugar and eggs into the bowl until smooth.
4. Add vanilla, oil, wheat bran, buttermilk, and bananas and whisk it well.
5. Whisk the salt, cinnamon, baking soda, baking powder, flour, all-purpose flour, and whole-wheat flour into the bowl.
6. Make a well in the middle of the dry ingredients and then add wet ingredients and stir well.
7. Add chocolate chips and stir well. Place batter into the muffin cups and sprinkle with walnuts. Bake it for fifteen to twenty-five minutes until golden brown.
8. Let cool it for five minutes.
9. Serve and enjoy!

NUTRITION FACTS:
Calories; 200kcal, carbs; 34.1g, protein; 4.8g, fat; 7g, fiber; 3.9g

303. BANANA BREAD

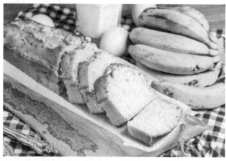

Preparation time: 15 minutes

Cooking time: 1 hour

Serving: 10

INGREDIENTS:
- White whole-wheat flour – 1 ¾ cups
- Baking powder – 1 ½ tsp
- Ground cinnamon – one tsp
- Salt – half tsp
- Baking soda – ¼ tsp
- Sugar – ¾ cup
- Unsalted butter or coconut oil – ¼ cup, softened
- Eggs – two
- Ripe bananas – 1 ½ cups, mashed
- Buttermilk – ¼ cup
- Vanilla extract – one tsp
- Walnuts or chocolate chips – half cup, chopped

DIRECTIONS:
1. Preheat the oven to 350°F-180°C.
2. Let coat the loaf pan with cooking spray.
3. Whisk the baking soda, salt, cinnamon, flour, and baking powder into the bowl.
4. Add butter and sugar into the bowl and beat it well using an electric mixer over medium-high heat.
5. Add eggs and beat it well. Add flour mixture and beat on low speed and then fold in chocolate chips or walnuts.
6. Place batter into the pan. Bake for forty-five to fifty-five minutes.
7. Serve and enjoy!

NUTRITION FACTS:
Calories; 221kcal, carbs; 39.4g, protein; 4.7g, fat; 5.9g, fiber; 3.1g

304. CHOCOLATE-RASPBERRY OATMEAL

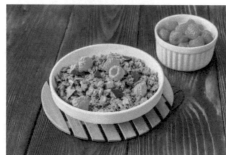

Preparation time: 10 minutes

Cooking time: 10 minutes

Serving: 4

INGREDIENTS:
- Regular rolled oats – 1 ½ cups
- Unsweetened cocoa powder – two tbsp
- Salt – ¼ tsp
- Unsweetened almond milk – three cups
- Fresh red raspberries – one cup
- Chocolate syrup – four tsp

DIRECTIONS:
1. Add salt, cocoa powder, and oats into the saucepan. Add almond milk and stir well. Let boil it over medium flame. Lower the heat and simmer for five to seven minutes.
2. Remove from the flame. Let stand for two minutes.
3. Place oatmeal mixture into the serving bowls.
4. Top with ¼ cup of raspberries.
5. Drizzle with one tsp chocolate syrup.

NUTRITION FACTS:
Calories; 157kcal, carbs; 26.2g, protein; 5.4g, fat; 4.7g, fiber; 6.6g

305. CHAI CHIA PUDDING

Preparation time: 10 minutes

Chill time: 8 hours

Serving: 1

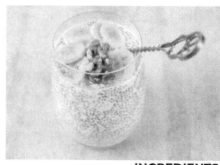

INGREDIENTS:
- Unsweetened almond milk – half cup
- Chia seeds – two tbsp
- Pure maple syrup – two tsp
- Vanilla extract – ¼ tsp
- Ground cinnamon – ¼ tsp
- Pinch of ground cardamom
- Pinch of ground cloves
- Banana – half cup, sliced
- Unsalted pistachios – one tbsp, chopped, roasted

DIRECTIONS:
1. Add cloves, cardamom, cinnamon, vanilla, maple syrup, chia, and almond milk into the bowl and stir well.
2. Cover with a lid and place it into the refrigerator for eight hours.
3. When ready to serve, combine it well. Place half of the pudding into the glass and top with half of pistachios and bananas.
4. Then, add the remaining pudding and top with remaining pistachios and bananas.
5. Serve and enjoy!

NUTRITION FACTS:
Calories; 264kcal, carbs; 38.2g, protein; 6.3g, fat; 11.2g, fiber; 10.8g

306. APPLE CINNAMON OATMEAL

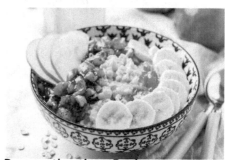

Preparation time: 5 minutes

Cooking time: 40 minutes

Serving: 4

INGREDIENTS:
- Crisp apples – four
- Steel-cut oats – one cup

- Water – four cups
- Brown sugar – three tbsp
- Ground cinnamon – half tsp
- Salt – ¼ tsp
- Nonfat plain Greek yogurt – half cup

DIRECTIONS

1. Firstly, cut two apples with a box grater.
2. Add oats into the saucepan and cook over medium-high flame until toasted, for two minutes.
3. Then, add shredded apples and water and boil it.
4. Then, lower the heat and cook for ten minutes.
5. During this, chop two apples.
6. When oats have cooked, add salt, cinnamon, two tbsp brown sugar, chopped apples and stir well for fifteen to twenty minutes.
7. Place between four bowls.
8. Top with ¾ tsp brown sugar and two tbsp yogurt.

NUTRITION FACTS:

Calories; 282kcal, carbs; 59.1g, protein; 8g, fat; 2.7g, fiber; 6.3g

307. APPLE BUTTER BRAN MUFFINS

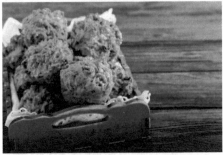

Preparation time: 5 minutes

Cooking time: 40 minutes

Serving: 12

INGREDIENTS:

- Raisins – half cup
- Whole-wheat flour – ¾ cup
- All-purpose flour – ¾ cup
- Baking powder – 2 ½ tsp
- Salt – ¼ tsp
- Ground cinnamon – half tsp
- Unprocessed wheat bran – ¾ cup
- Egg – one, beaten
- Low-fat milk – half cup
- Spiced apple butter – half cup
- Brown sugar – half cup
- Canola oil – ¼ cup
- Molasses – three tbsp
- Apple – one cup, diced, peeled

DIRECTIONS:

1. Preheat the oven to 375°F-190°C.
2. Let coat twelve muffin cups with cooking spray.
3. Add raisins into the bowl and cover with hot water and keep it aside.
4. Whisk the cinnamon, salt, baking powder, flour, all-purpose flour, and whole-wheat flour into the bowl. Then, add bran and stir well.
5. Whisk the molasses, oil, brown sugar, apple butter, egg, and milk into the bowl. Make a well in the dry ingredients and place in the wet ingredients. Then, drain the raisins and add them to the bowl with diced apple. Stir well.
6. Place batter into the pan. Bake for eighteen to twenty-two minutes.
7. Let cool the pan for five minutes.
8. Serve and enjoy!

NUTRITION FACTS:

Calories; 204kcal, carbs; 37.6g, protein; 3.9g, fat; 5.7g, fiber; 3.7g

308. PINEAPPLE RASPBERRY PARFAITS

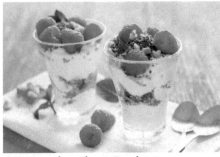

Preparation time: 5 minutes

Serving: 4

INGREDIENTS:

- Nonfat peach yogurt – two cups
- Raspberries – half pint
- Pineapple chunks – 1 ½ cups

DIRECTIONS:

1. Place pineapple, raspberries, and yogurt into the four glasses.
2. Serve and enjoy!

NUTRITION FACTS:

Calories; 155kcal, carbs; 33g, protein; 5.7g, fat; 0.5g, fiber; 2.9g

309. BERRY CHIA PUDDING

Preparation time: 5 minutes

Chill time: 8 hours

Serving: 2

INGREDIENTS:

- Blackberries, raspberries or diced mango – 1 ¾ cups
- Unsweetened almond milk – one cup
- Chia seeds – ¼ cup
- Pure maple syrup – one tbsp
- Vanilla extract – ¾ tsp
- Whole-milk plain Greek yogurt – half cup
- Granola – ¼ cup

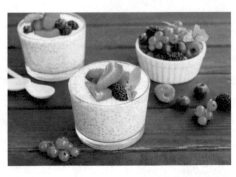

DIRECTIONS:

1. Add milk and 1 ¼ cups fruit into the blender and blend until smooth.
2. Transfer it to the medium bowl. Add vanilla, syrup, and chia and combine well. Place it into the refrigerator for eight hours.
3. Place pudding into the two bowls. Layering each serving with two tbsp granola, ¼ cup yogurt, and remaining ¼ cup of fruit.
4. Serve!

NUTRITION FACTS:

Calories; 343kcal, carbs; 39.4g, protein; 13.8g, fat; 15.4g, fiber; 14.9g

310. SPINACH AVOCADO SMOOTHIE

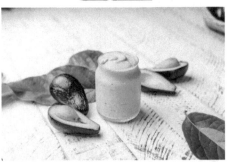

Preparation time: 5 minutes

Serving: 1

INGREDIENTS:

- Nonfat plain yogurt – one cup
- Fresh spinach – one cup
- Banana – one, frozen
- Avocado – ¼
- Water – two tbsp
- Honey – one tsp

DIRECTIONS:

1. Mix the honey, water, avocado, banana, spinach, and yogurt into the blender and blend until smooth.
2. Serve and enjoy!

NUTRITION FACTS:

Calories; 357kcal, carbs; 57.8g, protein; 17.7g, fat; 8.2g, fiber; 7.8g

311. STRAWBERRY PINEAPPLE SMOOTHIE

Preparation time: 5 minutes

Serving: 1

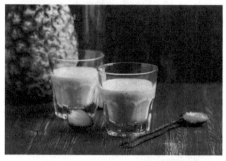

INGREDIENTS:

- Frozen strawberries – one cup
- Fresh pineapple – one cup, chopped
- Unsweetened almond milk – ¾ cup, chilled
- Almond butter – one tbsp

DIRECTIONS:

1. Mix the almond butter, almond milk, pineapple, and strawberries into the blender and process until smooth.
2. Add almond milk more if required.
3. Serve and enjoy!

NUTRITION FACTS:

Calories; 255kcal, carbs; 39g, protein; 5.6g, fat; 11.1g, fiber; 7.8g

312. PEACH BLUEBERRY PARFAITS

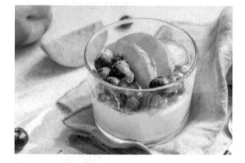

Preparation time: 10 minutes

Serving: 2

INGREDIENTS:

- Vanilla, Peach or blueberry fat-free yogurt – six ounce
- Sweetener multigrain clusters cereal – one cup
- Peach – one, pitted and sliced
- Fresh blueberries – half cup
- Ground cinnamon – ¼ tsp

DIRECTIONS:

1. Add half of the yogurt into the two glasses.
2. Top with half of the cereal. Top with half of cinnamon, blueberries, and peaches. Place remaining blueberries, peaches, cereal, and yogurt.
3. Serve and enjoy!

NUTRITION FACTS:

Calories; 166kcal, carbs; 34g, protein; 11g, fat; 1g, fiber; 7g

313. RASPBERRY YOGURT CEREAL BOWL

Preparation time: 5 minutes

Serving: 1

INGREDIENTS:

- Nonfat plain yogurt – one cup
- Wheat cereal – half cup, shredded
- Fresh raspberries – ¼ cup
- Mini chocolate chips – two tsp
- Pumpkin seeds – one tsp
- Ground cinnamon – ¼ tsp

DIRECTIONS:

1. Add yogurt into the bowl.
2. Top with cinnamon, pumpkin seeds, chocolate chips, raspberries, and shredded wheat.
3. Serve and enjoy!

NUTRITION FACTS:

Calories; 290kcal, carbs; 47.8g, protein; 18.4g, fat; 4.6g, fiber; 6g

314. AVOCADO TOAST

Preparation time: 10 minutes

Serving: 1

INGREDIENTS:

- Mixed salad greens – one cup
- Red-wine vinegar – one tsp
- Extra-virgin olive oil – one tsp
- Pinch of salt
- Pinch of pepper
- Sprouted whole-wheat bread – two slices, toasted
- Plain hummus – ¼ cup
- Alfalfa sprouts – ¼ cup
- Avocado – ¼, sliced
- Unsalted sunflower seeds – two tsp

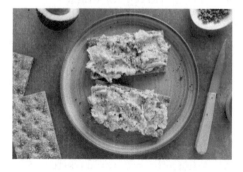

DIRECTIONS:

1. Firstly, toss greens with pepper, salt, oil, and vinegar into the bowl.
2. Spread each slice of toast with two tbsp hummus and top with greens, sprouts, avocado, and spinach.
3. Sprinkle with sunflower seeds.
4. Serve and enjoy!

NUTRITION FACTS:

Calories; 429kcal, carbs; 46.4g, protein; 16.2g, fat; 21.9g, fiber; 15.1g

315. LOADED PITA POCKETS

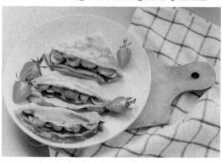

Preparation time: 5 minutes

Serving: 1

INGREDIENTS:

- Whole wheat pita – one, halved
- Low-fat cottage cheese – half cup
- Walnut halves – four, chopped
- Banana – one, sliced

DIRECTIONS:

1. Fill each pita with banana, walnuts, and cottage cheese.

NUTRITION FACTS:

Calories; 307kcal, carbs; 46g, protein; 21g, fat; 8.5g, fiber; 11g

316. HOMESTYLE PANCAKE MIX

Preparation Time: 10 minutes

Cooking Time: 30 minutes

Servings: 16

INGREDIENTS:

- 6 cups whole-wheat pastry flour
- 1 ½ cups (210 g) cornmeal
- 1/2 cup (100 g) sugar
- 1 1/2 cups (102 g) non-fat dry milk
- 2 tablespoons (28 g) baking powder

DIRECTIONS:

1. Merge all ingredients and store them in a tightly covered jar. To cook, attach 1 cup of water to 1 cup of the mix; use less water if you want a thicker pancake. Stir only until lumps disappear.
2. Coat a non-stick skillet or griddle with non-stick vegetable oil spray and preheat until drops of cold water bounce and sputter.
3. Drop the batter to the desired size and cook until bubbles form and edges begin to dry. Turn only once.

317. MULTIGRAIN PANCAKES

Preparation Time: 10 minutes

Cooking Time: 30 minutes

Servings: 6

INGREDIENTS:
- 1 ½ cup whole-wheat pastry flour
- 1/4 cup (35 g) cornmeal
- 1/4 cup (20 g) rolled oats
- 2 tablespoons oat bran
- 2 tablespoons wheat germ
- 2 tablespoons (18 g) toasted wheat cereal, such as Wheatena
- 1 teaspoon baking soda
- 1/2 teaspoon baking powder
- 1 teaspoon vanilla extract
- 1 1/2 cups (355 ml) skim milk
- 2 egg whites

DIRECTIONS:
1. Mix all dry ingredients. Add milk to make the batter. The thicker batter makes thicker pancakes. Set aside to rest for half an hour. Beat the egg whites until stiff peaks form.
2. Gently, fold into the batter after it has rested. Spoon onto the moderate griddle and cook until bubbles break. Turn and cook until done. Bake more slowly than with regular pancakes because of the heavy batter.

NUTRITION FACTS:
Calories: 303 Fat: 14 g Carbs: 15 g Sugar: 10 g Fiber: 2 g Protein: 30 g Sodium: 387 mg

318. CINNAMON–OAT BRAN PANCAKES

Preparation Time: 10 minutes

Cooking Time: 30 minutes

Servings: 6

INGREDIENTS:
- 3/4 cup (75 g) oat bran
- 3/4 cup whole-wheat pastry flour
- 1 tablespoon sugar
- 1/2 teaspoon baking powder
- 1/2 teaspoon cinnamon
- 1/4 teaspoon baking soda
- 1 1/4 cup (295 ml) buttermilk
- 1 tablespoon (15 ml) canola oil
- 1/2 cup (55 g) finely chopped pecans

DIRECTIONS:
1. In a medium mixing bowl, combine all dry ingredients. Set aside.
2. In another mixing bowl, combine the buttermilk and oil. Add to dry ingredients, stirring until just combined. Stir in the pecans.
3. Cook on the hot griddle. Set 1/4 cup of the batter for each pancake.

NUTRITION FACTS:
Calories: 297 Fat: 11 Carbs: 18 g Sugar: 15 g Fiber: 1 g Protein: 34 g Sodium: 528 mg

319. WHOLE-WHEAT BUTTERMILK PANCAKES

Preparation Time: 10 minutes

Cooking Time: 30 minutes

Servings: 6

INGREDIENTS:
- 1 cup whole-wheat flour
- 1/2 teaspoon baking soda
- 1/4 teaspoon cinnamon
- 1 1/4 cup (295 ml) buttermilk
- 2 eggs
- 3 tablespoons (45 ml) canola oil

DIRECTIONS:
1. Blend all dry ingredients. Merge the wet ingredients except for oil. Mix both mixtures. It will be slightly lumpy. Heat oil in a cast-iron skillet.
2. Pour 1/4 of the batter into the pan. When the pancake bubbles, turn and cook for 1-2 minutes more.

NUTRITION FACTS:
Calories: 207 Fat: 16 Carbs: 5 g Sugar: 2 g Fiber: 1 g Protein: 12 g Sodium: 366 mg

320. CORNMEAL PANCAKES

Preparation Time: 10 minutes

Cooking Time: 30 minutes

Servings: 6

INGREDIENTS:
- 1 cup (235 ml) boiling water
- 3/4 cup (105 g) cornmeal
- 1 1/4 cup (295 ml) buttermilk
- 2 eggs
- 1 cup whole-wheat pastry flour
- 1 tablespoon baking powder
- 1/4 teaspoon baking soda
- 1/4 cup (60 ml) canola oil

DIRECTIONS:
1. Pour water over the cornmeal, stir until thick. Add the buttermilk; beat in the eggs. Mix flour, baking powder, and baking soda.
2. Add to the cornmeal mixture. Stir in canola oil. Bake on a hot griddle.

NUTRITION FACTS:
Calories: 280 Fat: 16 Carbs: 5 g Sugar: 1 g Fiber: 0 g Protein: 29 g Sodium: 508 mg

321. OVEN-BAKED PANCAKE

Preparation Time: 10 minutes

Cooking Time: 30 minutes

Servings: 6

INGREDIENTS:
- 3 eggs
- 1/2 cup whole-wheat pastry flour
- 1/2 cup (120 ml) skim milk
- 1/4 cup (55 g) unsalted butter, divided
- 2 tablespoons (26 g) sugar
- 2 tablespoons (18 g) slivered almonds, toasted
- 2 tablespoons (30 ml) lemon juice

DIRECTIONS:
1. Set the eggs with an electric mixer at medium speed until well blended. Gradually add flour, beating until smooth. Add milk and 2 tablespoons (28 g) melted butter; beat until the batter is smooth.
2. Pour the batter into a 10-inch (25 cm) skillet coated with non-stick vegetable oil spray. Bake at 400°F for 15 minutes until the pancake is puffed and golden brown.
3. Sprinkle with sugar and toasted almonds. Combine the remaining butter and lemon juice; heat until butter melts. Serve over the hot pancake.

NUTRITION FACTS:
Calories: 429 Fat: 47 gCarbs: 5 gSugar: 1 gFiber: 1 gProtein: 27 g

322. BAKED PANCAKE

Preparation Time: 10 minutes

Cooking Time: 30 minutes

Servings: 4

INGREDIENTS:
- 1 ½ cup whole-wheat pastry flour
- 1 ½ cup (355 ml) skim milk
- 4 eggs, slightly beaten
- 1/4 cup (55 g) unsalted butter
- 1 cup (170 g) sliced strawberries

DIRECTIONS:
1. Gradually, add flour and milk to the eggs. Melt the butter in 9 x 13-inch (23 x 33 cm) pan.
2. Pour the batter over melted butter. Bake at 400°F-200°C for about 30 minutes.
3. Serve with fresh sliced strawberries.

NUTRITION FACTS:
Calories: 270 Fat: 11 g Carbs: 4 g Sugar: 1 g Fiber: 1 g Protein: 39 g Sodium: 664 mg

323. WHEAT WAFFLES

Preparation Time: 10 minutes

Cooking Time: 30 minutes

Servings: 8

INGREDIENTS:
- 2 cups whole-wheat pastry flour
- 4 teaspoons (18 g) baking powder
- 2 tablespoons (40 g) honey
- 1 ¾ cup (410 ml) skim milk
- 4 tablespoons (60 ml) canola oil
- 2 eggs

DIRECTIONS:
1. Mix all dry ingredients. Stir in the remaining ingredients. For lighter waffles, separate the eggs. Beat the egg whites and carefully fold in.
2. Set into a waffle iron coated with non-stick vegetable oil spray.

NUTRITION FACTS:
Calories: 389 Fat: 20 g Carbs: 1 g Sugar: 0 g Fiber: 1 g Protein: 49 g Sodium: 381 mg

324. OATMEAL WAFFLES

Preparation Time: 10 minutes

Cooking Time: 30 minutes

Servings: 5

INGREDIENTS:
- 1 ½ cup whole-wheat pastry flour
- 1 cup (80 g) quick-cooking oats
- 1 tablespoon baking powder
- 1 teaspoon cinnamon
- 2 tablespoons (30 g) brown sugar
- 3 tablespoons (42 g) unsalted butter
- 1 ½ cup (355 ml) skim milk
- 2 eggs, slightly beaten

DIRECTIONS:
1. In a bowl, merge all dry ingredients and set aside. Melt the butter, add milk and eggs. Mix well and then add to the flour mixture. Stir until well blended.
2. Set into a waffle iron coated with non-stick vegetable oil spray.

NUTRITION FACTS:
Calories: 224 Fat: 14 g Carbs: 15 g Sugar: 10 g Fiber: 5 g Protein: 12 g

325. BRAN APPLESAUCE MUFFINS

Preparation Time: 10 minutes

Cooking Time: 30 minutes

Servings: 12

INGREDIENTS:
- 3/4 cup (30 g) bran flakes cereal, crushed
- 1/2 cup (100 g) sugar
- 1 teaspoon baking soda
- 1 teaspoon cinnamon
- 1/2 teaspoon nutmeg
- 1 cup (245 g) applesauce
- 1/2 cup (120 ml) canola oil
- 1 teaspoon vanilla extract
- 2 eggs
- 1/2 cup (75 g) raisins
- 1 tablespoon sugar
- 1/2 teaspoon cinnamon

DIRECTIONS:
1. Heat the oven to 400°F-200°C.
2. Set 12 muffin cups with baking paper or sprinkle with non-stick vegetable oil spray.
3. In a bowl, combine all ingredients except the sugar and cinnamon; mix well. Set the batter into the prepared muffin cups, filling 2/3 full. In a bowl, combine the sugar and cinnamon; sprinkle over the top of each muffin. Bake at 400°F for 20 minutes or until a toothpick inserted in the center comes out clean. Immediately remove from pan. Serve warm.

NUTRITION FACTS:
Calories: 270 Fat: 11 g Carbs: 4 g Sugar: 1 g Fiber: 1 g Protein: 39 g Sodium: 664 mg

326. OAT BRAN MUFFINS

Preparation Time: 10 minutes

Cooking Time: 15-17 minutes

Servings: 12

INGREDIENTS:
- 2 ¼ cup (225 g) oat bran
- 1 tablespoon baking powder
- 1/4 cup (35 g) raisins
- 1/4 cup (28 g) chopped pecans
- 2 eggs
- 2 tablespoons (28 ml) olive oil
- 1/4 cup (85 g) honey
- 1 ¼ cup (295 ml) water

DIRECTIONS:
1. Preheat the oven to 425°F-220°C.
2. Put all dry ingredients, raisins, and pecans in a mixing bowl. Beat the eggs, olive oil, honey, and water lightly.
3. Attach this mixture to the dry ingredients and stir until moistened. Line muffin pans with paper liners or spray with non-stick vegetable oil spray and fill about half full. Bake for 15-17 minutes.

NUTRITION FACTS:
Calories: 270 Fat: 11 g Carbs: 4 g Sugar: 1 g Fiber: 1 g Protein: 39 g Sodium: 664 mg

327. ORANGE BRAN MUFFINS

Preparation Time: 10 minutes

Cooking Time: 25 minutes

Servings: 12

INGREDIENTS:
- 2 ½ cups (300 g) whole-wheat pastry flour
- 1 tablespoon baking soda
- 3 cups (177 g) raisin bran cereal
- 1/2 cup (100 g) sugar
- 1 teaspoon cinnamon
- 1 ½ tablespoon orange peel
- 2 cups (460 g) plain fat-free yogurt
- 2 eggs, beaten
- 1/2 cup (120 ml) cooking oil

DIRECTIONS:
1. In a bowl, merge flour and baking soda. Add the cereal, sugar, cinnamon, and orange peel, mixing well.
2. Briefly, but thoroughly mix in the yogurt, beaten eggs, and cooking oil. Set into muffin tins lined with paper liners or sprayed with non-stick vegetable oil spray.
3. Bake for 20 minutes in a 375°F-190°C oven.

NUTRITION FACTS:
Calories: 270 Fat: 11 g Carbs: 4 g Sugar: 1 g Fiber: 1 g Protein 39 g

328. PASTA FRITTERS

Preparation Time: 10 minutes

Cooking Time: 30 minutes

Servings: 6

INGREDIENTS:
- 2 cups (280 g) leftover spaghetti
- 1/4 cup (25 g) chopped scallions
- 1/2 cup (56 g) shredded zucchini
- 78 ml canola oil
- 1 egg
- 1 cup whole-wheat pastry flour
- 1 teaspoon black pepper
- 1 cup (235 ml) water

DIRECTIONS:
1. About 35 minutes before serving, coarsely chop the cooked spaghetti, onions, and shred zucchini; set aside. In a 12-inch (30 cm) skillet, over high heat, heat canola oil until very hot.
2. Meanwhile, prepare the batter. In a bowl, with a wire whisker or fork, mix the egg, flour, pepper, and water.
3. Stir in the spaghetti mixture. Drop it into hot oil in the skillet by 1/4 cup into 4 mounds about 2 inches (5 cm) apart. With a spatula, flatten each to make 3-inch (7.5 cm) pancake.
4. Set the fritters until golden brown on both sides; drain them on paper towels. Keep warm. Repeat

with the remaining mixture, adding more oil to the skillet if needed.

NUTRITION FACTS:

Calories: 178 Fat: 4 g Carbs: 7 g Fiber: 2 g Protein: 27 g

329. CINNAMON HONEY SCONES

Preparation Time: 10 minutes

Cooking Time: 20 minutes

Servings: 5

INGREDIENTS:

- 1 ¾ cup (220 g) whole-wheat pastry flour
- 1 ½ teaspoon baking powder
- ¼ teaspoon cinnamon
- 6 tablespoons (85 g) unsalted butter, softened
- 1 tablespoon (20 g) honey
- ½ cup (120 ml) skim milk
- 1 egg

DIRECTIONS:

1. Preheat the oven to 450°F-230°C.
2. Line a baking sheet with aluminum foil.
3. In a bowl, merge the flour, baking powder, and cinnamon with a wooden spoon. Work the butter into the mixture by hand until it is yellow.
4. Add honey and milk, then the egg. Stir with a wooden spoon until thoroughly mixed.
5. Scoop a spoonful of dough and drop it onto the baking sheet. Leave 1 inch (2.5 cm) between each. Bake for 15 minutes or until golden brown. Cool for 5 minutes.

NUTRITION FACTS:

Calories: 179 Fat: 13 g Carbs: 6 g Sugar: 3 g Fiber: 1 g Protein: 10 g Sodium: 265 mg

330. OATMEAL RAISIN SCONES

Preparation Time: 10 minutes

Cooking Time: 20-25 minutes

Servings: 5

INGREDIENTS:

- 2 cups whole-wheat pastry flour
- 3 tablespoons (45 g) brown sugar
- 1 teaspoon baking powder
- ½ teaspoon baking soda
- ½ cup unsalted butter, chilled
- 1 ½ cup (120 g) rolled oats
- ½ cup (75 g) raisins
- 1 cup (235 ml) buttermilk
- 2 tablespoons cinnamon
- 2 tablespoons (26 g) sugar

DIRECTIONS:

1. Heat the oven to 375°F-190°C.
2. Merge flour, brown sugar, baking powder, and baking soda. Divide in the butter until the mixture resembles coarse crumbs.
3. Stir in oats and raisins. Add the buttermilk and mix with a fork until the dough forms a ball. Set out on a lightly floured board and knead for 6-8 minutes. Pat the dough into ½-inch (1 cm) thickness. Divide 8-10 rounds or wedges and place them on an ungreased baking sheet. Sprinkle with sugar and cinnamon.
4. Bake for 20-25 minutes.

NUTRITION FACTS:

Calories: 329 Fat: 17 g Carbs: 9 g Sugar: 3 g Fiber: 5 g Protein: 37 g Sodium: 430 mg

331. WHOLE GRAIN SCONES

Preparation Time: 10 minutes

Cooking Time: 30 minutes

Servings: 5

INGREDIENTS:

- 1 egg
- ½ cup (100 g) sugar
- 5 tablespoons (75 ml) canola oil
- teaspoon lemon peel
- ½ cup (40 g) rolled oats
- ¼ cup (25 g) wheat bran
- 1 ½ cup whole-wheat pastry flour
- 2 tablespoons poppy seeds
- 1 tablespoon baking powder
- ½ teaspoon cinnamon
- ½ cup (120 ml) skim milk

Lemon Topping:
- 3 tablespoons (45 ml) lemon juice
- ¼ cup (25 g) confectioners' sugar

DIRECTIONS:

1. Preheat the oven to 375°F-190°C.
2. Set the egg, sugar, and oil together in a bowl. Mix the lemon peel and all the dry ingredients in a separate bowl. Stir with a wooden spoon until all of them are evenly dispersed throughout.
3. Slowly, add the dry ingredients into the egg, sugar, and oil. Mix to create a thick dough. Add the milk and mix well. Coat a baking sheet with non-stick vegetable oil spray.
4. Bake until the crust is barely golden brown and the dough is dry. Detach from the oven and let cool for 10 minutes. With a fork, mix the lemon topping ingredients until the sugar is completely melded in. Drizzle 1 tablespoon over each scone.

NUTRITION FACTS:

Calories: 280 Fat: 16 g Carbs: 5 g Sugar: 1 g Fiber: 0 g Protein: 29 g Sodium: 508 mg

GRANOLA

Preparation Time: 10 minutes

Cooking Time: 30 minutes

Servings: 30

INGREDIENTS:

- 6 cups (480 g) rolled oats
- 6 cups rolled wheat
- 2 cups (290 g) sunflower seeds
- 4 ounces (113 g) sesame seeds
- 2 cups (190 g) peanuts
- 3 cups (255 g) coconut
- 1 cup (112 g) wheat germ
- 1 ½ cup (355 ml) canola oil
- 1 cup (340 g) honey
- ½ cup (170 g) molasses
- 1 tablespoon (15 ml) vanilla extract
- 1 cup (145 g) raisins

DIRECTIONS:

1. Merge all dry ingredients in a large bowl. Put aside.
2. Heat the oil, honey, molasses, and vanilla together and mix with the dry ingredients. Spread the mixture on baking sheets.
3. Bake at 350°F-180°C until light brown. Stir frequently to brown evenly. Detach from the oven and add the raisins or any other dried fruit.

NUTRITION FACTS:

Calories: 270 Fat: 11 g Carbs: 4 g Sugar: 1 g Fiber: 1 g

332. TOASTY NUT GRANOLA

Preparation Time: 10 minutes

Cooking Time: 35 minutes

Servings: 30

INGREDIENTS:

- 6 cups (480 g) rolled oats
- 1 cup (110 g) chopped pecans
- ¾ cup (84 g) wheat germ
- ½ cup (115 g) firmly packed brown sugar
- ½ cup (40 g) shredded coconut
- ½ cup (72 g) sesame seeds
- ½ cup (120 ml) canola oil
- ½ cup (170 g) honey
- 1 ½ teaspoon vanilla extract

DIRECTIONS:

1. Toast the oats in a 9 x 13-inch (23 x 33 cm) pan at 350°F-180°C for 10 minutes.
2. Merge the remaining ingredients in a large bowl and add the toasted oats.
3. Bake on 2 baking sheets at 350°F-180°C for 20-25 minutes. Stir when cool and store in the refrigerator.

NUTRITION FACTS:

Calories: 270 Fat: 11 g Carbs: 4 g Sugar: 1 g Fiber: 1 g Protein: 39 g Sodium: 664 mg

333. BREAKFAST BARS

Preparation Time: 10 minutes

Cooking Time: 30 minutes

Servings: 30

INGREDIENTS:
- 1 cup (80 g) quick-cooking oats
- 1/2 cup whole-wheat flour
- 1/2 cup (58 g) crunchy wheat-barley cereal, such as Grape-Nuts
- 1/2 teaspoon cinnamon
- 1 egg
- 1/4 cup (60 g) applesauce
- 1/4 cup (85 g) honey
- 3 tablespoons (45 g) brown sugar
- 2 tablespoons (28 ml) canola oil
- 1/4 cup (36 g) sunflower seeds, unsalted
- 1/4 cup (30 g) chopped walnuts
- 7 ounces (198 g) dried fruit

DIRECTIONS:
1. Preheat the oven to 325°F-170°C. Set a 9-inch (23 cm) square baking pan with aluminum foil. Spray the foil with non-stick vegetable oil.
2. In a bowl, stir together the oats, flour, cereal, and cinnamon. Add the egg, applesauce, honey, brown sugar, and oil. Merge well.
3. Stir in the sunflower seeds, walnuts, and dried fruit. Spread the mixture evenly in the prepared pan.
4. Bake for 30 minutes or until firm and lightly browned around the edges. Let cool. Use the foil to lift from the pan. Cut into bars and store in the refrigerator.

NUTRITION FACTS:
Calories: 280 Fat: 16 Carbs: 5 g Sugar: 1 g Fiber: 0 g Protein: 29 g

334. WHOLE-WHEAT COFFEE CAKE

Preparation Time: 10 minutes

Cooking Time: 30-45 minutes

Servings: 12

INGREDIENTS:
For the cake:
- 1 ¾ cup (210 g) whole-wheat pastry flour
- 1 teaspoon baking powder
- 1 teaspoon baking soda
- 1/2 cup (112 g) unsalted butter, softened
- 1 cup (133 g) sugar
- 2 eggs
- 1 teaspoon vanilla extract
- 1 cup (230 g) sour cream

For the Bran Nut Filling:
- 1 cup (75 g) packed brown sugar
- 1/2 cup bran flakes (20 g) cereal
- 1/2 cup (60 g) chopped walnuts
- 1 teaspoon cinnamon

DIRECTIONS:
For the cake:
1. Merge flour, baking powder, and baking soda; set aside.
2. In a large bowl, beat the butter, sugar, eggs, and vanilla until light and fluffy. At low speed stir in the sour cream alternately with the flour mixture until blended.

For the Bran Nut Filling:
1. Combine all filling ingredients in a small bowl. To assemble the cake, spread 1/3 of the sour cream mixture in a 9-inch (23 cm) square pan coated with non-stick vegetable oil spray.
2. Sprinkle on about 1/2 cup of the filling. Repeat layering twice. Bake in a preheated oven at 350°F-180C, for 30-45 minutes. Cool slightly.

NUTRITION FACTS:
Calories: 224 Fat: 14g Carbs: 15g Sugar: 10g Fiber: 5g Protein: 12g

335. CRUNCHY BREAKFAST TOPPING

Preparation Time: 10 minutes

Cooking Time: 30 minutes

Servings: 12

INGREDIENTS:
- 1/4 cup (55 g) unsalted butter
- 1 ¼ cup (140 g) wheat germ
- 1/2 cup packed brown sugar
- 1/2 cup (47 g) ground almonds
- 1 tablespoon grated orange peel
- 1/2 teaspoon cinnamon

DIRECTIONS:
1. Melt the butter in a 9 x 13-inch (23 x 33 cm) baking pan into the oven for about 4 minutes.
2. Add the remaining ingredients and mix well. Bake until deep golden brown. Stir.
3. Cool and store in the refrigerator for up to 3 months.

NUTRITION FACTS:
Calories: 178 Fat: 4 g Carbs: 7 g Fiber: 2 g Protein: 27 g

336. PEAR PANCAKES

Preparation time: 10 minutes

Cooking time: 20 minutes

Servings: 4

INGREDIENTS:
- One cup whole wheat flour
- ¼ teaspoon baking soda
- ¼ teaspoon baking powder
- One cup pears
- Two eggs
- One cup milk

DIRECTIONS:
1. In a bowl, combine all ingredients and mix well
2. In a skillet, heat olive oil
3. Pour ¼ of the batter and cook each pancake for 1-2 minutes per side
4. When ready, remove from heat and serve

NUTRITION FACTS:
calories 277 fat 19gcarbs 56g protein 13.8g

337. ALMOND PANCAKES

Preparation time: 10 minutes

Cooking time: 30 minutes

Servings: 4

INGREDIENTS:
- One cup whole wheat flour
- ¼ teaspoon baking soda
- ¼ teaspoon baking powder
- One cup almonds
- Two eggs
- One cup milk

DIRECTIONS:
1. In a bowl, combine all ingredients and mix well
2. In a skillet, heat olive oil
3. Pour ¼ of the batter and cook each pancake for 1-2 minutes per side
4. When ready, remove from heat and serve

NUTRITION FACTS:
calories 234g fat 20gcarbs 4.0g protein 10g

338. AVOCADO PANCAKES

Preparation time: 10 minutes

Cooking time: 20 minutes

Servings: 4

INGREDIENTS:
- One cup whole wheat flour
- ¼ teaspoon baking soda
- ¼ teaspoon baking powder
- Two eggs
- One cup milk
- 1 cup mashed avocado

DIRECTIONS:
1. In a bowl, combine all ingredients and mix well
2. In a skillet, heat olive oil
3. Pour ¼ of the batter and cook each pancake for 1-2 minutes per side

4. When ready, remove from heat and serve

NUTRITION FACTS:

calories 310 fat 18gcarbs 34g protein 7g

339. STRAWBERRY PANCAKES

Preparation time: 10 minutes

Cooking time: 20 minutes

Servings: 4

INGREDIENTS:
- One cup whole wheat flour
- ¼ teaspoon baking soda
- ¼ teaspoon baking powder
- One cup strawberries
- Two eggs
- One cup milk

DIRECTIONS:
1. In a bowl, combine all ingredients and mix well
2. In a skillet, heat olive oil
3. Pour ¼ of the batter and cook each pancake for 1-2 minutes per side
4. When ready, remove from heat and serve

NUTRITION FACTS:

calories 102 fat 4.7gcarbs 12g protein 3g

340. CARAMBOLA PANCAKES

Preparation time: 10 minutes

Cooking time: 30 minutes

Servings: 4

INGREDIENTS:
- One cup whole wheat flour
- ¼ teaspoon baking soda
- ¼ teaspoon baking powder
- Two eggs
- One cup milk
- One cup carambola

DIRECTIONS:
1. In a bowl, combine all ingredients and mix well
2. In a skillet, heat olive oil
3. Pour ¼ of the batter and cook each pancake for 1-2 minutes per side
4. When ready, remove from heat and serve

NUTRITION FACTS:

calories 774 fat 35gcarbs 108g protein 5.89g

341. GINGER MUFFINS

Preparation time: 10 minutes

Cooking time: 20 minutes

Servings: 8-12

INGREDIENTS:
- Two eggs
- One tablespoon olive oil
- One cup milk
- Two cups whole wheat flour
- One teaspoon baking soda
- ¼ teaspoon baking soda
- One teaspoon ginger
- One teaspoon cinnamon
- ¼ cup molasses

DIRECTIONS:
1. In a bowl, combine all dry ingredients
2. In another bowl, combine all dry ingredients
3. Combine wet and dry ingredients
4. Fold in ginger and mix well
5. Pour mixture into 8-12 prepared muffin cups, fill 2/3 of the cups
6. Bake for 18-20 minutes at 375°F-190°C.
7. When ready, remove from the oven and serve

NUTRITION FACTS:

calories 18707 fat 6.4gcarbs 29.0g protein 6.1g

342. CARROT MUFFINSC

Preparation time: 10 minutes

Cooking time: 20 minutes

Servings: 8-12

INGREDIENTS:
- Two eggs
- One tablespoon olive oil
- One cup milk
- Two cups whole wheat flour
- One teaspoon baking soda
- ¼ teaspoon baking soda
- One teaspoon cinnamon
- One cup carrots

DIRECTIONS:
1. In a bowl, combine all dry ingredients
2. In another bowl, combine all dry ingredients
3. Combine wet and dry ingredients
4. Pour mixture into 8-12 prepared muffin cups, fill 2/3 of the cups
5. Bake for 18-20 minutes at 375°F-190°C.
6. When ready, remove from the oven and serve

NUTRITION FACTS:

calories 342 fat 12.89gcarbs 50.3g protein 6.85

343. BLUEBERRY MUFFINS

Preparation time: 10 minutes

Cooking time: 20 minutes

Servings: 8-12 minutes

INGREDIENTS:
- Two eggs
- One tablespoon olive oil
- One cup milk
- Two cups whole wheat flour
- One teaspoon baking soda
- ¼ teaspoon baking soda
- One teaspoon cinnamon
- One cup blueberries

DIRECTIONS:
1. In a bowl, combine all dry ingredients
2. In another bowl, combine all dry ingredients
3. Combine wet and dry ingredients
4. Pour mixture into 8-12 prepared muffin cups, fill 2/3 of the cups
5. Bake for 18-20 minutes at 375°F-190°C.
6. When ready, remove from the oven and serve

NUTRITION FACTS:

calories 467 fat 13gcarbs 68g protein 6g

344. COCONUT MUFFINS

Preparation time: 10 minutes

Cooking time: 20 minutes

Servings: 8-12

INGREDIENTS:
- Two eggs
- One tablespoon olive oil
- One cup milk
- Two cups whole wheat flour
- One teaspoon baking soda
- ¼ teaspoon baking soda
- One teaspoon cinnamon
- One cup coconut flakes

DIRECTIONS:
1. In a bowl, combine all dry ingredients
2. In another bowl, combine all dry ingredients
3. Combine wet and dry ingredients
4. Pour mixture into 8-12 prepared muffin cups, fill 2/3 of the cups
5. Bake for 18-20 minutes at 375°F-190°C.
6. When ready, remove from the oven and serve

NUTRITION FACTS:

calories 130 fat 12gcarbs 0g protein 1g

345. RAISIN MUFFIN

Preparation time: 10 minutes

Cooking time: 20minutes

Servings: 8-12

INGREDIENTS:
- Two eggs

- One tablespoon olive oil
- One cup milk
- Two cups whole wheat flour
- One teaspoon baking soda
- ¼ teaspoon baking soda
- One teaspoon cinnamon
- One cup raisins

DIRECTIONS:
1. In a bowl, combine all dry ingredients
2. In another bowl, combine all dry ingredients
3. Combine wet and dry ingredients
4. Pour mixture into 8-12 prepared muffin cups, fill 2/3 of the cups
5. Bake for 18-20 minutes at 375°F-190°C.
6. When ready, remove from the oven and serve

NUTRITION FACTS:
calories 502 fat 17gcarbs 79g protein 3.9g

346. PARMESAN OMELETE

Preparation time: 5 minutes

Cooking time: 10 minutes

Servings: 1

INGREDIENTS:
- Two eggs
- ¼ teaspoon salt
- ¼ teaspoon black pepper
- One tablespoon olive oil
- ¼ cup parmesan cheese
- ¼ teaspoon basil

DIRECTIONS:
1. In a bowl, combine all ingredients and mix well
2. In a skillet, heat olive oil and pour the egg mixture
3. Cook for 1-2 minutes per side
4. When ready, remove the omelet from the skillet and serve

NUTRITION FACTS:
calories 291 fat 21.7gcarbs 1.9g protein 22g

347. ASPARAGUS OMELET

Preparation time: 5 minutes

Cooking time: 10 minutes

Servings: 1

INGREDIENTS:
- Two eggs
- ¼ teaspoon salt
- ¼ teaspoon black pepper
- One tablespoon olive oil
- ¼ cup cheese
- ¼ teaspoon basil
- One cup asparagus

DIRECTIONS:
1. In a bowl, combine all ingredients and mix well
2. In a skillet, heat olive oil and pour the egg mixture
3. Cook for 1-2 minutes per side
4. When ready, remove the omelet from the skillet and serve

NUTRITION FACTS:
calories 102.5 fat 5.1gcarbs 3.3g protein 10.3g

348. ONION OMELET

Preparation time: 5 minutes

Cooking time: 10 minutes

Servings: 1

INGREDIENTS:
- Two eggs
- ¼ teaspoon salt
- ¼ teaspoon black pepper
- One tablespoon olive oil
- ¼ cup cheese
- ¼ teaspoon basil
- One cup red onion

DIRECTIONS:
1. In a bowl, combine all ingredients and mix well
2. In a skillet, heat olive oil and pour the egg mixture
3. Cook for 1-2 minutes per side
4. When ready, remove the omelet from the skillet and serve

NUTRITION FACTS:
calories 200 fat 15gcarbs 4.6 protein 7.2g

349. OLIVE OMELETE

Preparation time: 5 minutes

Cooking time: 10 minutes

Servings: 1

INGREDIENTS:
- Two eggs
- ¼ teaspoon salt
- ¼ teaspoon black pepper
- One tablespoon olive oil
- ¼ cup cheese
- ¼ teaspoon basil
- ½ cup olives

DIRECTIONS:
1. In a bowl, combine all ingredients and mix well
2. In a skillet, heat olive oil and pour the egg mixture
3. Cook for 1-2 minutes per side
4. When ready, remove the omelet from the skillet and serve

NUTRITION FACTS:
calories 183 fat 13.8carbs 4g protein 15g

350. TOMATO OMELET

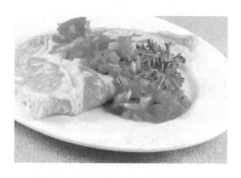

Preparation time: 5 minutes

Cooking time: 10 minutes

Servings: 1

INGREDIENTS:
- Two eggs
- ¼ teaspoon salt
- ¼ teaspoon black pepper
- One tablespoon olive oil
- ¼ cup cheese
- ¼ teaspoon basil
- One cup tomatoes

DIRECTIONS:
1. In a bowl, combine all ingredients and mix well
2. In a skillet, heat olive oil and pour the egg mixture
3. Cook for 1-2 minutes per side
4. When ready, remove the omelet from the skillet and serve

NUTRITION FACTS:
calories 456 fat 33gcarbs 13g protein 18.4g

351. MORNING BAGEL

Preparation time: 5 minutes

Cooking time: 5 minutes

Servings: 1

INGREDIENTS:
- One bagel
- One tablespoon cream cheese
- 2-3 tomato slices
- 1-2 onion slices

DIRECTIONS:
1. Slice bagel and spread cream cheese over half
2. Place tomato slices and onion over one half
3. Top with the other half and serve

NUTRITION FACTS:
calories 289 fat 2gcarbs 56g protein 11g

352. OATMEAL CUSTARD

Preparation time: 5 minutes

Cooking time: 5 minutes

Servings: 1

INGREDIENTS:
- ½ cup oatmeal
- ¼ cup coconut milk
- ¼ teaspoon cinnamon
- ¼ pear

DIRECTIONS:
1. In a mug, combine oats, milk, pear, and almonds
2. Microwave for 3-4 minutes
3. When ready, remove and serve

NUTRITION FACTS:
calories 140 fat 2.5g carbs 28g protein 5g

353. SCRAMBLED EGGS

Preparation time: 10 minutes

Cooking time: 10 minutes

Servings: 3

INGREDIENTS:
- Six eggs
- ½ cup low-fat milk
- ¼ teaspoon salt
- ¼ teaspoon pepper
- One tablespoon butter
- ½ cup cream cheese
- ½ cup parmesan cheese

DIRECTIONS:
1. In a bowl, whisk together eggs, salt, milk, and pepper
2. In a skillet, pour the egg mixture and sprinkle cream cheese and cook for 2-3 minutes per side
3. Remove and serve with parmesan cheese

NUTRITION FACTS: calories 179 fat 13 carbs 1.6g protein 17g

354. FRENCH TOAST

Preparation time: 5 minutes

Cooking time: 10 minutes

Servings: 2

INGREDIENTS:
- Two bread slices
- One teaspoon unsalted butter
- One egg
- ½ almond milk

DIRECTIONS:
1. In a bowl, combine all ingredients for the dipping
2. Place the bread slices in the bowl and let the bread soak for 3-4 minutes
3. Fry in a skillet for 2-3 minutes per side

4. When ready, remove from the skillet and serve

NUTRITION FACTS:
calories 229 fat 11g carbs 25g protein 8g

355. SIMPLE PIZZA RECIPE

Preparation time: 10 minutes

Cooking time: 15 minutes

Servings: 6-8

INGREDIENTS:
- One pizza crust
- ½ cup tomato sauce
- ¼ black pepper
- One cup pepperoni slices
- One cup mozzarella cheese
- One cup olives

DIRECTIONS:
1. Spread tomato sauce on the pizza crust
2. Place all the toppings on the pizza crust
3. Bake the pizza at 425°F-220°C for 12-15 minutes
4. When ready, remove pizza from the oven and serve

NUTRITION FACTS:
calories 266 fat 10g carbs 33g protein 11g

356. ZUCCHINI PIZZA

Preparation time: 10 minutes

Cooking time: 15 minutes

Servings: 6-8

INGREDIENTS:
- One pizza crust
- ½ cup tomato sauce
- ¼ black pepper
- One cup zucchini slices
- One cup mozzarella cheese
- One cup olives

DIRECTIONS:
1. Spread tomato sauce on the pizza crust
2. Place all the toppings on the pizza crust
3. Bake the pizza at 425°F-220°C for 12-15 minutes
4. When ready, remove pizza from the oven and serve

NUTRITION FACTS:
calories 121 fat 13g carbs 31g protein 11g

357. LEEKS FRITATTA

Preparation time: 10 minutes

Cooking time: 20 minutes

Servings: 2

INGREDIENTS:
- ½ lb. Leek
- One tablespoon olive oil
- ½ red onion
- ¼ teaspoon salt
- Two eggs
- 2 oz. Cheddar cheese
- One garlic clove
- ¼ teaspoon dill

DIRECTIONS:
1. In a bowl, whisk eggs with salt and cheese
2. In a frying pan, heat olive oil and pour egg mixture
3. Add remaining ingredients and mix well
4. Serve when ready

NUTRITION FACTS:
calories 225 fat 14.3g carbs 9.7g protein 15g

358. MUSHROOM FRITATTA

Preparation time: 10 minutes

Cooking time: 20 minutes

Servings: 2

INGREDIENTS:
- ½ lb. Mushrooms
- One tablespoon olive oil
- ½ red onion
- ¼ teaspoon salt
- Two eggs
- 2 oz. Cheddar cheese
- One garlic clove
- ¼ teaspoon dill

DIRECTIONS:
1. In a bowl, whisk eggs with salt and cheese
2. In a frying pan, heat olive oil and pour egg mixture
3. Add remaining ingredients and mix well
4. Serve when ready

NUTRITION FACTS:
calories 195 fat 12,6g carbs 12g protein 9g

359. PEAS FRITATTA

Preparation time: 10 minutes

Cooking time: 20 minutes

Servings: 2

INGREDIENTS:
- One cup peas
- One tablespoon olive oil
- ½ red onion
- ¼ teaspoon salt

- Two eggs
- 2 oz. Cheddar cheese
- One garlic clove
- ¼ teaspoon dill

DIRECTIONS:

1. In a bowl, whisk eggs with salt and cheese
2. In a frying pan, heat olive oil and pour egg mixture
3. Add remaining ingredients and mix well
4. Serve when ready

NUTRITION FACTS:

calories 205 fat 11gcarbs 12g protein 11g

360. VITAMINS PACKED GREEN JUICE

Preparation Time: 10 minutes

Cooking Time: 0 minutes

Servings: 2

INGREDIENTS:

- 6 pears, cored and chopped
- 3 celery stalks
- 3 C. fresh kale
- 2 tbsp. fresh parsley

DIRECTIONS:

1. Place all the ingredients in a blender and pulse until well combined.
2. Through a cheesecloth-lined strainer, strain the juice and transfer into 2 glasses.
3. Serve immediately.

NUTRITION FACTS:

calories: 209; carbs: 50.5g; Protein: 5.1g; Fat: 0.9g; Sugar: 26.2g; Sodium: 66mg; Fiber: 15.2g

361. HEALTHIER BREAKFAST JUICE

Preparation Time: 10 minutes

Cooking Time: 0 minutes

Servings: 2

INGREDIENTS:

- 2 large Granny Smith apples, cored and sliced
- 4 medium carrots, peeled and chopped
- 2 medium grapefruit, peeled and seeded
- 1 C. fresh kale
- 1 tsp. fresh lemon juice

DIRECTIONS:

1. Place all the ingredients in a blender and pulse until well combined.
2. Through a cheesecloth-lined strainer, strain the juice and transfer into 2 glasses.
3. Serve immediately.

NUTRITION FACTS:

calories: 265; carbs: 67g; Protein: 4.2g; Fat: 0.7g; Sugar: 47.1g; Sodium: 101mg; Fiber: 11.7g

362. SUMMER PERFECT SMOOTHIE

Preparation Time: 10 minutes

Cooking Time: 0 minutes

Servings: 2

INGREDIENTS:

- 2 C. frozen peaches, pitted
- ½ C. rolled oats
- ¼ tsp. ground cinnamon
- 1½ C. plain yogurt
- ½ C. fresh orange Juice

DIRECTIONS:

1. In a high-speed blender, add all the ingredients and pulse until smooth and creamy.
2. Transfer the smoothie into 2 serving glasses and serve immediately.

NUTRITION FACTS:

calories: 328; carbs: 56g; Protein: 15g; Fat: 4.1g; Sugar: 41g; Sodium: 131mg; Fiber: 5g

363. FILLING BREAKFAST SMOOTHIE

Preparation Time: 10 minutes

Cooking Time: 0 minutes

Servings: 4

INGREDIENTS:

- 2 oz. rolled oats
- 4 apples, peeled, cored and chopped roughly
- 4 scoops unsweetened vegan protein powder
- 1 tsp. stevia powder
- 1 tsp. ground cinnamon
- 1 tsp. ground nutmeg
- 17 oz. plain yogurt
- 2 C. milk

DIRECTIONS:

1. In a high-speed blender, add all the ingredients and pulse until smooth and creamy.
2. Transfer the smoothie into 4 serving glasses and serve immediately.

NUTRITION FACTS:

calories: 437; carbs: 55.6g; Protein: 38.7g; Fat: 6.6g; Sugar: 37.5g; Sodium: 409mg; Fiber: 7.3g

364. BRIGHT GREEN BREAKFAST BOWL

Preparation Time: 10 minutes

Cooking Time: 0 minutes

Servings: 2

INGREDIENTS:

- 2 C. fresh spinach
- 1 medium avocado, peeled, pitted and chopped roughly
- 2 scoops unsweetened vegan protein powder
- 3 tbsp. maple syrup
- 2 tbsp. fresh lemon juice
- 1 C. milk
- ¼ C. ice cubes

DIRECTIONS:

1. In a high-speed blender, place all ingredients and pulse until creamy.
2. Pour into 2 serving bowls and serve immediately with your favorite topping.

NUTRITION FACTS:

calories: 471; carbs: 36.2g; Protein: 32.2g; Fat: 23.5g; Sugar: 24.3g; Sodium: 357mg; Fiber: 8g

365. QUICKEST BREAKFAST PORRIDGE

Cooking Time: 4 minutes

Preparation Time: 10 minutes

Servings: 4

INGREDIENTS:

- 2 C. milk
- 3 large apples, peeled, cored and grated
- ½ tsp. vanilla extract
- Pinch of ground cinnamon
- 1 banana, peeled and sliced
- ½ small apple, cored and sliced

DIRECTIONS:

1. In a large pan, add the milk, grated apples, vanilla extract and cinnamon and mix well.
2. Place the pan over medium-low heat and cook for about 3-4 minutes, stirring occasionally.
3. Transfer the porridge into the serving bowls.
4. Top with the banana and apple slices and serve.

NUTRITION FACTS:

calories: 194; carbs: 40.9g; Protein: 5.9g; Fat: 3g; Sugar: 30g; Sodium: 60mg; Fiber: 6g

366. HALLOWEEN MORNING OATMEAL

Preparation Time: 10 minutes

Cooking Time: 2 minutes

Servings: 2

INGREDIENTS:

- 2 C. hot water
- 1/3 C. pumpkin puree
- 1/3 C. rolled oats
- 1 tsp. ground cinnamon
- 1 tsp. ground ginger
- ¼ tsp. ground nutmeg
- 2 scoops unsweetened vanilla vegan protein powder
- 1 tbsp. maple syrup
- 1 small banana, peeled and sliced

DIRECTIONS:

1. In a microwave-safe bowl, place water, pumpkin puree, oats, chia seeds and spices and mix well.
2. Microwave on High for about 2 minutes.
3. Remove the bowl of oatmeal from the microwave and stir in the protein powder and maple syrup.
4. Top with banana slices and serve immediately.

NUTRITION FACTS:

calories: 268;carbs: 34.4g; Protein: 28.4g; Fat: 2.4g; Sugar: 14.8g; Sodium: 269mg; Fiber: 5g

 AUTHENTIC BULGUR PORRIDGE

Preparation Time: 10 minutes

Cooking Time: 15 minutes

Servings: 2

INGREDIENTS:

- 2/3 C. milk
- 1/3 C. bulgur, rinsed
- Pinch of salt
- 1 ripe banana, peeled and mashed
- 1 large apple, peeled, cored and chopped

DIRECTIONS:

1. In a pan, add the soy milk, bulgur and salt over medium-high heat and bring to a boil.
2. Reduce the heat to low and simmer for about 10 minutes.
3. Remove the pan of bulgur from heat and immediately, stir in the mashed banana.
4. Serve warm with the topping of chopped apple.

NUTRITION FACTS:

calories: 231;carbs: 50.6g; Protein: 6.5g; Fat: 2.4g; Sugar: 22.6g; Sodium: 121mg; Fiber: 8.5g

 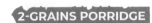 **2-GRAINS PORRIDGE**

Preparation Time: 10 minutes

Cooking Time: 20 minutes

Servings: 3

INGREDIENTS:

- 2 C. milk
- 2 C. water
- 1 C. old-fashioned oats
- 1/3 C. dried quinoa, rinsed
- 3 tbsp. maple syrup
- ½ tsp. vanilla extract
- 1 large banana, peeled and sliced
- 1 small apple, peeled, cored and chopped

DIRECTIONS:

1. In a pan, mix together all the ingredients except for banana and apple over medium heat and bring to a gentle boil.
2. Cook for about 20 minutes, stirring occasionally.
3. Remove from the heat and serve warm with the garnishing of banana and apple.

NUTRITION FACTS:

calories: 384;carbs: 72g; Protein: 12.2g; Fat: 6.5g; Sugar: 32.9g; Sodium: 87mg; Fiber: 7g

 SAVORY CREPES

Preparation Time: 10 minutes

Cooking Time: 20 minutes

Servings: 4

INGREDIENTS:

- 1¼ C. chickpea flour
- 1½ C. water
- ¼ tsp. red chili powder
- Salt, as required

DIRECTIONS:

1. In a blender, add all the ingredients and pulse until well combined.
2. Heat a lightly greased nonstick skillet over medium-high heat.
3. Add the desired amount of the mixture and tilt the pan to spread it evenly.
4. Cook for about 3 minutes.
5. Carefully, flip the crepe and cook for about 1-2 minutes.
6. Repeat with the remaining mixture.
7. Serve warm.

NUTRITION FACTS:

calories: 229;carbs: 38.1g; Protein: 12.1g; Fat: 3.8g; Sugar: 6.7g; Sodium: 55mg; Fiber: 11g

 EGG-FREE OMELET

Preparation Time: 15 minutes

Cooking Time: 12 minutes

Servings: 4

INGREDIENTS:

- 1 C. chickpea flour
- ¼ tsp. ground turmeric
- ¼ tsp. red chili powder
- Pinch of ground cumin
- Pinch of sea salt
- 1½-2 C. water
- 1 medium onion, chopped finely
- 2 medium tomatoes, chopped finely
- 2 tbsp. fresh cilantro, chopped
- 2 tbsp. olive oil, divided

DIRECTIONS:

1. In a large bowl, add the flour, spices, and salt and mix well.
2. Slowly, add the water and mix until well combined.
3. Fold in the onion, tomatoes and cilantro.
4. In a large non-stick frying pan, heat ½ tbsp. of the oil over medium heat.
5. Add ½ of the tomato mixture and tilt the pan to spread it.
6. Cook for about 5-7 minutes.
7. Place the remaining oil over the "omelet" and carefully flip it over.
8. Cook for about 4-5 minutes or until golden brown.
9. Repeat with the remaining mixture.

NUTRITION FACTS:

calories: 267;carbs: 35.7g; Protein: 10.6g; Fat: 10.3g; Sugar: 8.3g; Sodium: 86mg; Fiber: 10.2g

371. **SUMMER TREAT SALAD**

Preparation Time: 15 minutes

Cooking Time: 0 minutes

Servings: 4

INGREDIENTS:

- 2 large avocados, peeled, pitted and chopped
- 1 large apple, peeled, pitted and chopped
- 1 large peach, peeled, pitted and chopped
- 1 C. cantaloupe, peeled and chopped
- 1 shallot, chopped finely
- 1 seedless cucumber, peeled and chopped
- ¼ C. fresh lime juice
- ¼ C. fresh mint, chopped
- 6 C. lettuce leaves, torn

DIRECTIONS:

1. In a large salad bowl, add all the ingredients and toss to coat well.
2. Set aside for at least 10-20 minutes before serving.

NUTRITION FACTS:

calories: 262;carbs: 28.7g; Protein: 3.7g; Fat: 17.1g; Sugar: 14.9g; Sodium: 20mg; Fiber: 9.5g

372. SECRETLY AMAZING SALAD

Preparation Time: 15 minutes
Cooking Time: 35 minutes
Servings: 6

INGREDIENTS:

For Lentils:
- 4 C. water
- 2 C. dried green lentils, rinsed
- 2 large garlic cloves, halved lengthwise
- 2 tbsp. olive oil

For Dressing:
- 1 garlic clove, minced
- ¼ C. fresh lemon juice
- 2 tbsp. olive oil
- 1 tsp. maple syrup
- 1 tsp. Dijon mustard
- Salt and freshly ground black pepper, to taste

For Salad:
- 1½ (15-oz.) cans chickpeas, rinsed and drained
- 2 large avocados, peeled, pitted and chopped
- 2 C. radishes, trimmed and sliced
- ¼ C. fresh mint leaves, chopped

DIRECTIONS:

For lentils:
1. in a medium pot, add all ingredients over medium-high heat and bring to a boil.
2. Reduce the heat to low and simmer for about 25-35 minutes or until the lentils are cooked through and tender.
3. Drain the lentils and discard the garlic cloves.

For dressing:
1. add all ingredients in a small bowl and beat until well combined.
2. In a large serving bowl, add lentils, chickpeas, radishes, avocados and mint and mix.
3. Add the dressing and toss to coat well.
4. Serve immediately.

NUTRITION FACTS:
calories: 561;carbs: 66.4g; Protein: 24.9g; Fat: 22.2g; Sugar: 3.2g; Sodium: 96mg; Fiber: 29.2g

373. DOUBLE CHOCOLATE SCONES

Preparation Time: 10 minutes
Cooking Time: 25 minutes
Servings: 8

INGREDIENTS:

- 125g | 1 cup all-purpose flour
- 97g | ¾ cup wholewheat flour
- 25g | ¼ cup cocoa powder
- 62g | ¼ heaping cup natural cane sugar (you can sub this for any granulated sugar or coconut sugar)
- ½ teaspoon salt
- 1 tablespoon ground flax
- 1 tablespoon baking powder
- ¼ packed cup coconut oil (it needs to be hard)
- 1 teaspoon vanilla extract
- 207mls | ¾ cup + 2 tablespoons cup of non-dairy milk
- 130g | ¾ cup dairy-free chocolate chips or chunks (i like to use semi-sweet, but you can use any kind you have to hand).
- A little sugar for sprinkling

For the drizzle (optional)
- 43g | ¼ cup dairy-free chocolate
- 2 tablespoons non-dairy milk

DIRECTIONS:

1. Pre-heat the oven to 400°F-200°C.
2. Use parchment paper or a silicone baking mat to line a baking sheet.
3. In a large mixing basin, combine the flour and baking powder.
4. Mix in the coconut oil with your fingertips or a pastry cutter until the mixture resembles bread crumbs.
5. Stir in all of the remaining dry ingredients, including the chocolate.
6. Add the vanilla extract to the milk and mix to blend, then add the liquid to the dry ingredients and swirl to combine.
7. It's now simpler to get your hands into the dough and shape it into a ball. Don't be too rough with it since the less you handle it, the better your scones will be.
8. Place on the prepared tray and press or roll into a 1 inch thick round.
9. Divide the mixture into 8 equal wedges and divide them so that they all have some space between them.
10. sprinkle with sugar and bake for 20 - 25 minutes, or until cooked through (if you're not sure, insert a toothpick or skewer and it should come out largely clean).
11. allow cooling on a cooling rack.
12. optional chocolate drizzling
13. place the chocolate and milk in a small dish and gently melt in a microwave or over a saucepan of boiling water.
14. drizzle the melted chocolate mixture over the cooled scones using a spoon.

NUTRITION FACTS:
calories: 285 |carbs: 41 g | protein: 6 g | fat: 12 g | cholesterol: 90 mg

374. BANANA AND BLUEBERRY FRITTERS

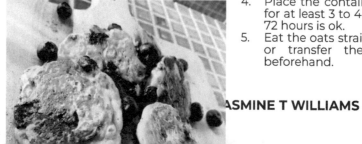

Preparation Time: 10 minutes
Cooking Time: 5 minutes
Servings: 6

INGREDIENTS:

- Two ripe bananas
- ¼ - ½ cup buckwheat flour (or plain flour)
- ¼ cup blueberries
- Pinch of cinnamon (optional)
- One tablespoon coconut oil for frying

DIRECTIONS:

1. After mashing the bananas, add the flour and cinnamon.
2. Stir in the blueberries until they are evenly distributed.
3. Heat the coconut oil in a nonstick frying pan over high heat.
4. Reduce the heat to medium-low and pour one tablespoon of batter into the frying pan for each fritter.
5. Fry fritters until both sides are golden brown.
6. Remove the fritters from the pan and set them aside to cool slightly before serving.

NUTRITION FACTS:
calories: 62 |carbs: 13 g | protein: 1 g | fat: 2 g | cholesterol: 18 mg

375. STRAWBERRY OVERNIGHT OATS

Preparation Time: 5 minutes
Cooking Time: 0 minutes
Servings: 1

INGREDIENTS:

- ½ cup (50 grams) rolled or old-fashioned oats, use certified gluten-free oats if necessary
- 1 tablespoon chia
- ¾ cup (180 ml) non-dairy milk
- ½ teaspoon vanilla extract
- 1 tablespoon maple syrup (optional), use real maple syrup, not pancake syrup
- 1 tablespoon strawberry jam (optional - but recommended)
- Around ½ cup (60 grams) fresh strawberries, chopped

DIRECTIONS:

1. Add the oats and chia to a jar (or another covered container).
2. 2. Stir in the milk, vanilla extract, and optional maple syrup.
3. Pour in the strawberry jam, followed by the cut strawberries.
4. Place the container in the fridge for at least 3 to 4 hours, but up to 72 hours is ok.
5. Eat the oats straight from the jar, or transfer them to a bowl beforehand.

NUTRITION FACTS:

calories: 388 |carbs: 61 g | protein: 14 g | fat: 10 g | cholesterol: 386 mg

376. STRAWBERRY BANANA PEANUT BUTTER SMOOTHIE

Preparation Time: 5 minutes

Cooking Time: 5 minutes

Servings: 1

INGREDIENTS:

- 2 cups (approx 288 grams) strawberries, fresh or frozen
- 1 medium frozen banana, fresh and not frozen if using frozen strawberries
- 2 tablespoons peanut butter, or any other nut or butter
- 1 cup (240 ml) plant milk, of choice

Optional
- 1 tablespoon maple syrup, or a medjool date
- 1 tablespoon flax
- 1 tablespoon chia

DIRECTIONS:

1. In a blender, combine all of the ingredients.
2. Blend until completely smooth.
3. Check the sweetness and, if required, add the optional maple syrup or date, then mix again to combine.

NUTRITION FACTS:

calories: 465 |carbs: 60 g | protein: 18 g | fat: 21 g | cholesterol: 276 mg

HIGH FIBER DIET

LUNCH

377. PEA SOUP

Preparation time: 5 minutes

Cooking time: 25 minutes

Serving: 5

INGREDIENTS:
- Peas – 500g
- Potatoes – 150g
- Zucchini – two
- Vegetable stock – 1 liter
- Full fat coconut milk – 400ml, full-fat
- Coconut oil – 2 tbsp
- Onion – one tsp
- Ginger – 20g
- Lemongrass stalk – two
- Garlic – one clove
- Salt – ½ tsp
- Pepper – ½ tsp

DIRECTIONS:
1. Slice the zucchini. Dice the garlic, potato, ginger, and onion.
2. Add coconut oil into the pan and add potatoes to it and cook for one to two minutes. When potatoes are softened, add lemongrass, ginger, garlic, and onion and cook for one to two minutes more.
3. Add zucchini, pepper, and salt and cook for two minutes more.
4. Then, add vegetable stock and peas and bring to a boil.
5. Lower the heat and simmer for few minutes. Add coconut milk.
6. Place soup into the handheld blender and blend on low flame until creamy and smooth.
7. Transfer it to the bowl. Garnish with pine nuts, peas, and fresh coriander leaves.

NUTRITION FACTS:

Calories; 347kcal, fat ; 23g, Carbohydrate; 31g, Protein; 9g, Fiber; 7g

378. GUACAMOLE

Preparation time: 10 minutes

Cooking time: 0 minutes

Serving: 4

INGREDIENTS:
- Avocados – two
- Red onion – one
- Coriander leaves – ¼ cup
- Limes – two
- Salt – ¼ tsp
- Optional:
- Green chili jalapeño – one
- Cherry tomatoes – half cup
- Pepper – ¼ tsp

DIRECTIONS:
1. Let chop the coriander, chili, and onion.
2. Mash the avocados with a fork until creamy.
3. Combine the chopped veggies into the mashed avocado.
4. Add lemon juice and salt over it.
5. Combine it well.
6. Sprinkle with pepper and salt.

NUTRITION FACTS:

Calories; 189kcal, fat ; 15g, Carbohydrate; 16g, Protein; 3g, Fiber; 9g

CABBAGE SOUP

Preparation time: 10 minutes

Cooking time: 30 minutes

Serving: 8

INGREDIENTS:
- Extra-virgin olive oil – 2 tbsp
- Onions – 2 cups, chopped
- Carrot – one cup, chopped
- Celery – one cup, chopped
- Poblano or green bell pepper – one cup, chopped
- Garlic – four cloves, minced
- Cabbage – eight cups, sliced
- Tomato paste – one tbsp
- Chipotle chilies in adobo sauce – 1 tbsp, minced
- Ground cumin – one tsp
- Ground coriander – half tsp
- Vegetable broth or chicken broth – four cups, low-sodium
- Water – four cups
- Pinto or black beans – 30 ounces, rinsed, low-sodium
- Salt – ¾ tsp
- Fresh cilantro – half cup, chopped
- Lime juice – 2 tbsp

DIRECTIONS:
1. Add oil into the pot and place it over medium flame.
2. Then, add garlic, bell pepper, celery, carrots, and onions and cook for ten to twelve minutes.
3. Add cabbage and cook for ten minutes until softened.
4. Add coriander, cumin, chipotle, and tomato paste and cook for one minute more.
5. Add salt, beans, water, and broth and cover with a lid. Bring to a boil over high heat. Lower the heat and simmer for ten minutes.
6. Remove from the flame.
7. Add lime juice and fresh coriander leaves.

NUTRITION FACTS:

Calories; 167kcal, fat ; 3.8g, Carbohydrate; 27.1g, Protein; 6.5g, Fiber; 8.7g

379. CAULIFLOWER AND POTATO CURRY SOUP

Preparation time: 10 minutes

Cooking time: 1 hour

Serving: 8

INGREDIENTS:
- Ground coriander – 2 tsp
- Ground cumin – 2 tsp
- Ground cinnamon – 1 ½ tsp
- Ground turmeric – 1 ½ tsp
- Salt – 1 ¼ tsp
- Ground pepper – ¾ tsp
- Cayenne pepper – 1/8 tsp
- Cauliflower – six cups, cut into small florets
- Extra-virgin olive oil – 2 tbsp
- Onion – one, chopped
- Carrot – one, diced
- Garlic – three cloves, minced
- Fresh ginger – 1 ½ tsp, grated
- Red chili powder – one, minced
- Tomato sauce – 14 ounces, salt-less
- Vegetable broth – four cups, low-sodium
- Potatoes – three cups, diced, peeled
- Lime zest – two tsp
- Lime juice – 2 tbsp
- Coconut milk – 14 ounces

DIRECTIONS:
1. Preheat the oven to 450°F-230°C.
2. Mix the cayenne, pepper, salt, turmeric, and cinnamon, cumin, and coriander leaves into the bowl.
3. Toss cauliflower with one tbsp oil into the big bowl. Sprinkle with one tsp spice mixture. Spread onto the rimmed baking sheet.
4. Cook for 15 to 20 minutes. Keep it aside.
5. Meanwhile, add one tbsp oil into the pot and heat it over medium-high flame. Add carrot and onion and cook for three to four minutes.
6. Lower the heat and cook for three to four minutes more.
7. Then, add the remaining spice mixture, chili, garlic, and ginger and cook for one minute more.
8. Add tomato sauce and stir well. Let simmer for one minute.
9. Add lime zest, lime juice, sweet potatoes, and broth, and bring to a boil over high flame.
10. Lower the heat and simmer for 35 to 40 minutes.
11. Add roasted cauliflower and coconut milk and stir well.
12. Simmer until cooked well.

NUTRITION FACTS:
Calories; 272kcal, fat ; 14.8g, Carbohydrate; 33.4g, Protein; 5.3g, Fiber; 7.2g

380. SWEET POTATO AND BLACK BEAN CHILI

Preparation time: 10 minutes

Cooking time: 30 minutes

Serving: 4

INGREDIENTS:
- Extra-virgin olive oil – 1 tbsp plus 2 tsp
- Sweet potato – one, peeled and diced
- Onion – one, diced
- Garlic – four cloves, minced
- Chili powder – two tbsp
- Ground cumin – four tsp
- Chipotle chili – ½ tsp, ground
- Salt – ¼ tsp
- Water – 2 ½ cups
- Black beans – 30 ounces, rinsed
- Tomatoes – 14 ounces, diced
- Lime juice – 4 tsp
- Fresh cilantro – half cup, chopped

DIRECTIONS:
1. Add oil into the Dutch oven and place it over medium-high flame.
2. Add onion and sweet potatoes and cook for four minutes until softened.
3. Add salt, chipotle, cumin, chili powder, and garlic and cook for a half-minute.
4. Add water and bring to a simmer. Lower the heat and cook for 10 to 12 minutes.
5. Add lime juice, tomatoes, and beans and simmer over high heat.
6. Lower the heat and simmer for five minutes more.
7. Remove from the flame.
8. Garnish with fresh cilantro leaves.

NUTRITION FACTS:
Calories; 323kcal, fat ; 7.6g, Carbohydrate; 54.7g, Protein; 12.5g, Fiber; 15.6g

381. WHITE BEAN CHILI

Preparation time: 10 minutes

Cooking time: 1 hour

Serving: 6

INGREDIENTS:
- Avocado oil or canola oil – ¼ cup
- Anaheim or poblano chilies – 2 cups, seeded and chopped
- Onion – one, chopped
- Garlic – four cloves, minced
- Quinoa – half cup, rinsed
- Dried oregano – four tsp
- Ground cumin – four tsp
- Salt – one tsp
- Ground coriander – half tsp
- Ground pepper – half tsp
- Vegetable broth – four cups, low-sodium
- White beans – 30 ounces, rinsed
- Zucchini – one, diced
- Fresh cilantro – ¼ cup, chopped
- Lime juice – 2 tbsp

DIRECTIONS:
1. Add oil into the pot and place it over medium flame.
2. Add garlic, onion, and chilies, and cook for five to seven minutes.
3. Then, add pepper, coriander, salt, cumin, oregano, and quinoa and cook for one minute.
4. Add beans and broth and stir well. Bring to a boil and simmer for twenty minutes.
5. Add zucchini and cook for 10 to 15 minutes.
6. Garnish with lime juice and fresh cilantro leaves.
7. Top with lime wedges.

NUTRITION FACTS:
Calories; 283kcal, fat ; 11.7g, Carbohydrate; 36.7g, Protein; 9.7g, Fiber; 8.4g

382. CHICKPEA STEW

Preparation time: 10 minutes

Cooking time: 30-40 minutes

Serving: 8

INGREDIENTS:
- Spinach – 10 ounces
- Canola oil – 1 ½ tbsp
- Onion – one, chopped
- Ginger – one-piece, peeled and minced
- Jalapeno pepper – half, seeded and chopped
- Garlic – three cloves, minced
- Curry powder – one tbsp
- Carrots – three, peeled and thinly sliced
- Cauliflower – half head, broken into bite-size florets
- Chickpeas – 30 ounces, low-sodium, rinsed
- Tomatoes – 28 ounces, drained, diced, salt-free
- Half-and-half – half cup, fat-free
- Coconut milk – 1/3 cup

DIRECTIONS:
1. Place spinach into the microwave-safe bowl and then add one tbsp water and cover it. Let microwave it for one to two minutes.
2. Transfer it to the colander and drain it.
3. When cooled, chop it and keep it aside.
4. Add oil into the skillet and heat it.
5. Add onion and cook for eight minutes.
6. Add curry powder, garlic, jalapeno, and ginger and cook for a half-minute. Then, add 2 tbsp water and carrots and cook for ten minutes.
7. Add cauliflower and cook for five to ten minutes more.
8. Add coconut milk, half-and-half, tomatoes, and chickpeas, and stir well. Bring to a boil. Then, lower the heat and simmer for 15

minutes.
9. Then, add reserved spinach and stir well.

NUTRITION FACTS:

Calories; 249kcal, fat ; 6.5g, Carbohydrate; 38.8g, Protein; 11.2g, Fiber; 10g

383. VEGGIE SANDWICH

Preparation time: 10 minutes
Cooking time: 0 minutes
Serving: 8

INGREDIENTS:
- Sprouted-grain bread – two slices, toasted
- Avocado – ¼, mashed
- Hummus – one tbsp
- Salt – one pinch
- Cucumber – four slices
- Tomato – two slices
- Carrot – 2 tbsp, shredded
- Clementine – one, peeled

DIRECTIONS:
1. Place one slice of bread onto the plate and spread avocado and hummus.
2. Sprinkle with salt. Fill the sandwich with carrot, tomato, and cucumber.
3. Cut in half and serve with Clementine.

NUTRITION FACTS:
Calories; 315kcal, fat ; 10.1g, Carbohydrate; 48.6g, Protein; 11.4g, Fiber; 12.5g

384. BEAN AND VEGGIE TACO BOWL

Preparation time: 20 minutes
Cooking time: 8 minutes
Serving: 1

INGREDIENTS:
- Olive oil – one tsp
- Green bell pepper – half, cored, and sliced
- Red onion – half, sliced
- Cooked brown rice – half cup
- Black beans – ¼ cup, rinsed
- Sharp cheddar cheese – ¼ cup, shredded
- Pico de gallo or salsa – ¼ cup
- Cilantro – 2 tbsp

DIRECTIONS:
1. Add oil into the skillet and place it over medium flame.
2. Add onion and bell pepper and cook for 5 to 8 minutes.
3. Mound rice and beans into the bowl. Top with cilantro, pico de gallo, cheese, and vegetables.
4. Top with hot sauce and lime wedges.

NUTRITION FACTS:
Calories; 435kcal, fat ; 15.5g, Carbohydrate; 59.6g, Protein; 16.4g, Fiber; 9.6g

385. COBB SALAD

Preparation time: 10 minutes
Cooking time: 0 minutes
Serving: 1

INGREDIENTS:
- Iceberg lettuce – three cups, chopped
- Chicken thighs – one, diced, roasted
- Celery – one stalk, diced
- Carrot – one, diced
- Egg – one, hard-boiled, diced
- Blue cheese – one tbsp, crumbled
- Honey and mustard vinaigrette – 2 tbsp

DIRECTIONS:
1. Place blue cheese, egg, carrot, celery, chicken, and lettuce into the salad bowl.
2. Drizzle with dressing.

NUTRITION FACTS:
Calories; 481kcal, fat ; 16.7g, Carbohydrate; 67.6g, Protein; 17.3g, Fiber; 13.4g

386. ASPARAGUS SOUP

Preparation time: 5 minutes
Cooking time: 10 minutes
Serving: 4

INGREDIENTS:
- Olive oil – one tbsp
- Shallots – one cup, chopped
- Garlic – three cloves, minced
- Asparagus – two pounds, chopped into one inch pieces
- Vegetable stock – six cups
- Salt – one tsp

DIRECTIONS:
1. Add olive oil into the pot and cook over medium flame. Add garlic and shallot and cook for three to five minutes until softened.
2. Add salt, vegetable stock, and asparagus stalks and then boil it.
3. Cover the pot with a lid and simmer on a low flame.
4. When done, transfer the cooled soup into the blender and blend until creamy.
5. Add asparagus tops and cook for five minutes until tender.
6. Serve and enjoy!

NUTRITION FACTS:
Calories; 205kcal,carbs; 18g, protein; 7g, fat; 0g, fiber; 11g

387. CREAMY CARROT SOUP

Preparation time: 5 minutes
Cooking time: 20 minutes
Serving: 4-6

INGREDIENTS:
- Olive oil – two tbsp
- Carrots – four cups, chopped
- Onion – one, chopped
- Garlic – three cloves, minced
- Curry powder – one tbsp
- Chicken broth – three cups
- Carrot juice – 1 ½ cups

DIRECTIONS:
1. Add oil into the pot and cook over medium flame.
2. Add onion and carrots and cook for six to eight minutes.
3. Then, add curry powder and garlic and cook for one minute more.
4. Add half tsp salt and broth and simmer over low flame for fifteen minutes.
5. Add carrot juice and combine well. Let cool it. Transfer it to the blender and blend until smooth.
6. Place soup back in the pot and sprinkle with pepper and salt.
7. Add cream and combine well.
8. Serve and enjoy!

NUTRITION FACTS:
Calories; 176kcal,carbs; 21.7g, protein; 6.8g, fat; 8.3g, fiber; 5.2g

388. MUSHROOM BARLEY SOUP

Preparation time: 5 minutes
Cooking time: 30 minutes
Serving: 4

INGREDIENTS:
- Olive oil – two tbsp
- Carrots – one cup, chopped
- Onion – one cup, chopped
- White mushrooms – 1lb, sliced
- Smoked ham – 1 ½ cups, chopped
- Chicken broth – 28 ounces,
- Stewed tomatoes – 14 ounces, seedless
- Quick cooking barley – half cup

DIRECTIONS:
1. Add olive oil into the pot and cook over medium-high flame.
2. Add onion and carrots and cook for five minutes.
3. Add mushrooms and cook for five minutes more.
4. Add ham and cook for one to two minutes and stir well.
5. Add barley, tomatoes, and

chicken broth and stir well.
6. Let boil it. Then, lower the heat and simmer for twenty minutes.
7. Serve and enjoy!

NUTRITION FACTS:

Calories; 200kcal, carbs; 30.8g, protein; 5.8g, fat; 7.3g, fiber; 4.8g

389. BROCCOLI SOUP

Preparation time: 5 minutes

Cooking time: 45 minutes

Serving: 4

INGREDIENTS:

- Olive oil – two tbsp
- Leek – one, chopped
- Celery stalk – one, chopped
- Garlic – two cloves, minced
- Potatoes – three, unpeeled, chopped
- Salt – ½ tsp
- Bay leaf – one
- Vegetable broth – three cups
- Broccoli florets – 1 ½ cups

DIRECTIONS:

1. Add oil into the pan and cook over medium-high flame.
2. Add bay leaf, salt, potatoes, garlic, leek, and celery and cook until browned.
3. Add stock and boil it. Then, lower the heat and simmer for thirty minutes.
4. Add broccoli florets and simmer for fifteen minutes until tender.
5. Remove from the flame. Let cool it.
6. Discard bay leaf and then add to the blender and blend until smooth.
7. Serve and enjoy!

NUTRITION FACTS:

Calories; 361kcal, carbs; 33g, protein; 12g, fat; 23g, fiber; 12g

390. CHICKEN AND ASPARAGUS PASTA

Preparation time: 5 minutes

Cooking time: 20 minutes

Serving: 4

INGREDIENTS:

- Whole wheat penne pasta – 1lb
- Olive oil – two tbsp
- Chicken breast halves – 1lb, boneless and sliced into strips
- Poultry seasoning – half tsp
- Garlic – four cloves, minced
- Asparagus, frozen – 1 ½ cups, thawed, cut into 1 inch pieces
- Peas, frozen – one cup, thawed
- Parmesan cheese – ¼ cup, grated

DIRECTIONS:

1. Add water and salt into the pot and boil it. Then, add pasta and cook until al dente.
2. Add one tbsp olive oil into the pan and cook over medium flame. Add chicken and poultry seasoning and cook until golden.
3. Remove cooked chicken from the pan.
4. Then, add peas, asparagus, garlic, and the remaining tbsp of olive oil and cook until tender.
5. Add chicken back with asparagus mixture and cook for two minutes.
6. Add pasta to the bowl and toss with chicken mixture.
7. Sprinkle with parmesan cheese.

NUTRITION FACTS:

Calories; 625kcal, carbs; 76g, protein; 34g, fat; 23g, fiber; 9g

391. RED BEANS AND RICE

Preparation time: 5 minutes

Cooking time: 35 minutes

Serving: 4

INGREDIENTS:

- Olive oil – one tbsp
- Onion – one, chopped
- Stalks celery – three, chopped
- Garlic cloves – three, minced
- Tomato sauce – 14 ounce
- Oregano – half tsp
- Thyme – half tbsp
- Beef stock – 14 ounce
- Red beans – 28 ounce, drained and rinsed
- Brown rice – four cups, cooked

DIRECTIONS:

1. Add olive oil into the pan and cook over medium flame.
2. Add garlic, celery, and onions and cook and stir well.
3. Add thyme, oregano, and tomato paste and stir well.
4. Add beef broth and simmer for thirty-five minutes.
5. Add red beans and cook it well.
6. Place over brown rice.

NUTRITION FACTS:

Calories; 413kcal, carbs; 76.3g, protein; 21.1g, fat; 2.5g, fiber; 10.1g

392. BEEF STIR FRY

Preparation time: 5 minutes

Cooking time: 35 minutes

Serving: 2-3

INGREDIENTS:

- Orange juice – ¼ cup
- Low-sodium soy sauce – ¼ cup
- Rice vinegar – two tbsp
- Water – ¼ cup
- Canola oil – two tbsp
- Beef round steak – eight ounce, thinly sliced
- Garlic – three cloves, minced
- Peas – six ounce
- Broccoli florets – one bunch
- Edamame – eight ounce, shelled
- Cornstarch – 1 ½ tsp, dissolved in ¼ cup hot water

DIRECTIONS:

1. Mix the water, rice vinegar, soy sauce, and orange juice into the bowl and keep it aside.
2. Add one tbsp canola oil into the pan and cook over medium flame.
3. Add beef and cook for two minutes. Transfer the beef to another plate.
4. Add one tbsp of oil into another pan and cook over medium flame.
5. Add garlic and cook for one minute. Add edamame, broccoli, and peas and cook for three minutes.
6. Add soy sauce mixture and cook for five minutes until tender.
7. Place sliced beef back in the pan.
8. Meanwhile, add cornstarch to the water and dissolve it. Add it to the pan and combine it well.
9. Serve and enjoy!

NUTRITION FACTS:

Calories; 368kcal, carbs; 27g, protein; 37g, fat; 13g, fiber; 3g

393. SOUTH WESTERN SALAD

Preparation Time: 20 minutes

Cooking Time: 0 minutes

Servings: 6

INGREDIENTS:

For Dressing:
- 2 tbsp. fresh lime juice
- 2 tbsp. maple syrup
- 1 tbsp. Dijon mustard
- ½ tsp. ground cumin
- 1 tsp. garlic powder
- Salt and freshly ground black pepper, to taste
- ¼ C. extra-virgin olive oil

For Salad:
- 2 C. fresh mango, peeled, pitted and cubed
- 2 tbsp. fresh lime juice, divided
- 2 avocados, peeled, pitted and cubed
- Pinch of salt
- 1 C. cooked quinoa
- 2 (14-oz.) cans black beans, rinsed and drained
- 1 small red onion, chopped
- ½ C. fresh cilantro, chopped
- 6 C. romaine lettuce, shredded

DIRECTIONS:

1. For dressing: in a blender, add all the ingredients except oil and pulse until well combined.
2. While the motor is running,

HIGH FIBER DIET - LUNCH

gradually add the oil and pulse until smooth.
3. For salad: in a bowl, add the mango and 1 tbsp. of lime juice and toss to coat well.
4. In another bowl, add the avocado, a pinch of salt and remaining lime juice and toss to coat well.
5. In a large serving bowl, add the mango, avocado and remaining salad ingredients and mix.
6. Place the dressing and toss to coat well.
7. Serve immediately.

NUTRITION FACTS:

calories: 555;carbs: 71.5g; Protein: 18.1g; Fat: 24.4g; Sugar: 13g; Sodium: 69mg; Fiber: 19.7g

 ## 394. VEGAN-FRIENDLY PLATTER

Preparation Time: 10 minutes

Cooking Time: 30 minutes

Servings: 4

INGREDIENTS:

- 1 tbsp. olive oil
- 2 small onions, chopped
- 5 garlic cloves, chopped finely
- 1 tsp. of dried oregano
- 1 tsp. ground cumin
- ½ tsp. ground ginger
- Salt and freshly ground black pepper, to taste
- 2 cups tomatoes, peeled, seeded and chopped
- 2 (13½-oz.) cans black beans, rinsed and drained
- ½ C. homemade vegetable broth

DIRECTIONS:

1. In a pan, heat the olive oil over medium heat and cook the onion for about 5-7 minutes, stirring frequently.
2. Add the garlic, oregano, spices, salt and black pepper and cook for about 1 minute.
3. Add the tomatoes and cook for about 1-2 minutes.
4. Add in the beans and broth and bring to a boil.
5. Reduce the heat to medium-low and simmer, covered for about 15 minutes.
6. Serve hot.

NUTRITION FACTS:

calories: 327;carbs: 54.1g; Protein: 19.1g; Fat: 5.1g; Sugar: 4g; Sodium: 595mg; Fiber: 18.8g

 ## 395. BROCCOLI SALAD

Preparation time: 10 minutes

Cooking time: 0 minutes

Serving: 4

INGREDIENTS:

- Mayonnaise – half cup
- Whole-grain mustard – one tbsp
- Cider vinegar – one tbsp
- Clove garlic – one, grated
- Sugar – one tsp
- Ground pepper – ¼ tsp
- Broccoli crowns – four cups, chopped
- Cauliflower – one cup, chopped
- Red onion – ¼ cup, chopped
- Sunflower seeds – three tbsp, toasted

DIRECTIONS:

1. Add pepper, sugar, garlic, vinegar, mustard, and mayonnaise into the bowl and whisk it well.
2. Add sunflower seeds, onion, broccoli, and cauliflower and stir well.
3. Serve and enjoy!

NUTRITION FACTS:

Calories; 246kcal,carbs; 7.7g, protein; 5.4g, fat; 2.8g, fiber; 22g

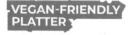 ## 396. BEEF AND BEAN SLOPPY JOES

Preparation time: 10 minutes

Cooking time: 20 minutes

Serving: 4

INGREDIENTS:

- Extra-virgin olive oil – one tbsp
- Ground beef – 12 ounce
- No-salt-added black beans – one cup, rinsed
- Onion – one cup, chopped
- Chili powder – two tsp
- Garlic powder – half tsp
- Onion powder – half tsp
- Pinch of cayenne pepper
- Tomato sauce – one cup
- Ketchup – three tbsp
- Worcestershire sauce – one tbsp
- Spicy brown mustard – two tsp
- Brown sugar – one tsp
- Whole-wheat hamburger buns – four, split and toasted

DIRECTIONS:

1. Add oil into the skillet and cook over medium-high flame.
2. Add beef and cook for three to four minutes until browned.
3. Transfer the beef to the bowl using a slotted spoon.
4. Add onion and beans to the pan and cook until softened for five minutes.
5. Add cayenne, onion powder, garlic powder, and chili powder and cook for thirty seconds.
6. Add brown sugar, mustard, Worcestershire sauce, ketchup, and tomato sauce and stir well.
7. Place beef back in the pan and simmer for five minutes.
8. Serve and enjoy!

NUTRITION FACTS:

Calories; 411kcal,carbs; 43.8g, protein; 25.8g, fat; 15g, fiber; 8.4g

 ## 397. SWEET POTATO AND PEANUT SOUP

Preparation time: 15 minutes

Cooking time: 20 minutes

Serving: 6

INGREDIENTS:

- Canola oil – two tbsp
- Yellow onion – 1 ½ cups, diced
- Garlic – one tbsp, minced
- Fresh ginger, one tbsp, minced
- Red curry paste – four tsp
- Serrano chili – one, ribs and seeds removed, minced
- Sweet potatoes – 1lb, peeled and cubed
- Water – three cups
- Coconut milk – one cup
- Unsalted dry-roasted peanuts – ¾ cup
- White beans – 15 ounce, rinsed
- Salt – ¾ tsp
- Ground pepper – ¼ tsp
- Fresh cilantro – ¼ cup, chopped
- Lime juice – two tbsp
- Unsalted roasted pumpkin seeds – ¼ cup
- Lime wedges – to garnish

DIRECTIONS:

1. Add oil into the pot and heat over medium-high flame.
2. Add onion and cook for minutes until softened.
3. Add Serrano, curry paste, ginger, and garlic and stir and cook for one minute. Add water and sweet potatoes and boil it.
4. Lower the heat and cook over medium-low flame for ten to twelve minutes.
5. Transfer half of the soup to the blender and then add peanut and coconut milk and blend until smooth. Place it back in the pot with the remaining soup.
6. Add pepper, salt, and beans and stir well.
7. When done, remove from the flame.
8. Add lime juice and fresh cilantro leaves.
9. Serve and enjoy!

NUTRITION FACTS:

Calories; 345kcal,carbs; 37.4g, protein; 12.6g, fat; 19.4g, fiber; 8.4g

 ## 398. BEET SALAD

Preparation time: 15 minutes

Baking time: 1 hour and 10 minutes

Serving: 6

INGREDIENTS:
- Beets – 2lb, scrubbed
- Extra-virgin olive oil – three tbsp
- Balsamic vinegar – two tbsp
- Salt – ¼ tsp
- Ground pepper – ¼ tsp
- Feta cheese – 1/3 cup, crumbled
- Fresh dill – two tbsp, chopped

DIRECTIONS:
1. Preheat the oven to 400°F-200°C.
2. Wrap beets in the foil and put them onto the rimmed baking sheet.
3. Bake for one hour and ten minutes until tender.
4. Let cool it. Peel and cut into cubes.
5. Whisk the pepper, salt, vinegar, and oil into the bowl.
6. Add feta and beets and toss to combine.
7. Top with dill.

NUTRITION FACTS:
Calories; 155kcal, carbs; 15.8g, protein; 3.7g, fat; 9g, fiber; 4.3g

399. BROCCOLI CASSEROLE

Preparation time: 10 minutes

Baking time: 1 hour and 5 minutes

Serving: 6

INGREDIENTS:
- Whole-wheat sandwich bread – two slices
- Broccoli florets – 2lb
- Butter – three tbsp
- Extra-virgin olive oil – two tbsp
- Onion – two cups, diced
- Garlic – four cloves, minced
- All-purpose flour – 1/3 cup
- Chicken broth – 3 ½ cups, low-sodium
- Cream cheese – six ounce, low-fat
- Worcestershire sauce – two tsp
- Ground pepper – ¾ tsp
- Salt – half tsp
- Colby jack cheese – two cups, shredded

DIRECTIONS:
1. Preheat the oven to 300°F-150°C.
2. Let coat the baking dish with cooking spray.
3. Add bread into pieces and then add to the food processor until crumbs form.
4. Place breadcrumbs onto the baking sheet and bake for ten minutes.
5. During this, add water to the pot and boil it. Add broccoli and steam it for four to six minutes. Let chop it and place it onto the baking dish.
6. Elevate the temperature to 350°F-180°C.
7. Add oil and one tbsp butter into the saucepan and cook over medium-high flame. Add garlic and onion and cook for three to five minutes.
8. Place flour over the vegetables and cook for one minute.
9. Add chicken broth and stir well. Let cook for three minutes.
10. Add salt, pepper, Worcestershire sauce, and cream cheese and stir well. Cook for two minutes.
11. Remove from the flame. Add cheese and stir well.
12. Place cheese sauce onto the broccoli.
13. Melt two tbsp butter and mix with breadcrumbs into the bowl.
14. Place over the broccoli mixture and top with a half cup of cheese.
15. Bake for twenty-five to thirty minutes.
16. Serve and enjoy!

NUTRITION FACTS:
Calories; 225kcal, carbs; 13.1g, protein; 10.9g, fat; 15.1g, fiber; 3.2g

400. CHICKEN FAJITA BOWLS

Preparation time: 10 minutes

Baking time: 30 minutes

Serving: 4

INGREDIENTS:
- Chili powder – two tsp
- Ground cumin – two tsp
- Salt – ¾ tsp
- Garlic powder – half tsp
- Smoked paprika – half tsp
- Ground pepper – ¼ tsp
- Olive oil – two tbsp
- Chicken tenders – 1 ¼ lbs
- Yellow onion – one, sliced
- Red bell pepper – one, sliced
- Green bell pepper – one, sliced
- Stemmed kale – four cup, chopped
- Black beans – 15 ounce, rinsed
- Plain Greek yogurt – ¼ cup, low-fat
- Lime juice – one tbsp
- Water – two tsp

DIRECTIONS:
1. Preheat the oven to 425°F-220°C.
2. Mix the ground pepper, paprika, garlic powder, half tsp salt, cumin, and chili powder into the bowl.
3. Transfer one tsp of the spice mixture to the bowl and keep it aside.
4. Whisk one tbsp oil into the remaining spice mixture into the big bowl.
5. Then, add green bell pepper, onion, and chicken and toss to combine.
6. Remove the pan from the oven. Place chicken mixture onto the pan and cook for fifteen minutes.
7. Mix the black beans, kale, one tbsp olive oil, and ¼ tsp into the bowl. Toss to combine.
8. When done, remove the pan from the oven. Add vegetables and chicken and stir well.
9. Place beans and kale over it and cook for five to seven minutes more.
10. During this, add water, lime juice, and yogurt to the spice mixture and stir well.
11. Place mixture into the four bowls.
12. Drizzle with yogurt dressing.

NUTRITION FACTS:
Calories; 343kcal, carbs; 23.7g, protein; 42.7g, fat; 9.9g, fiber; 8.2g

401. PUMPKIN SOUP

Preparation time: 5 minutes

Cooking time: 20 minutes

Serving: 4

INGREDIENTS:
- Olive oil – one tbsp
- Onion – ¼ cup, chopped
- Curry powder – one tbsp
- Pumpkin puree – 15 ounce
- Vegetable broth – two cups
- Maple syrup – two tbsp
- Salt – half tbsp
- Unsweetened coconut milk – 14 ounces
- Sour cream – four tsp, optional

DIRECTIONS:
1. Add oil into the pot and cook over medium flame.
2. Add onion and cook for five minutes until softened.
3. Add pumpkin puree and curry powder and stir well.
4. Add broth and whisk it well.
5. Add maple syrup and sprinkle with salt.
6. Let simmer for ten minutes.
7. Add soup in the blender and blend until smooth.
8. Place soup back to the pot and lower the heat.
9. Add coconut milk but do not boil it. Just heat it.
10. Top with sour cream.

NUTRITION FACTS:
Calories; 630kj, carbs; 4.1g, protein; 5.4g, fat; 6.1g, fiber; 3.4g

402. HIGH-FIBER DUMPLINGS

Preparation Time: 10 minutes

Cooking Time: 10 minutes

Servings: 8

INGREDIENTS:
- 200 g cream quark
- 60 g psyllium husks
- 10 g bamboo fibers

- 1 bowl Vegetable broth
- 2 eggs

DIRECTIONS:

1. Take a bowl and add the psyllium husks along with the bamboo fibers. Mix well with a spoon.
2. Put the eggs in the same bowl, add the cream curd and vegetable stock. Knead well, it's best done by hand. Alternatively, the kneading hooks of the mixer can be used.
3. Set a large saucepan with water and bring to a boil on the stove. In the meantime, moisten your hands with water and roll the dough into 12 balls.
4. Put the balls in the hot water and cook for 10 minutes, then serve. High-fiber vegetables like beans and matching sauces also taste great.

NUTRITION FACTS:

Calories: 75 Carbs: 0.1 g Protein: 13.4 g Fat: 1.7 g Sugar: 0 g Sodium: 253 mg

403. PIZZA MADE WITH BAMBOO FIBERS

Preparation Time: 10 minutes

Cooking Time: 20 minutes

Servings: 4

INGREDIENTS:

- 2 eggs
- 60 g bamboo fibers
- 80 g sour cream
- 40 g olive oil
- 150 g grated Gouda cheese
- Salt and pepper

DIRECTIONS:

1. First, preheat the oven to 360°F-180°C and cover a baking sheet with baking paper.
2. Take a bowl and beat in the eggs. Whisk briefly with a fork, then add the remaining ingredients and knead everything well. This is best done by hand, but you can also work with the dough hook on the mixer.
3. Finally, flavor with salt and pepper to taste, then place the dough on the baking tray and roll out evenly. If necessary, flour the dough with a little bamboo fiber so that the dough does not stick to the rolling pin.
4. Bake the tray for 10 minutes on the lower rack. The pizza base can now be topped with delicious low-carb foods, depending on your taste. Then bake for another 10 minutes on the lower rack and then enjoy hot.

NUTRITION FACTS:

Calories: 599 Fat: 19 g Carbs: 9 g Sugar: 4 g Fiber: 2 g Protein: 97 g

Sodium: 520 mg

404. VEGETARIAN HAMBURGERS

Preparation Time: 10 minutes

Cooking Time: 30 minutes

Servings: 4

INGREDIENTS:

- 90 g protein flour
- 120 ml egg white
- 100 g carrots, grated
- 2 tablespoons coconut oil
- 100 g low-fat quark
- 2 eggs
- 6 g baking powder
- 20 g gold linseed (alternatively other nuts and grains)
- Preferred spices (Worcester sauce, soy sauce, salt or chili)
- Preferred topping (tomatoes, cucumbers, radishes, ...)

DIRECTIONS:

1. First, preheat the oven to 360°F-180°C and line 6-7 muffin tins with paper cases.
2. Take a bowl and add 50 g of flour along with the egg white and carrots, and then stir well. Divide the dough into 6-7 parts and shape a meatball from each one.
3. Now, put 2 tablespoons of coconut oil in a non-stick pan and heat over medium heat until it has melted. Put the meatballs in the hot pan and fry vigorously on both sides.
4. Take a separate bowl, add the remaining flour along with the low-fat quark, eggs, baking powder and gold linseed.
5. Mix well, then pour into the prepared muffin cups. Bake in the oven for 25 minutes, let the finished rolls cool down well. Finally, cut the rolls in half with a sharp knife, top with a meatball of your choice and season. Then, skewer the finished burger with a toothpick and enjoy.

NUTRITION FACTS:

Calories: 178 Fat: 4 g Carbs: 7 g Fiber: 2 g Protein: 27 g

405. PORK STEAKS WITH AVOCADO

Preparation Time: 10 minutes

Cooking Time: 30 minutes

Servings: 8

INGREDIENTS:

For the salsa:
- 6 limes
- 3 tablespoons fruity olive oil
- 1 ½ dried chili pepper
- Salt and freshly ground pepper
- 2 mangoes (ripe, but still firm)
- 2 shallots
- 2 avocados
- A bunch of coriander

For the steaks:
- 4 pork neck steaks (approximately 150 g each)
- 1 teaspoon ground anise
- 1 teaspoon ground cumin
- Salt
- freshly ground pepper
- 2 tablespoons clarified butter

DIRECTIONS:

For the salsa:
1. Halve the limes and squeeze them thoroughly, measure out 10 tablespoons of lime juice. Place in a small bowl.
2. Add olive oil and stir well with a whisker. Crumble the chili pepper and mix into the dressing together with salt and pepper.
3. Now, peel the mangoes with a vegetable peeler, remove the stone and dice the pulp. Finely chop the shallots with a sharp knife.
4. Take a separate bowl, add the mangoes and shallots; stir well.
5. Remove the stone and skin from the avocados, dice the meat and then fill the mango mixture. Immediately, pour the dressing over it so that the avocado doesn't tarnish. Mix gently.
6. Finally, wash the coriander thoroughly under running water and dry it carefully. Remove the tender leaves and also add to the salsa. Mix again.

For the steaks:
1. Preheat the oven to 140°F-60°C. Rinse the steaks under running water and dry them carefully with a little kitchen roll. Sprinkle the anise, cumin, salt and pepper over them. Place the clarified butter in a pan and heat over medium heat until melted. Set the steaks in the hot pan and fry briefly while turning for 3 minutes.
2. Put the steaks on a piece of aluminum foil and seal it tightly around the steak. Place in the oven and let rest briefly for 3 minutes.
3. Arrange on a plate with the meat juice and salsa. Enjoy immediately!

NUTRITION FACTS:

Calories: 303 Fat: 14 g Carbs: 15 g Sugar: 10 g Fiber: 2 g Protein: 30 g Sodium: 387 mg

406. CHICKEN WITH ASPARAGUS SALAD

Preparation Time: 10 minutes

Cooking Time: 30 minutes

Servings: 4

INGREDIENTS:
- 800 g green asparagus
- 1/2 bunch spring onions
- 3 tablespoons white wine vinegar
- Salt
- Pepper
- 1 teaspoon mustard
- 1/2 teaspoon honey
- 8 tablespoons olive oil
- 4 chicken breast fillets (approximately 200 g each)
- 250 g sliced breakfast bacon
- 2 tablespoons clarified butter
- Basil leaves for garnishing

DIRECTIONS:
1. First, preheat the oven to 360°F-180°C and place baking paper on a baking sheet.
2. Take the asparagus and peel only the bottom stick.
3. Remove the woody ends, then wash thoroughly. Halve the asparagus lengthways and cut so that oblique pieces are created. Now, wash the spring onions and cut them into large pieces.
4. Take a bowl, pour the white wine vinegar into it. Also, attach 2 tablespoons of water along with mustard, honey, salt and pepper. Stir well.
5. Finally, slowly add 6 tablespoons of olive oil, spoon by spoon. Stir.
6. Take the meat, rinse under running water and dry with a little kitchen roll, then season with salt and pepper on both sides.
7. Take the bacon slices and wrap the meat in them.
8. Put the clarified butter in a non-stick pan and heat over medium fire until the fat has melted. Set the chicken breasts in the hot pan, first placing them to the point where the ends of the bacon slice meet. Turn after 2 minutes and fry again briefly for 2 minutes.
9. Remove from the pan and place on the tray so that the meat can cook in the oven for another 15 minutes.
10. In the meantime, set the remaining olive oil in a pan and heat over medium fire. Put the vegetables in the hot oil and fry briefly. Meanwhile, salt and pepper. After 4 minutes, take the vegetables out of the pan and add them to the vinegar mixture, mix well.
11. Finally, arrange the meat with the asparagus salad on a plate and enjoy immediately.

NUTRITION FACTS:

Calories: 315 Fat: 9 g Carbs: 30 g Sugar: 6 g Fiber: 4 g Protein: 28 g Sodium: 677 mg

 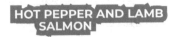

HOT PEPPER AND LAMB SALMON

Preparation Time: 10 minutes

Cooking Time: 20 minutes

Servings: 6

INGREDIENTS:

For the Meat:
- 700 g lamb salmon
- 2 garlic cloves
- 1/2 bunch mint
- 2 sprigs rosemary
- 1/2 bunch oregano
- 10 peppercorns
- 4 tablespoons olive oil
- Salt
- Pepper

For the Peperonat:
- 1 small zucchini
- 2 red peppers
- 2 yellow peppers
- 1 onion
- 3 garlic cloves
- 3 tomatoes
- 1 chili pepper
- 3 tablespoon small capers
- 2 tablespoons olive oil
- Salt
- Pepper
- 2 tablespoons chopped parsley

DIRECTIONS:

For the Meat:
1. First, rinse the meat under running water and dry it with a little kitchen roll, then carefully remove the tendons and fat. Peel and cut the garlic to make fine slices.
2. Wash the rosemary, oregano and mint, pat dry carefully. Then, chop the leaves and needles (not too fine). Put the peppercorns in the mortar and press lightly. Take a bowl, add the herbs and peppercorns.
3. Attach 2 tablespoons of olive oil and stir well, then rub the meat with the mixture. Finally, wrap it in foil and refrigerate for 4 hours.
4. Preheat the oven to 70°C, placing a baking dish in it that will be used for the meat later.
5. Now, take the meat and remove the marinade with the back of a knife, then season with salt and pepper. Set the remaining oil in a pan and heat over medium fire.
6. Place the meat in the hot oil and fry briefly while turning for 2 minutes. Put it in the pan into the oven and cook for another 40 minutes.

For the Peperonata:
1. Wash the zucchini thoroughly and dice with the skin. Halve and core the peppers, wash them too. Cut so that narrow strips are created. First, peel the onion and garlic then process into fine cubes.
2. Score the tomatoes, pour hot water, at that time peel them and remove the seeds. Cut the pulp into small pieces. Alternatively, canned tomatoes can also be used here. Halve and core the chili pepper, wash it well and cut into small pieces. Finally, rinse the capers in a sieve and let them drain.
3. Now, pour olive oil over the pan and heat over medium fire. Put the onion in the hot oil and fry briefly, then add the peppers, zucchini, garlic and chili. Cook for 5 minutes, stirring evenly. Attach tomatoes and season with salt and pepper.
4. Let everything fry for 10 minutes, stir in the capers and cook for another 5 minutes.

NUTRITION FACTS:

Calories: 599 Fat: 19 g Carbs: 9 g Sugar: 4 g Fiber: 2 g Protein: 97 g Sodium: 520 mg

 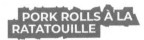

PORK ROLLS À LA RATATOUILLE

Preparation Time: 10 minutes

Cooking Time: 30 minutes

Servings: 8

INGREDIENTS:

For the Ratatouille:
- 2 yellow peppers
- 2 red peppers
- 2 small zucchini
- 2 red onions
- 3 garlic cloves
- 250 g cherry tomatoes
- A bunch of thyme
- 3 tablespoons olive oil
- Salt
- Freshly ground pepper
- 250 ml vegetable stock
- 3 tablespoons tomato paste

For the Pork Rolls:
- 2 bunches basil
- 30 g Parmesan cheese
- 30 g pine nuts
- 5 tablespoons olive oil
- Salt
- Freshly ground pepper
- 75 g sun-dried tomatoes in oil
- 8 small pork schnitzel (approximately 75 g each)

DIRECTIONS:

For the Ratatouille:
1. First, preheat the oven to 360°F-180°C.
2. Halve and core the peppers, wash thoroughly and cut so that narrow strips are formed.
3. Wash the zucchini as well, then cut into cubes with the skin on. First, peel the onion and garlic then cut into strips. Clean the tomatoes thoroughly, cut them in half.
4. Rinse the thyme under running water and pat dry carefully, remove the leaves. Take a bowl, add the vegetables with the thyme and mix well.
5. Flavor with salt, pepper and olive oil; mix again. Take the frying pan from the oven and distribute the

vegetable mixture in it. Bake for 20 minutes.

For the Pork Rolls:
1. Now, rinse the basil with water and shake dry, pluck the leaves and chop finely. Coarsely or finely grate the Parmesan with the grater to taste.
2. Take a small pan, add the pine nuts and briefly toast them without adding any further fat, then put them in the blender. Also, add half of the chopped basil along with the Parmesan and 3 tablespoons of olive oil. Puree everything into a pesto, then season with salt and pepper.
3. Wash the tomatoes and cut them to make strips. Clean the pork as well, dry it with a little kitchen roll and then plate with a meat tenderizer or a saucepan. Sprinkle with salt and pepper, spread some pesto on top.
4. Spread the sun-dried tomatoes and the remaining basil on top, roll into roulades and set. Add the remaining oil to a pan and heat over medium fire, place the rolls in the hot oil and fry on all sides for 5 minutes.
5. Take a small bowl, add the vegetable stock and tomato paste. Stir.
6. Add the cherry tomatoes and the mixture to the cooked vegetables in the oven. Put the meat on it and bake for another 15 minutes. Enjoy served on a plate with the remaining pesto.

NUTRITION FACTS:

Calories: 280 Fat: 16 Carbs: 5 g Sugar: 1 g Fiber: 0 g Protein: 29 g

409. PEPPER FILLET WITH LEEK

Preparation Time: 10 minutes

Cooking Time: 30 minutes

Servings: 8

INGREDIENTS:

For the Vegetables:
- 50 g sun-dried tomatoes
- 100 g pine nuts
- 4 large leeks
- 2 tablespoon raisins
- 2 cups Peppercorns
- 2 tablespoons olive oil
- Salt
- Freshly ground pepper

For the Meat:
- 2 tablespoons black pepper
- 4 tablespoons sesame seeds
- 1 teaspoon salt
- 4 sprigs rosemary
- 4 beef fillet steaks (approximately 180 g each)
- 4 tablespoons sunflower oil

DIRECTIONS:

1. Place the tomatoes in a heat-resistant bowl and pour boiling water over them. Let stand for 10 minutes, then take out the tomatoes and chop with a sharp knife.
2. Now, put the pine nuts in a small pan and briefly toast them without adding any further fat, stirring well. Set aside and wash the leek thoroughly and cut so that rings are formed. Rinse the raisins under cold running water.
3. Take a non-stick pan and pour in olive oil. Heat on high and add the leek. Saute briefly, add tomatoes and raisins over low heat and stir well. Cook for 10 minutes, season with salt and pepper. Add the pine nuts then carefully stir in.
4. At the same time, put the peppercorns in the mortar and coarsely crush them, stir in a small bowl with salt and sesame seeds.
5. Rinse off the rosemary and steaks then dry them with a little paper towel. Place the steaks with the edges in the pepper mixture so that the spices stick to the edges.
6. Now, heat oil in a non-stick pan on a high level and sear the meat on both sides for 3 minutes. Immediately, wrap in a piece of aluminum foil, covering a sprig of rosemary with it.
7. After resting for 5 minutes, remove the steaks and arrange on a plate with the leek vegetables. Garnish with meat juice and enjoy instantly.

NUTRITION FACTS:

Calories: 504 Fat: 39 g Carbs: 10 g Sugar: 1 g Fiber: 2 g Protein: 28 g Sodium: 75mg

410. LAMB CHOPS WITH BEANS

Preparation Time: 10 minutes

Cooking Time: 50 minutes

Servings: 8

INGREDIENTS:

- 1 kg lamb chops
- 2 lemons juice
- Salt
- Pepper
- 150 ml olive oil (approximately)
- 6 garlic cloves
- 6 sprigs rosemary
- 6 sprigs thyme
- 2 onions
- 12 cocktail tomatoes
- 300 g green beans
- 2 shallots
- 70 g bacon
- 2 teaspoons butter
- Savory to taste

DIRECTIONS:

1. First, rinse the lamb chops briefly under running water and carefully dry them with a little kitchen roll. Pour the lemon juice into a small bowl, add 100 ml of olive oil, salt and pepper; stir well. Take the garlic and remove the peel. Cut so that thin slices are formed, also add to the lemon marinade.
2. Now, put the marinade together with the chops in a freezer bag, squeeze out the air and seal.
3. Set aside for at least 2 hours and let it soak in.
4. Preheat the oven to 360°F-180°C. Rinse the rosemary, thyme and pat dry. Take a baking dish and grease it with olive oil. Spread the herb sprigs in it.
5. Add the onions and cut into 4 parts, place them in the mold as well. Wash the tomatoes thoroughly and cut in half depending on the size, then add to the onions.
6. Set the meat out of the marinade and place it on top of the vegetables. Spread the soak and a little olive oil on top. Bake on the middle rack for 40 minutes.
7. In the meantime, take the beans and cut the ends, then wash. Set the water to a boil in a saucepan, season with salt and add the beans. Cook for 8 minutes. Meanwhile, take the shallots and remove the skin, cut into small cubes. Finely dice the bacon as well.
8. Put the butter in a pan and heat over medium fire until it has melted.
9. Place the shallots and bacon in the hot oil and fry until everything takes on a brown color.
10. Add the beans with a little savory, stir well.
11. Salt and pepper, then serve with the lamb and the bed of vegetables. Enjoy hot.

NUTRITION FACTS:

Calories: 413 Fat: 20 g Carbs: 7 g Sugar: 1 g Fiber: 1 g Protein: 50 g Sodium: 358 mg

411. FILLET OF BEEF ON SPRING VEGETABLES

Preparation Time: 10 minutes

Cooking Time: 30 minutes

Servings: 8

INGREDIENTS:

- 500 g green asparagus
- 2 bulbs kohlrabi
- 1 bunch flat-leaf parsley
- 1 bunch tarragon
- Salt
- Pepper
- 4 beef fillet steaks (approximately 150 g each)
- 4 tablespoons olive oil
- 300 ml cream

DIRECTIONS:

1. Wash the asparagus, peel only the bottom stick with the vegetable peeler. Divide off the woody ends, then cut the asparagus in half. Now, peel the kohlrabi with the knife, cut so that narrow sticks are formed.
2. Rinse the herbs under running water, dry them carefully and remove the leaves. Finely chop with a sharp knife. Take a bowl, pour in 2/3 of the herbs, set aside the rest for now.
3. After that, add the vegetables to the herbs in the bowl, season with salt and pepper and mix well. Put the mixture in a roasting tube (must be closed on one side).
4. Take a large saucepan, pour water up to 1/3 full. Set on the stove and bring to a boil.
5. In the meantime, rinse the steaks with water and dry them carefully with a little kitchen roll.
6. Season with salt and pepper on both sides. Put the oil in a pan and heat over medium fire.
7. Set the meat in the hot oil and fry briefly on all sides for 3 minutes. Place it on the vegetables in the roasting tube.
8. Pour the oil out of the pan and add in the cream. Bring to the boil briefly so that the roasting loosens, then pour over the meat in the roasting tube.
9. Now, close the hose and add it to the boiling water. Cook gently over low heat and cover for 12 minutes.
10. Finally, arrange the meat with the bed of vegetables on a plate and garnish with the remaining herbs.

NUTRITION FACTS:

Calories: 209 Fat: 10 g Carbs: 21 g Sugar: 13 g Fiber: 8 g Protein: 11 g Sodium: 644 mg

 412. BOLOGNESE WITH ZUCCHINI NOODLES

Preparation Time: 10 minutes

Cooking Time: 50 minutes

Servings: 4-8

INGREDIENTS:

- 4 zucchini (approximately 200 g each)
- Salt
- 1 onion
- 3 garlic cloves
- 2 tablespoons coconut oil
- 4 tablespoons tomato paste
- 3 tablespoons balsamic vinegar
- 600 g chunky tomatoes (canned)
- 4 sprigs rosemary
- 1 handful basil leaves
- 1/2 tbsp. Dried oregano
- 1/4 tsp. Dried thyme
- Freshly ground black pepper
- 600 g mixed minced meat
- 2 tablespoons olive oil

DIRECTIONS:

1. First, wash the zucchini and cut them into thin, narrow slices.
2. For preparing the Bolognese, peel the onion and garlic; cut into fine cubes. Set the oil in a saucepan and heat over medium fire. Put the onion in the hot oil and fry until it becomes translucent.
3. Stir well and fry briefly before adding the tomato paste. Cook them together again, pour in the balsamic vinegar until the bottom can no longer be seen. Bring to a boil, add the tomatoes.
4. Wash the rosemary, and basil then dry them carefully. Pluck the needles and leaves, chop and add to the Bolognese. Season with the remaining herbs to taste.
5. Reduce the heat and simmer gently for 30 minutes before stirring in the minced meat. Cook for another 15 minutes, then cook over high heat for 5 minutes.
6. At the same time, attach olive oil to the zucchini noodles and mix well.
7. Put the oiled zucchini in a pan and cook only briefly over medium heat without becoming too soft.
8. Arrange with the Bolognese on a plate and enjoy hot.

NUTRITION FACTS:

Calories: 75 Carbs: 0.1 g Protein: 13.4 g Fat: 1.7 g Sugar: 0 g Sodium: 253 mg

 413. CHICKEN WITH CHICKPEAS

Preparation Time: 10 minutes

Cooking Time: 30 minutes

Servings: 4

INGREDIENTS:

- 12 sun-dried tomatoes in oil
- 2 garlic cloves
- 2 zucchini
- 500 g chickpeas (canned, drained weight)
- 4 tablespoons olive oil
- 100 ml poultry stock
- 2 bags saffron threads
- Salt
- Freshly ground black pepper
- 1/4 teaspoon ground coriander
- 4 chicken breasts (approximately 200 g each)
- 1 tbsp. Ras el Hanout

DIRECTIONS:

1. First, get the sun-dried tomatoes out of the oil and dry them with a little kitchen roll, then cut them so that narrow strips are formed.
2. Take the garlic, remove the skin and cut into slices.
3. Wash the zucchini and cut into cubes with the skin on.
4. Rinse the chickpeas in a colander and drain well.
5. Set a saucepan, add 2 tablespoons of olive oil. Warmth on medium heat, add the tomatoes with garlic to the hot oil. Fry briefly for 1 minute.
6. Place the zucchini with chickpeas, stir well and fry briefly together before deglazing with the broth. Add saffron threads, coriander, salt and pepper. Bring to a boil.
7. Set the heat, cover the saucepan and let the vegetables simmer for 5 minutes.
8. In the meantime, rinse the meat under running water and dry it with a little kitchen roll. Set the remaining oil in a pan and heat over medium fire.
9. For now, sprinkle the meat on both sides with salt, pepper and Ras el Hanout, then add to the hot oil and fry for 7 minutes, turning.
10. Serve the meat with the vegetables on a large plate and enjoy hot.

NUTRITION FACTS:

Calories: 329 Fat: 17 g Carbs: 9 g Sugar: 3 g Fiber: 5 g Protein: 37 g Sodium: 430 mg

414. HAM WITH CHICORY

Preparation Time: 10 minutes

Cooking Time: 30 minutes

Servings: 4-8

INGREDIENTS:

- 4 sprigs chicory (approximately 200 g each)
- 150 g Emmental cheese
- 8 sage leaves
- 40 g butter
- 3 tablespoons orange juice
- Salt
- Pepper
- 8 slices Black Forest ham

DIRECTIONS:

1. First, preheat the oven to 400°F-200°C.
2. Wash and clean the chicory and cut it lengthways in half. Remove the stalk with a knife.
3. Shred the cheese coarsely or finely with a grater to taste.
4. Rinse the sage leaves under running water and gently shake dry.
5. Put the butter in a pan and heat over medium fire. Extinguish with orange juice and so froth the butter. Add the sage.
6. Place the chicory with the cut side in the hot oil. Reduce the heat and fry for 5 minutes.
7. Remove the chicory, cover with a sage leaf and sprinkle with salt and pepper.
8. Chop the ham and put it on the

baking dish. Sprinkle with cheese and drizzle with liquid orange and butter. Bake in the oven for 20 minutes, then serve hot.

NUTRITION FACTS:

Calories: 75 Carbs: 0.1 g Protein: 13.4 g Fat: 1.7 g Sugar: 0 g Sodium: 253 mg

415. PORK MEDALLIONS WITH ASPARAGUS AND COCONUT CURRY

Preparation Time: 10 minutes

Cooking Time: 30 minutes

Servings: 4-8

INGREDIENTS:

- 1 kg white asparagus
- 500 g carrots
- 2 onions
- 1 red chili pepper
- 40 g butter
- 3-4 tablespoons curry powder
- 250 ml vegetable stock
- 400 ml coconut milk
- 2–3 tablespoons lime juice
- Salt
- Pepper
- 1 tablespoon chopped coriander
- 4 pork medallions (125 g each)
- 2-3 tablespoons oil

DIRECTIONS:

1. First, peel the asparagus and remove the woody ends, wash well and cut into bite-sized pieces. Then, peel the carrots, wash and cut them into slices. Now, take the onions, remove the skin and cut them into cubes. Divide the chili in half, take out the seeds and carefully dice.
2. Put the butter in a pan and heat over medium fire until it has melted.
3. Put the onions and chili in the hot oil and saute until translucent. Add asparagus, carrots and fry everything for 5 minutes, stirring regularly.
4. Pour the curry over it and fry briefly before adding the broth. Set the heat, cover the saucepan and simmer for 15 minutes.
5. Add in the coconut milk and cook for 3 more minutes. Pour in lime juice, salt and pepper to taste. Sprinkle on 1/2 tablespoon of coriander; stir well.
6. Now, take the meat and season with salt and pepper on both sides. Put the oil in a pan and heat over medium fire.
7. Place the medallions in the hot oil and fry briefly on both sides for about 3-5 minutes.
8. Arrange medallions with curry on a plate, garnish with coriander and serve hot.

NUTRITION FACTS:

Calories: 432 Fat: 12 g Carbs: 12 g Sugar: 5 g Fiber: 3 g Protein: 57 g Sodium: 566 mg

416. LAMB WITH CARROT AND BRUSSELS SPROUTS SPAGHETTI

Preparation Time: 10 minutes

Cooking Time: 30 minutes

Servings: 4-8

INGREDIENTS:

- 250 g Brussels sprouts
- 300 g carrots
- 5 tablespoons sesame oil
- 3 tablespoons soy sauce
- 1 lime juice
- A pinch of sugar
- Salt
- 600 g loosened saddle of lamb
- Pepper
- 2 tablespoons butter
- 2 tablespoons sesame seeds

DIRECTIONS:

1. First, preheat the oven to 210°F-100°C.
2. Take the Brussels sprouts, wash and clean. Then, cut them into strips.
3. For preparing the marinade, place 3 tablespoons of sesame oil together with soy sauce, sugar, salt and lime juice in a bowl; merge well.
4. Put the vegetable spaghetti in the marinade and let it steep for a moment.
5. In the meantime, flavor the lamb with salt and pepper. Pour the remaining oil into a coated pan and heat on high.
6. Set the meat in the hot oil and sear it on all sides, then put it in the oven and let it cook gently for 10 minutes.
7. After that, melt the butter in the same pan and fry the marinated vegetables for about 3-4 minutes. Arrange on a plate with the sliced lamb and garnish with sesame seeds.

NUTRITION FACTS:

Calories: 270 Fat: 11 g Carbs: 4 g Sugar: 1 g Fiber: 1 g Protein: 39 g Sodium: 664 mg

417. CABBAGE WRAP

Preparation Time: 10 minutes

Cooking Time: 30 minutes

Servings: 4-8

INGREDIENTS:

- 1 head white cabbage
- Salt
- 100 ml milk
- 1 roll (from the day before)
- 350 g mixed minced meat
- 1 egg freshly ground pepper
- 2 tablespoons clarified butter
- 250 ml meat stock
- 1 tablespoon flour
- 4 tablespoons cream

DIRECTIONS:

1. First, separate the large outer leaves (12-16 pieces) from the cabbage and cut out the strong leaf veins with a knife. Set a saucepan with water and bring to a boil. Salt well and add the large cabbage leaves with the rest of the cabbage. Cook everything for 5-10 minutes.
2. Heat the milk in a saucepan. Put the roll on it and soak for a few minutes.
3. Squeeze out the bun and place in a bowl. Also add the minced meat, egg, pepper and salt. Mix everything well until a batter is formed.
4. Cut the cooked cabbage (not the large leaves) and add to the dough, mix again.
5. Take 3-4 cabbage leaves and stack them on top of each other. Spread some batter on top, then roll the leaves and fix with toothpicks, roulade needles, or kitchen twine.
6. Put the clarified butter in a pan and heat over medium fire until it melts. Then, place the cabbage rolls in the hot oil and fry them lightly brown.
7. Extinguish with the broth, cover the pan and simmer the cabbage rolls over low heat for 25 minutes. Take out the cabbage rolls and briefly keep them warm.
8. Now, stir in the flour in a little cream and add everything to the sauce. Bring to a boil briefly.
9. Arrange on plates with the cabbage rolls.

NUTRITION FACTS:

Calories: 329 Fat: 17 g Carbs: 9 g Sugar: 3 g Fiber: 5 g Protein: 37 g

418. VEAL WITH ASPARAGUS

Preparation Time: 10 minutes

Cooking Time: 30 minutes

Servings: 4-8

INGREDIENTS:

- 800 g green asparagus
- Salt
- 3-4 tablespoons rapeseed oil
- A pinch of sugar
- Pepper
- 1/2 fresh lemon zest, grated
- Oil for frying
- 8 slices veal from the back (60 g each)
- 8 slices Parma ham
- 8 sage leaves
- 125 ml white wine
- 1 tablespoon butter

DIRECTIONS:

1. First, peel the lower part of the sticks with a vegetable peeler, then remove the woody ends. Wash the asparagus thoroughly.
2. At the same time, fill a saucepan with water and bring it to a boil. Salt well, add the asparagus, and cook for 8 minutes, they must not become too soft. Drain them and rinse directly with ice water.
3. Place the asparagus on a piece of kitchen roll to dry, then put them in a baking dish.
4. Take a small bowl and add the oil, salt, pepper, sugar 0and lemon zest. Mix everything well and pour over the asparagus stalks. Let sit in the marinade for 25 minutes.
5. Put the oil in a pan and heat over medium fire. Detach the asparagus from the marinade and place them in the hot oil. Fry while turning.
6. Now, pepper the meat and cover it with Parma ham and a sage leaf. Secure everything with a toothpick.
7. Put the oil in a pan, heat it and place the meat in it. Fry briefly on medium heat and turning for 3 minutes.
8. Serve with the asparagus on a plate. Extinguish the now-empty pan with white wine so that the roasting residue dissolves, then stir in the butter and briefly bring to a boil.
9. Pour the sauce over the asparagus and meat. Enjoy hot.

NUTRITION FACTS:

Calories: 599 Fat: 19 g Carbs: 9 g
Sugar: 4 g Fiber: 2 g Protein: 97 g
Sodium: 520 mg

419. SALMON WITH SESAME SEEDS AND MUSHROOMS

Preparation Time: 10 minutes

Cooking Time: 30 minutes

Servings: 4-8

INGREDIENTS:

- 500 g salmon fillet
- 4 tablespoons fish sauce
- 200 g mushrooms
- 400 g fresh spinach leaves
- 2 tablespoons vegetable oil
- 2 tablespoons sesame oil
- 1 tablespoon sesame seeds
- 1 teaspoon sambal oelek

DIRECTIONS:

1. First, take the salmon, rinse under running water, dry with a little kitchen roll, and then cut so that strips are formed. Take a bowl, pour in the fish sauce. Soak the salmon in the sauce for 10 minutes.
2. In the meantime, it is best to carefully clean the mushrooms with a brush, cut them to make slices. Rinse and dry the spinach under the tap.
3. Now, take a wok, add the vegetable and sesame oil. Heat on high, add the mushrooms to the hot oil, and fry briefly. Put the spinach in the wok and fry until it collapses.
4. Now, move the vegetables away from the center to the edge of the wok and reduce the heat.
5. Place the salmon on the resulting surface and fry gently while turning.
6. Arrange it with the vegetables on a plate, carefully refine with sambal oelek to taste.

NUTRITION FACTS:

Calories: 599 Fat: 19 g Carbs: 9 g
Sugar: 4 g Fiber: 2 g Protein: 97 g
Sodium: 520 mg

420. STUFFED TROUT WITH MUSHROOMS

Preparation Time: 10 minutes

Cooking Time: 30 minutes

Servings: 4-8

INGREDIENTS:

- 4 ready-to-cook trout
- 1 lemon juice
- Salt
- Pepper
- 1/2 bunch dill
- 500 g mushrooms
- 2 tablespoons butter
- 2 tablespoons freshly chopped parsley
- 3 tablespoons chopped almonds
- 4 tablespoons oil

DIRECTIONS:

1. First, preheat the oven to 425°F-220°C.
2. Take the lemon juice and use it to drizzle the trout inside and out. Wash the dill, shake dry and chop.
3. Salt and pepper the trout and refine each with 1 tablespoon of dill. It is best to carefully clean the mushrooms with a brush and cut them into slices.
4. Then, put them in a bowl. Also add the butter, almonds and parsley. Stir everything well.
5. Now, distribute the filling over the trout's abdominal cavities. Fix the abdomen with wooden skewers, wrap the trout well in aluminum foil coated with oil. Let it cook in the oven for 20 minutes.
6. Finally, put the fish on a plate and enjoy hot.

NUTRITION FACTS:

Calories: 413 Fat: 20 g Carbs: 7 g
Sugar: 1 g Fiber: 1 g Protein: 50 g
Sodium: 358 mg

421. SALMON WITH BASIL AND AVOCADO

Preparation Time: 10 minutes

Cooking Time: 30 minutes

Servings: 4-8

INGREDIENTS:

- 1 avocado
- 1 teaspoon pickled capers
- 3 garlic cloves
- A handful of basil leaves
- 1 tablespoon fresh lemon zest
- 4 salmon fillets (approximately 200 g each)
- Coconut oil for greasing the tray

DIRECTIONS:

1. Preheat the oven at 360°F-180°C and use a brush to spread coconut oil on a baking sheet.
2. Divide the avocado in half, then remove the core and skin.
3. Mash the pulp with a fork in a small bowl.
4. Put the capers in a colander and drain, chop finely.
5. Peel the garlic cloves and mash them with a press. Alternatively, chop them very finely with a sharp knife.
6. Then, wash the basil and shake it dry, pluck the leaves off and chop them too.
7. Attach everything to the avocado in the bowl, refine with lemon zest and mix well.
8. Wash the salmon, dry with a little kitchen roll, and place on the baking sheet. It is best to spread the avocado mixture over the fish with a spoon.
9. Put the tray in the oven and bake briefly for 10 minutes. Switch on the grill function and bake for another 4 minutes until the avocado takes on a light brown color.
10. Set the salmon fillets on a plate and enjoy hot.

NUTRITION FACTS:

Calories: 209 Fat: 10 g Carbs: 21 g
Sugar: 13 g Fiber: 8 g Protein: 11 g
Sodium: 644 mg

422. LEEK QUICHE WITH OLIVES

Preparation Time: 10 minutes

Cooking Time: 30 minutes

Servings: 4-8

INGREDIENTS:

- 140 g almonds
- 40 g walnuts
- 25 g coconut oil
- 1 teaspoon salt
- 1 leek
- 50 g spinach
- 2 sprigs rosemary
- 40 g fresh basil
- 30 g pine nuts
- 4 tablespoons extra-virgin olive oil
- 2 tablespoons lime juice

- 1/2 garlic clove
- 50 g pitted black olives
- 1 teaspoon red pepper berries

DIRECTIONS:

1. First, coarsely grind the almonds and walnuts in a food processor or blender, then put them in a small bowl together with the coconut oil and 1/2 teaspoon of salt.
2. Merge thoroughly, pour the mixture into a cake springform pan. Press the dough with your fingers at the same time and distribute it in the mold so that a border of 4 cm high is created. Put it in the freezer for 15 minutes.
3. Now, wash the leek, spinach and herbs, then pat dry. Slice the leek and place it in a bowl.
4. Stir in the remaining salt and set aside to draw.
5. Meanwhile, put the basil, pine nuts, olive oil, and lime juice in a blender. Pulse until you have a creamy puree.
6. Alternatively, a large mixing vessel or a hand blender can also be used here.
7. Now, peel the garlic clove and chop half. Remove the needles from the rosemary and also finely chop them.
8. Cut the spinach into narrow strips and halve the olives.
9. Add everything to the leek in the bowl, and then add the basil puree. Mix well.
10. Distribute the mixture to the base of the springform pan, sprinkle the pepper berries over it. Finally, cut the quiche into pieces and enjoy.

NUTRITION FACTS:

Calories: 270 Fat: 11 g Carbs: 4 g Sugar: 1 g Fiber: 1 g Protein: 39 g Sodium: 664 mg

 FRIED EGG ON ONIONS WITH SAGE

Preparation Time: 10 minutes

Cooking Time: 30 minutes

Servings: 4-8

INGREDIENTS:

- 275 g onions
- 1/2 bunch sage
- 3 tablespoons clarified butter
- 1 ½ tablespoon coconut flour
- Salt
- 1 teaspoon sweet paprika powder
- 8 eggs
- Freshly ground black pepper

DIRECTIONS:

1. First, remove the skin from the onions, then cut into thin rings. Rinse the sage under running water, pat dry and remove the leaves.
- Now, put 1 ½ tablespoon of clarified butter in a pan and heat over medium fire until it has melted. Place the sage leaves in the hot oil and fry until they are crispy. Place on kitchen paper to drain.
- Meanwhile, put the remaining clarified butter in the same pan and heat it, then place the onion rings in it.
- Scatter the coconut flour on top and fry for 10 minutes, stirring at regular intervals. Sprinkle salt and paprika too.
- Take the eggs and beat them one by one on the onions in the pan. Let the eggs sink to the bottom of the pan, if necessary use a wooden spoon to help.
- Now, cover the pan and fry everything for 10 minutes until the eggs are completely set.
- Arrange the fried eggs with the onions on flat plates, season with salt and pepper. Garnish with the roasted sage.

NUTRITION FACTS:

Calories: 179 Fat: 13 g Carbs: 6 g Sugar: 3 g Fiber: 1 g Protein: 10 g Sodium: 265 mg

 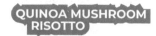 **QUINOA MUSHROOM RISOTTO**

Preparation Time: 10 minutes

Cooking Time: 30 minutes

Servings: 4-8

INGREDIENTS:

- 1 garlic clove
- 30 g hazelnuts
- Salt
- 1 fresh lemon zest, grated
- 2 shallots
- 650 g small mushrooms
- 1 bunch flat-leaf parsley
- 70 g quinoa
- 2 tablespoons olive oil
- Pepper
- 100 g baby spinach
- 30 g grated Parmesan cheese
- 20 g butter
- Red pepper to taste
- 500 ml hot water

DIRECTIONS:

1. First, peel the garlic clove and put it in a blender. Also add the hazelnuts, lemon zest and a little salt; mix until everything is finely ground. Put aside.
2. Peel the shallots, then cut them into fine cubes. It is best to carefully clean the mushrooms with a brush, chop them so that thin slices are formed.
3. Rinse and dab the parsley under running water, remove the leaves and chop with a sharp knife.
4. Put the quinoa in a colander and wash well under the tap; drain thoroughly.
5. Pour olive oil into a non-stick pan and warmth over medium heat. Put the shallots in it and fry until they turn slightly brown.
6. Add the mushrooms to the shallots and fry them together until they turn brown. Attach the quinoa, but at the same time pour in the hot water. Season with salt and pepper, stir well.
7. Cook over low heat until all the water has boiled away. The quinoa should be soft.
8. Now, add the parsley, spinach, Parmesan and butter; stir thoroughly.
9. Salt and pepper again and set with garlic and the hazelnut mixture.
10. Arrange on a plate and serve garnished with red pepper if necessary.

NUTRITION FACTS:

Calories: 166 Fat: 10 g Carbs: 17 g Sugar: 12 g Fiber: 2 g Protein: 7 g Sodium: 892 mg

425. VEGETARIAN LENTIL STEW

Preparation Time: 10 minutes

Cooking Time: 30 minutes

Servings: 4

INGREDIENTS:

- 50 g carrots
- 30 g parsnip or parsley root
- 30 g celery
- 1 leek
- 1 yellow pepper
- 250 g red lentils
- 1 ½ teaspoon ground cumin
- 3 tablespoons balsamic vinegar
- 3 tablespoons walnut oil
- 2-3 tablespoons maple syrup
- Salt and pepper
- A pinch of cayenne pepper
- 1/2 bunch flat-leaf parsley

DIRECTIONS:

1. Measure 1000 ml of water and pour into a saucepan. Warmth on high heat until boil.
2. In the meantime, cut the peppers in half, remove the seeds and wash them together with the leek. Peel the carrots, parsnips and celery.
3. Process everything into fine cubes, only use the white part of the leek.
4. Pour everything into the boiling water and bring to a boil. Then, add the lentils. Cook for 10 minutes, or until they are soft.
5. Ideally, most of the liquid has boiled away, if necessary drain. Season with cumin, balsamic vinegar, maple syrup, walnut oil, salt and pepper. Add the cayenne pepper to taste.
6. Turn off the stove and set the

vegetarian lentils stew aside briefly to steep.
7. In the meantime, rinse the parsley under the tap, pat dry, pluck the leaves off and sprinkle them into the stew.
8. Arrange in deep plates and enjoy hot.

NUTRITION FACTS:

Calories: 413 Fat: 20 g Carbs: 7 g Sugar: 1 g Fiber: 1 g Protein: 50 g Sodium: 358 mg

426. LEMON CHICKEN SOUP WITH BEANS

Preparation Time: 10 minutes

Cooking Time: 50 minutes

Servings: 4

INGREDIENTS:

- 1 onion
- 6 garlic cloves
- 600 g chicken breast
- 3 tablespoons olive oil
- 1 chicken broth
- 1 fresh lemon
- 250 g cooked white beans (canned)
- Salt
- Pepper
- 120 g Feta
- A bunch of chives

DIRECTIONS:

1. First, peel the onion, then the garlic cloves. Divide the onion in half and cut it into thin slices.
2. Rinse the meat under running water and dry it with a little paper towel.
3. Put the olive oil in a large saucepan and heat over medium fire, add the onion and garlic to the hot oil.
4. Fry until everything is soft, deglaze with the chicken stock. Also, add the meat and bring to a boil.
5. In the meantime, wash and dry the lemon, then rub and peel it with a grater, alternatively, you can also use a zester. Add the lemon zest to the broth and cook everything for 40 minutes before adding the beans. Salt and pepper, then cook again for 10 minutes.
6. Now, remove the meat and tear it into small pieces on a plate or board with 2 forks. Put the chicken back into the soup, then crumble the Feta over the soup.
7. Finally, rinse the chives with water, dry and cut them so that small rolls are created. Sprinkle into the soup, stir well and immediately enjoy hot.

NUTRITION FACTS:

Calories: 329 Fat: 17 g Carbs: 9 g Sugar: 3 g Fiber: 5 g Protein: 37 g

Sodium: 430 mg

427. CROWD PLEASING SALAD

Preparation Time: 15 minutes

Cooking Time: 0 minutes

Servings: 5

INGREDIENTS:

- 2 C. cooked quinoa
- 2 C. canned red kidney beans, rinsed and drained
- 5 C. fresh baby spinach
- ¼ C. tomatoes, peeled, seeded and chopped
- ¼ C. fresh dill, chopped
- ¼ C. fresh parsley, chopped
- 3 tbsp. fresh lemon juice
- Salt and freshly ground black pepper, to taste

DIRECTIONS:

1. In a large bowl, add all the ingredients and toss to coat well.
2. Serve immediately.

NUTRITION FACTS:

calories: 354; carbs: 62.7g; Protein: 16.6g; Fat: 4.8g; Sugar: 2.5g; Sodium: 331mg; Fiber: 11.5g

428. GREAT LUNCHEON SALAD

Preparation Time: 20 minutes

Cooking Time: 15 minutes

Servings: 4

INGREDIENTS:

For Salad:
- ½ C. homemade vegetable broth
- ½ C. couscous
- 3 C. canned red kidney beans, rinsed and drained
- 2 large tomatoes, peeled, seeded and chopped
- 5 C. fresh spinach, torn

For Dressing:
- 1 garlic clove, minced
- 2 tbsp. shallots, minced
- 2 tsp. lemon zest, grated finely
- ¼ C. fresh lemon juice
- 2 tbsp. extra-virgin olive oil
- Salt and freshly ground black pepper, to taste

DIRECTIONS:

1. In a pan, add the broth over medium heat and bring to a boil.
2. Add the couscous and stir to combine.
3. Cover the pan and immediately remove from the heat.
4. Set aside, covered for about 5-10 minutes or until all the liquid is absorbed.
5. For salad: in a large serving bowl, add the couscous and remaining ingredients and stir to combine.
6. For dressing: in another small bowl, add all the ingredients and beat until well combined.
7. Pour the dressing over salad and gently toss to coat well.
8. Serve immediately.

NUTRITION FACTS:

calories: 341; carbs: 53.2g; Protein: 15.7g; Fat: 8.5g; Sugar: 6.6g; Sodium: 670mg; Fiber: 13.5g

429. FLAVORS POWERHOUSE LUNCH MEAL

Preparation Time: 15 minutes

Cooking Time: 5 minutes

Servings: 2

INGREDIENTS:

- 1 large avocado
- 1¼ C. cooked chickpeas
- ¼ C. celery stalks, chopped
- 1 scallion (greed part), sliced
- 1 small garlic clove, minced
- 1½ tbsp. fresh lemon juice
- ½ tsp. olive oil
- Salt and freshly ground black pepper, to taste
- 1 tbsp. fresh cilantro, chopped

DIRECTIONS:

1. Cut the avocado in half and then remove the pit.
2. With a spoon, scoop out the flesh from each avocado half.
3. Then, cut half of the avocado flesh in equal-sized cubes.
4. In a large bowl, add avocado cubes and remaining ingredients except for sunflower seeds and cilantro and toss to coat well.
5. Stuff each avocado half with chickpeas mixture evenly.
6. Serve immediately with the garnishing of cilantro.

NUTRITION FACTS:

calories: 403; carbs: 0g; Protein: 9.8g; Fat: 22.6g; Sugar: 1.1g; Sodium: 546mg; Fiber: 13.8g

430. EYE-CATCHING SWEET POTATO BOATS

Preparation Time: 20 minutes

Cooking Time: 40 minutes

Servings: 2

INGREDIENTS:

For Sweet Potatoes:
- 1 large sweet potato, halved lengthwise
- ½ tbsp. olive oil
- Salt and freshly ground black pepper, to taste

For Filling:
- ½ tbsp. olive oil
- 1/3 C. canned chickpeas, rinsed and drained
- 1 tsp. curry powder
- 1/8 tsp. garlic powder

- 1/3 C. cooked quinoa
- Salt and freshly ground black pepper, to taste
- 1 tsp. fresh lime juice
- 1 tsp. fresh cilantro, chopped

DIRECTIONS:
1. Preheat the oven to 375°F-190°C.
2. Rub each sweet potato half with oil evenly.
3. Arrange the sweet potato halves onto a baking sheet, cut side down and sprinkle with salt and black pepper.
4. Bake for about 40 minutes or until sweet potato becomes tender.
5. Meanwhile, for filling: in a skillet, heat the oil over medium heat and cook the chickpeas, curry powder and garlic powder for about 6-8 minutes, stirring frequently.
6. Stir in the cooked quinoa, salt and black pepper and remove from the heat.
7. Remove from the oven and arrange each sweet potato halves onto a plate.
8. With a fork, fluff the flesh of each half slightly.
9. Place chickpeas mixture in each half and drizzle with lime juice.
10. Serve immediately with the garnishing of cilantro and sesame seeds.

NUTRITION FACTS:
calories: 286; carbs: 43g; Protein: 8.2g; Fat: 9.7g; Sugar: 6.6g; Sodium: 175mg; Fiber: 8g

431. MEXICAN ENCHILADAS

Preparation Time: 15 minutes

Cooking Time: 20 minutes

Servings: 8

INGREDIENTS:
- 1 (14-oz.) can red beans, drained, rinsed and mashed
- 2 C. cheddar cheese, grated
- 2 C. tomato sauce
- ½ C. onion, chopped
- ¼ C. black olives, pitted and sliced
- 2 tsp. garlic salt
- 8 whole-wheat tortillas

DIRECTIONS:
1. Preheat the oven to 350°F-180°C.
2. In a medium bowl, add the mashed beans, cheese, 1 C. of tomato sauce, onions, olives and garlic salt and mix well.
3. Place about 1/3 C. of the bean mixture along center of each tortilla.
4. Roll up each tortilla and place enchiladas in large baking dish.
5. Place the remaining tomato sauce on top of the filled tortillas.
6. Bake for about 15-20 minutes.
7. Serve warm.

NUTRITION FACTS:
calories: 358; carbs: 46.2g; Protein: 20.6g; Fat: 11.2g; Sugar: 4.5g; Sodium: 550mg; Fiber: 10.3g

432. UNIQUE BANANA CURRY

Preparation Time: 15 minutes

Cooking Time: 15 minutes

Servings: 3

INGREDIENTS:
- 2 tbsp. olive oil
- 2 yellow onions, chopped
- 8 garlic cloves, minced
- 2 tbsp. curry powder
- 1 tbsp. ground ginger
- 1 tbsp. ground cumin
- 1 tsp. ground turmeric
- 1 tsp. ground cinnamon
- 1 tsp. red chili powder
- Salt and freshly ground black pepper, to taste
- 2/3 C. plain yogurt
- 1 C. tomato puree
- 2 bananas, peeled and sliced
- 3 tomatoes, peeled, seeded and chopped finely

DIRECTIONS:
1. In a large pan, heat the oil over medium heat and sauté onion for about 4-5 minutes.
2. Add the garlic, curry powder and spices and sauté for about 1 minute.
3. Add the yogurt and tomato sauce and bring to a gentle boil.
4. Stir in the bananas and simmer for about 3 minutes.
5. Stir in the tomatoes and simmer for about 1-2 minutes.
6. Remove from the heat and serve hot.

NUTRITION FACTS:
calories: 318; carbs: 49.7g; Protein: 9g; Fat: 12.2g; Sugar: 24.2g; Sodium: 138mg; Fiber: 9.5g

433. ARMENIAN STYLE CHICKPEAS

Preparation Time: 15 minutes

Cooking Time: 15 minutes

Servings: 4

INGREDIENTS:
- 2 tbsp. olive oil
- 1 medium yellow onion, chopped
- 4 garlic cloves, minced
- 1 tsp. dried thyme, crushed
- 1 tsp. dried oregano, crushed
- ½ tsp. paprika
- 1 C. tomato, chopped finely
- 2½ C. canned chickpeas, rinsed and drained
- 5 C. Swiss chard, chopped
- 2 tbsp. water
- 2 tbsp. fresh lemon juice
- Salt and freshly ground black pepper, to taste
- 3 tbsp. fresh basil, chopped

DIRECTIONS:
1. In a skillet, heat the olive oil over medium heat and sauté the onion for about 6-8 minutes.
2. Add the garlic, herbs and paprika and sauté for about 1 minute.
3. Add the Swiss chard and 2 tbsp. water and cook for about 2-3 minutes.
4. Add the tomatoes and chickpeas and cook for about 2-3 minutes.
5. Add in the lemon juice, salt and black pepper and remove from the heat.
6. Serve hot with the garnishing of basil.

NUTRITION FACTS:
calories: 260; carbs: 34g; Protein: 12g; Fat: 8.6g; Sugar: 3.1g; Sodium: 178mg; Fiber: 9g

434. PROTEIN-PACKED SOUP

Preparation Time: 15 minutes

Cooking Time: 1 hour 10 minutes

Servings: 8

INGREDIENTS:
- 2 tbsp. olive oil
- 1½ lb. ground turkey
- Salt and freshly ground black pepper, to taste
- 1 large carrot, peeled and chopped
- 1 large celery stalk, chopped
- 1 large onion, chopped
- 6 garlic cloves, chopped
- 1 tsp. dried rosemary
- 1 tsp. dried oregano
- 2 large potatoes, peeled and chopped
- 8-9 C. chicken bone broth
- 4-5 C. tomatoes, peeled, seeded and chopped
- 2 C. dry lentils
- ¼ C. fresh parsley, chopped

DIRECTIONS:
1. In a large soup pan, heat the olive oil over medium-high heat and cook the turkey for about 5 minutes or until browned.
2. With a slotted spoon, transfer the turkey into a bowl and set aside.
3. In the same pan, add the carrot, celery onion, garlic and dried herbs over medium heat and cook for about 5 minutes.
4. Add the potatoes and cook for about 4-5 minutes.
5. Add the cooked turkey, tomatoes and broth and bring to a boil over high heat.
6. Reduce the heat to low and cook, covered for about 10 minutes.
7. Add the lentils and cook, covered for about 40 minutes.
8. Stir in black pepper and remove

from the heat.
9. Serve hot with the garnishing of parsley.

NUTRITION FACTS:

calories: 485; carbs: 44.6g; Protein: 43g; Fat: 16.5g; Sugar: 8.5g; Sodium: 452mg; Fiber: 16.6g

 435. ONE-POT DINNER SOUP

Preparation Time: 15 minutes

Cooking Time: 50 minutes

Servings: 4

INGREDIENTS:

- 1 tbsp. olive oil
- 1 C. yellow onion, chopped
- ½ C. carrots, peeled and chopped
- ½ C. celery, chopped
- 2 garlic cloves, minced
- 4 C. homemade vegetable broth
- 2½ C. sweet potatoes, peeled and chopped
- 1 C. red lentils, rinsed
- 1½ tbsp. fresh lemon juice
- Salt and freshly ground black pepper, to taste
- 2 tbsp. fresh cilantro, chopped

DIRECTIONS:

1. In a large Dutch oven, heat the oil over medium heat and sauté the onion, carrot and celery for about 5-7 minutes.
2. Add the garlic and sauté for about 1 minute.
3. Add the sweet potatoes and cook for about 1-2 minutes.
4. Add in the broth and bring to a boil.
5. Reduce the heat to low and simmer, covered for about 5 minutes.
6. Stir in the red lentils and gain bring to a boil over medium-high heat.
7. Reduce the heat to low and simmer, covered for about 25-30 minutes or until desired doneness.
8. Stir in the lemon juice, salt and black pepper and remove from the heat.
9. Serve hot with the garnishing of cilantro.

NUTRITION FACTS:

calories: 471; carbs: 61g; Protein: 19,3g; Fat: 5.6g; Sugar: 4.4g; Sodium: 836mg; Fiber: 19.7g

 436. 3-BEANS SOUP

Preparation Time: 15 minutes

Cooking Time: 45 minutes

Servings: 4

INGREDIENTS:

- ¼ C. olive oil
- 1 large onion, chopped
- 1 large sweet potato, peeled and cubed
- 3 carrots, peeled and chopped
- 3 celery stalks, chopped
- 3 garlic cloves, minced
- 2 tsp. dried thyme, crushed
- 1 tbsp. red chili powder
- 1 tbsp. ground cumin
- 4 large tomatoes, peeled, seeded and chopped finely
- 2 (16-oz.) cans great Northern beans, rinsed and drained
- 2 (15¼-oz.) cans red kidney beans, rinsed and drained
- 1 (15-oz.) can black beans, drained and rinsed
- 12 C. homemade vegetable broth
- 1 C. fresh cilantro, chopped
- Salt and freshly ground black pepper, to taste

DIRECTIONS:

1. In a Dutch oven, heat the oil over medium heat and sauté the onion, sweet potato, carrot and celery for about 6-8 minutes.
2. Add the garlic, thyme, chili powder and cumin and sauté for about 1 minute.
3. Add in the tomatoes and cook for about 2-3 minutes.
4. Add the beans and broth and bring to a boil over medium-high heat.
5. Cover the pan with lid and cook for about 25-30 minutes.
6. Stir in the cilantro and remove from heat.
7. Serve hot.

NUTRITION FACTS:

calories: 411; carbs: 69.7g; Protein: 22.7g; Fat: 5.7g; Sugar: 7.1g; Sodium: 931mg; Fiber: 18.9g

 437. CHICKEN AND QUINOA PITA

Preparation Time: 10 mins.

Cooking Time: 0 mins.

Servings: 4

INGREDIENTS:

- fat free cream cheese (1 cup, softened)
- fat free mayonnaise (1 tbs)
- cooked chicken (2 cups, cubed)
- tomatoes (1 cup, seeded, sliced)
- Quinoa (1 (14 oz) can, cooked)
- romaine lettuce leaves (4)
- alfalfa sprouts (2 cups, rinsed, drained)
- whole wheat pita bread (4 round)

DIRECTIONS:

1. In a bowl, combine mayonnaise and cream cheese until it is fully mixed.
2. Add chicken, tomatoes, Quinoa; mix well. Slice the pita bread to form a pocket.
3. Fill your pitas with lettuce and chicken. Top with alfalfa sprouts.
4. Serve.

NUTRITION FACTS:

331 calories, 23 g fat, 5 g carbs, 2 g fiber, 26 g protein

438. TURKEY FLORENTINE

Preparation Time: 15 mins.

Cooking Time: 18 mins.

Servings: 4

INGREDIENTS:

- olive oil (2 tbs)
- zucchinis (2 medium, seeded, thinly sliced)
- green onions (1/2 cups, sliced)
- turkey breast (2 cups, cubed)
- salt (1/2 tsp)
- thyme (1/2 tsp, ground)
- pimento (2 tbs, chopped)
- cooked long-grain rice (3 cups)
- fresh baby spinach (4 cups)
- low fat parmesan cheese (1/4 cup, freshly grated)

DIRECTIONS:

1. In a non-stick pan, heat olive oil over moderate heat. Add zucchini, turkey, and onions, stir ever now and then for 5 to 10 minutes.
2. Add salt, thyme, pimento, rice and spinach. Cook and stir for another 6 - 8 minutes or until heated through and spinach wilts.
3. Remove from heat, transfer to large serving bowl, and stir in cheese. Serve.

NUTRITION FACTS:

593 calories, 8 g fat, 11 g carbs, 4 g fiber, 12 g protein

439. CHICKEN LETTUCE WRAPS

Preparation Time: 15 mins.

Cooking Time: 0 mins.

Servings: 2

INGREDIENTS:

- Mayonnaise (1/4 cup, low fat)
- lemon juice (2 tsp)
- white beans (1/2 cup, canned, cooked, drained)
- feta cheese (1/3 cup, crumbled)
- pimentos (2 tbs, chopped)
- lettuce leaves (8 large, washed, and dried)
- chicken breast strips (1/2 lb cooked, preferably grilled)

DIRECTIONS:

1. In a medium bowl, combine mayonnaise and lemon juice. Stir

in beans, mashing slightly with fork.
2. Add cheese and pimentos and mix lightly. Spread lettuce leaves evenly with bean mixture. Top with chicken; roll up.
3. Serve.

NUTRITION FACTS:
338 calories, 10 g fat, 39g carbs, 9 g fiber, 26 g protein

440. COUSCOUS WITH TURKEY

Preparation Time: 20 mins.

Cooking Time: 26 mins.

Servings: 4

INGREDIENTS:
- extra-virgin olive oil (4 tbs)
- turkey thighs (1 lb boneless, skinless, chopped)
- onion (1, chopped)
- cloves garlic (3, minced)
- carrots (1 cup, shredded)
- smoked paprika (1 tsp)
- ground cinnamon (1/8 tsp)
- salt (1/2 tsp)
- dried fruits (1 cup chopped, pitted dates, apricots)
- turkey stock (4 cups, divided)
- butter (2 tablespoons)
- couscous (1 1/2 cups)
- Italian parsley (1/2 cup, chopped)

DIRECTIONS:
1. Set your oil to get hot on medium heat. Cook turkey and brown 3 to 4 minutes on each side.
2. Add onions, garlic, carrots, and season with spices and salt. Cook 6-8 minutes.
3. Stir the fruits into the turkey and vegetables, and 2 ½ cups of stock.
4. Allow to boil. Turn down the heat to low, cover and let it simmer for 10 minutes.
5. In a separate small saucepan, over medium heat, pour 1 ½ cups of stock and bring up to a boil then stir in the couscous.
6. Take the content off the heat and let it stand 5 minutes while the cover is on. Fluff with fork and serve with turkey.

NUTRITION FACTS:
469 calories, 24 g fat, 40 g carbs, 4 g fiber, 18 g protein

441. EASY TURKEY CHILI

Preparation Time: 25 mins.

Cooking Time: 50 mins.

Servings: 4-6

INGREDIENTS:
- olive oil (3 tbs)
- garlic cloves (4, minced)
- onion (1 medium, chopped)
- ground turkey (1 lb.)
- bay leaf (1)
- ground cumin (1 tsp)
- dried oregano (1 tsp)
- tomato (1, seeded and chopped)
- tomato sauce (1 14 oz.) can)
- Pork broth (1 cup
- salt (1 tsp)
- red beans (2 (14 oz.) cans, drained and rinsed)

DIRECTIONS:
1. Heat the oil over medium heat, in a large pot and cook the onions and garlic for 5 minutes.
2. Turn the heat from medium to high. Add oregano, bay leaf, turkey and cumin. Cook for 5-7 minutes or until turkey has browned.
3. Add broth, tomato sauce, tomato and salt. Once the pot is boiling, lower the heat to simmer. Let it simmer for about 20 minutes, covered.
4. If needed, add more water and beans and continue to simmer for 15 more minutes.
5. Serve.

NUTRITION FACTS:
193 calories, 13 g fat, 5 g carbs, 1 g fiber, 16 g protein

442. HAM, BEAN AND CABBAGE STEW

Preparation Time: 15 mins.

Cooking Time: 17 mins.

Servings: 4

INGREDIENTS:
- extra virgin olive oil (1 tbs)
- smoked ham (8 oz, chopped)
- onion (1 large, chopped)
- stalks celery (2, sliced)
- cloves garlic (5, chopped finely)
- chicken broth (4 cups)
- tomatoes (1 (28 oz) can, seedless, drained)
- whole wheat pasta (3 cups)
- coleslaw (8 oz)
- kidney beans (2 (14 oz) cans)
- dried basil (1 tsp)
- dried rosemary (1 tsp)

DIRECTIONS:
1. In a good size pot, heat olive oil over medium heat. Cook ham, onion, celery and garlic stirring occasionally, until vegetables are tender.
2. Stir in broth and tomatoes, breaking up tomatoes. Stir the pasta in, heat to boiling and turn down the heat low.
3. Cover and simmer about 10 minutes or until pasta is tender. Stir in coleslaw, beans, basil and oregano.
4. Bring stew to a boil and reduce heat to low. Simmer uncovered about 5-7 minutes or until cabbage is tender.

NUTRITION FACTS:
543 calories, 21 g fat, 47g carbs, 8 g fiber, 40 g protein

443. GRILLED FISH TACOS

Preparation Time: 25 mins.

Cooking Time: 6 mins.

Servings: 4

INGREDIENTS:
- Salt (1/4 tsp)
- Juice of 1/2 lemon
- olive oil (2 tbs)
- trout filets (4, rinsed and dried)
- red onion (1/2 cup, chopped)
- jicama (1/2 cup, peeled, chopped)
- red bell pepper (1/3 cup, chopped)
- fresh cilantro (2/3 cup, finely chopped)
- black beans (1 cup, drained and rinsed)
- Zest and juice (1/2 lime)
- plain yogurt (1 tbs, non-fat)
- whole wheat tortillas (8, warmed)

DIRECTIONS:
1. Combine your oil, lemon juice and salt.
2. Pour mixture over fish fillets and let marinate for 10 minutes. Put the fish on the grill over high heat.
3. Cook the fish on both side for 3 minutes. In another bowl, combine onion, bell pepper, jicama, cilantro, yogurt and zest and juice of lime to make a salsa.
4. Add your fish on top of a warm tortilla. Top with salsa and fold in half before serving.

NUTRITION FACTS:
356 calories, 9 g fat, 57g carbs, 17 g fiber, 15 g protein

444. PASTA WITH TURKEY AND OLIVES

Preparation Time: 20 mins.

Cooking Time: 30 mins.

Servings: 4

INGREDIENTS:
- whole wheat pasta (1 lb, uncooked)
- olive oil (2 tsp)
- onion (1 large, peeled, chopped finely)
- cloves garlic (4, peeled, finely chopped)
- turkey breast (1 lb, cut into chunks)
- basil (1 tsp, dried)
- rosemary (1 tsp, dried)
- black olives (12 med, pitted)

- green bell pepper (1 med, seeded and chopped)
- tomatoes (1 (14 oz) can, seedless, chopped)
- chicken broth (1 can)
- Romano cheese (1/2 cup, shredded)

DIRECTIONS:

1. Bring a salted water to boil in a large pot. Add pasta and cook until al dente follow instruction according to the package.
2. While pasta cooks, heat the oil in a large pan over medium heat. Add the garlic and onion. Cook for 6 minutes.
3. Add the turkey, rosemary and basil. Cook for about 8 minutes.
4. Stir in the olives, tomatoes and green pepper and cook for 2 minutes. In the pan add the chicken broth, heat the pan to a boil.
5. Reduce half of the liquid by boiling for 7 minutes. When pasta is done, add to sauce mixture.
6. Toss until pasta is evenly mixed with sauce. Top with cheese and serve.

NUTRITION FACTS:

165 calories, 4 g fat, 18 g carbs, 3 g fiber, 14 g protein

445. BANANA OAT SHAKEBANANA OAT SHAKE

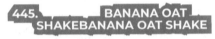

Preparation Time: 20 minutes

Cooking Time: 0 minutes

Servings: 2

INGREDIENTS:

- 1/2 cup cooked oatmeal, chilled
- 2/3 cup skim milk
- 2 tablespoons brown sugar
- 1 tablespoon wheat germ
- 1 1/2 teaspoons vanilla extract
- 1/2 frozen banana, cut into chunks

DIRECTIONS:

1. Blend the oatmeal for a few minutes in a blender.
2. Mix in the milk, brown sugar, wheat germ, vanilla extract, and 1/2 banana. Blend until the mixture is thick and smooth.
3. If desired, serve with ice.

NUTRITION FACTS:

calories: 173 |carbs: 33 g | protein: 6 g | fat: 1 g | cholesterol: 150 mg

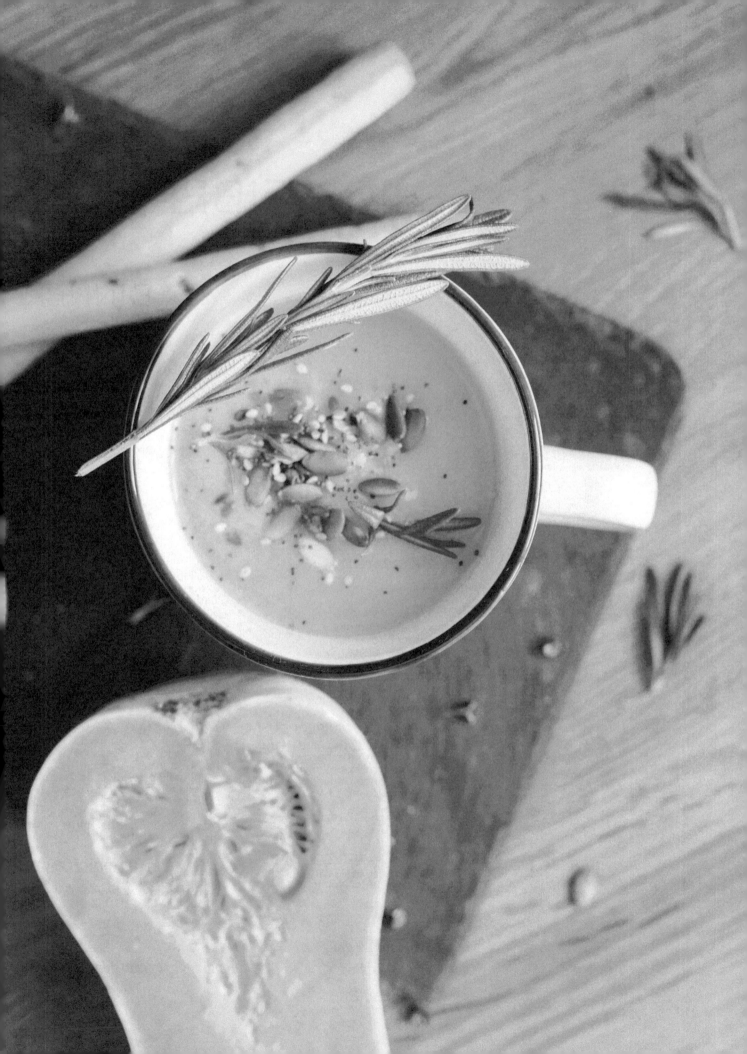

HIGH FIBER DIET

DINNER

446. GRILLED PEAR CHEDDAR POCKETS

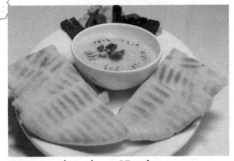

Preparation time: 15 minutes
Cooking time: 4 minutes
Serving: 1

INGREDIENTS:
- Dijon mustard – 2 tsp
- Whole grain flatbread – half
- Cheddar cheese – 2 slices
- Arugula – ¼ cup
- Red pear – 1/3, cored and cut into thick slices

DIRECTIONS:
1. Spread mustard over the inner side of the flatbread pocket.
2. Place cheese slices and fold them. Then, add pear slices and arugula.
3. Place it into the skillet and cook for 3 to 4 minutes.

NUTRITION FACTS:
Calories; 223kcal, fat ; 8.6g, Carbohydrate; 28.6g, Protein; 11.3g, Fiber; 6.8g

447. CHICKEN AND APPLE KALE WRAPS

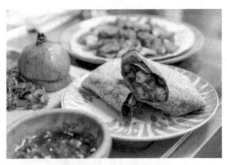

Preparation time: 10 minutes
Cooking time: 0 minutes
Serving: 1

Ingredients:
- Mayonnaise – 1 tbsp
- Dijon mustard – 1 tsp
- Kale leaves – three
- Chicken breast – three ounces, thinly sliced, cooked
- Red onion – six slices, thin
- Apple – one, cut into nine slices

DIRECTIONS:
1. Combine the mustard and mayonnaise into the bowl.
2. Spread onto the kale leaves—top with one-ounce chicken, three slices of apples, and two slices of onion.
3. Then, roll each kale leaf.
4. Cut in half.

NUTRITION FACTS:
Calories; 370kcal, fat ; 13.7g, Carbohydrate; 34.1g, Protein; 29.3g, Fiber; 6g

448. CAULIFLOWER RICE PILAF

Preparation time: 10 minutes
Cooking time: 10 minutes
Serving: 1

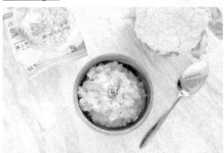

INGREDIENTS:
- Cauliflower florets – six cups
- Extra-virgin olive oil – three tbsp
- Garlic – two cloves, minced
- Salt – half tsp
- Almonds – ¼ cup, toasted, sliced
- Herbs – ¼ cup, chopped
- Lemon zest – 2 tsp

DIRECTIONS:
1. Add cauliflower florets into the food processor and blend until chopped.
2. Add oil into the skillet and place it over medium-high flame.
3. Then, add garlic and cook for a half-minute.
4. Add cauliflower rice and season with salt. Let cook for three to five minutes.
5. Remove from the flame.
6. Add lemon zest, herbs, and almonds and stir well.

NUTRITION FACTS:
Calories; 114kcal, fat ; 9.2g, Carbohydrate; 6.7g, Protein; 3g, Fiber; 2.8g

449. FRESH HERB AND LEMON BULGUR PILAF

Preparation time: 10 minutes

Cooking time: 40 minutes

Serving: 6

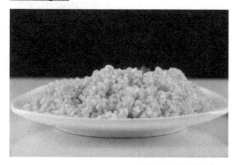

INGREDIENTS:

- Extra-virgin olive oil – 2 tbsp
- Onion – two cups, chopped
- Garlic – one clove, chopped
- Bulgur – 1 ½ cups
- Ground turmeric – half tsp
- Ground cumin – half tsp
- Vegetable or chicken broth – 2 cups, low-sodium
- Carrot – 1 ½ cups, chopped
- Fresh ginger – 2 tsp, grated or chopped
- Salt – one tsp
- Fresh dill – ¼ cup, chopped
- Fresh mint – ¼ cup, chopped
- Parsley – ¼ cup, chopped
- Lemon juice – three tbsp
- Walnuts – half cup, chopped, toasted

DIRECTIONS:

1. Add oil into the skillet and place it over medium flame.
2. Add onion and cook for 12 to 18 minutes.
3. Add garlic and cook for one minute.
4. Then, add cumin, turmeric, and bulgur and cook for one minute.
5. Add salt, ginger, carrot, and broth and bring to a boil over medium0high flame, about 15 minutes.
6. Remove from the flame.
7. Let rest for five minutes.
8. Add lemon juice, parsley, dill, and mint into the pilaf and stir well.
9. Garnish with walnuts.

NUTRITION FACTS:

Calories; 273kcal, fat ; 11.7g, Carbohydrate; 38.8g, Protein; 7.3g, Fiber; 7.7g

 CORN CHOWDER

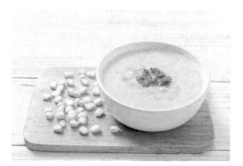

Preparation time: 10 minutes

Cooking time: 5 hours

Serving: 6

INGREDIENTS:

- Yellow split peas – ¾ cup, split
- Chicken broth – 28 ounces, low-sodium
- Water – one cup
- Corn kernels – 12 ounces, frozen
- Red sweet peppers – half cup, chopped and roasted
- Green chilies – 4 ounces, diced
- Ground cumin – one tsp
- Dried oregano – half tsp, crushed
- Dried thyme – half tsp, crushed
- Cream cheese – ½ cup

DIRECTIONS:

1. Rinse split peas underwater.
2. Mix the thyme, oregano, cumin, chilies, red peppers, corn, water, split peas, and chicken broth and cook on high heat for five to six hours.
3. Let cool it for ten minutes.
4. Transfer two cups of soup into the food processor and blend until smooth.
5. Add pureed soup into the slow cooker. Then, add cream cheese and whisk to combine—Cook for five minutes.
6. Serve!

NUTRITION FACTS:

Calories; 222kcal, fat ; 7.5g, Carbohydrate; 29.8g, Protein; 10.5g, Fiber; 7.7g

451. **STRAWBERRY AND RHUBARB SOUP**

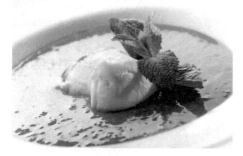

Preparation time: 5 minutes

Cooking time: 30 minutes

Serving: 4

INGREDIENTS:

- Rhubarb – four cups
- Water – three cups
- Strawberries – 1 ½ cups, sliced
- Sugar – ¼ cup
- Salt – 1/8 tsp
- Mint or basil – 1/3 cup, chopped
- Ground pepper – to taste

DIRECTIONS:

1. Add three cups of water and rhubarb into the saucepan.
2. Cook for five minutes until softened.
3. Transfer it to the bowl.
4. Add 2-inch ice water into the bowl and keep it aside with rhubarb.
5. Place it into the fridge for twenty minutes.
6. Transfer the rhubarb to the blender. Then, add salt, sugar, and strawberries and blend until smooth.
7. Place it back in the bowl. Add basil or mint.
8. Serve!

NUTRITION FACTS:

Calories; 95kcal, fat ; 0.5g, Carbohydrate; 23.1g, Protein; 1.6g, Fiber; 3.5g

452. **CHICKEN SANDWICHES**

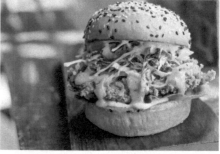

Preparation time: 5 minutes

Cooking time: 30 minutes

Serving: 4

INGREDIENTS:

- Red onion – four slices
- Red sweet pepper – one, seeded and quartered
- Chicken breast – six ounces, boneless, cut in half, horizontally
- Multi-grain sandwich round – four, split
- Basil pesto – 2 tbsp
- Kalamata olives – 2 tbsp, pitted and chopped
- Mozzarella cheese – 1/3 cup, shredded
- Feta cheese – ¼ cup, low-fat, crumbled

DIRECTIONS:

1. Heat the skillet over medium flame.
2. Let coat with pepper and red onion with non-stick cooking spray.
3. Add it to the pan and cook for six to eight minutes.
4. Remove from the skillet. Let coat the chicken with non-stick cooking spray.
5. Add chicken to the grill pan and cook for three to five minutes.
6. Remove from the skillet.
7. Pull chicken into shreds. Cut

pepper into strips.
8. To assemble the sandwiches: Spread the pesto onto the sandwich and sprinkle with olives. Place grilled onion slices. Top with pepper strips.
9. Place chicken over it. Sprinkle with feta cheese and mozzarella cheese.
10. Then, place skillet over medium-low flame.
11. Place the sandwich into the skillet and cook for three to four minutes.
12. Flip and cook for three to four minutes.
13. Serve!

NUTRITION FACTS:
Calories; 296kcal, fat ; 10g, Carbohydrate; 27.7g, Protein; 25.8g, Fiber; 6.2g

453. TEX-MEX BEAN TOSTADAS

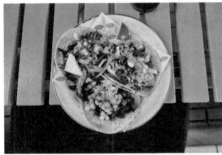

Preparation time: 10 minutes

Cooking time: 15 minutes

Serving: 4

INGREDIENTS:
- Tostada shells – four
- Pinto beans – 16 ounces, rinsed and drained
- Salsa – half cup, prepared
- Chipotle seasoning – ½ tsp
- Cheddar cheese – ½ cup, shredded
- Iceberg lettuce – 1 ½ cups
- Tomato – one cup, chopped
- Lime wedges – one

DIRECTIONS:
1. Preheat the oven to 350°F-180°C.
2. Place tostada shells onto the baking sheet and bake for three to five minutes.
3. Meanwhile, mix the seasoning, salsa, and bean into the bowl.
4. Mash the mixture with a potato masher.
5. Then, divide the bean mixture between tostada shells.
6. Top with half of the cheese. Bake for five minutes.
7. Top with chopped tomato and shredded lettuce.
8. Then, place the remaining cheese and lime wedges.

NUTRITION FACTS:
Calories; 230kcal, fat ; 6g, Carbohydrate; 33g, Protein; 12g, Fiber; 6g

454. FISH TACOS

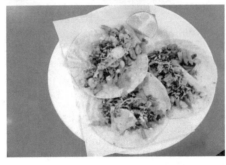

Preparation time: 10 minutes

Cooking time: 15 minutes

Serving: 4

INGREDIENTS:
- Tilapia fillets – 1lb
- Extra-virgin olive oil – 2 tsp
- Chipotle seasoning blend – 2 tsp
- Coleslaw mix – 2 cups
- Salad dressing – 2 tbsp, ranch
- Whole wheat tortillas – eight
- Avocado – half, thinly sliced
- Cilantro leaves – ¼ cup
- Lime – one, quartered

DIRECTIONS:
1. Preheat the oven to 450°F-230°C.
2. Place fillets onto the baking dish and brush the fish with oil.
3. Sprinkle with seasoning.
4. Bake for four to six minutes.
5. Meanwhile, mix the dressing and coleslaw into a bowl. Keep it aside.
6. Flake the fish into big chunks and place them into the tortillas.
7. Top with lime, cilantro, avocado, and coleslaw mixture.

NUTRITION FACTS:
Calories; 341kcal, fat ; 12g, Carbohydrate; 30.5g, Protein; 29.5g, Fiber; 21.2g

455. CUCUMBER ALMOND GAZPACHO

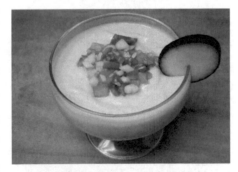

Preparation time: 20 minutes

Chill time: 2 hours

Serving: 5

INGREDIENTS:
- English cucumbers – two
- Yellow bell pepper – two cups, chopped
- Whole wheat bread – 2 cups
- Unsweetened almond milk – 1 ½ cups
- Almonds – ½ cup, toasted, slivered
- Olive oil – five tsp
- White-wine vinegar – 2 tsp
- Garlic – one clove
- Salt – half tsp

DIRECTIONS:
1. Dice unpeeled cucumber and mix with half a cup bell pepper.
2. Peel the remaining cucumbers and cut them into chunks.
3. Add remaining bell pepper, peeled cucumber, salt, garlic, vinegar, oil, six tbsp of almonds, almond milk, and bread into the blender and blend until smooth. Let chill for two hours.
4. Garnish with the remaining 2 tbsp almonds.
5. Drizzle with oil.

NUTRITION FACTS:
Calories; 201kcal, fat ; 11.8g, Carbohydrate; 19g, Protein; 6.3g, Fiber; 4.3g

456. PEA AND SPINACH CARBONARA

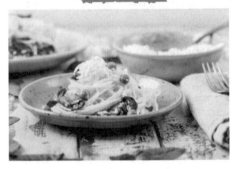

Preparation time: 5 minutes

Cooking time: 15 minutes

Serving: 4

INGREDIENTS:
- Extra-virgin olive oil – 1 ½ tbsp
- Panko breadcrumbs (whole-wheat) – half cup
- Garlic – one clove, minced
- Parmesan cheese – eight tbsp, grated
- Fresh parsley – three tbsp, chopped
- Egg yolks – three
- Egg – one
- Ground pepper – half tsp
- Salt – ¼ tsp
- Tagliatelle or linguine – 9 ounce
- Baby spinach – eight cups

- Peas – one cup

DIRECTIONS:
1. Add ten cups of water into the pot and boil it over high flame.
2. During this, add oil into the skillet and cook over medium-high flame.
3. Add garlic and breadcrumbs and cook for two minutes until toasted.
4. Transfer it to the small bowl. Add parsley and two tbsp parmesan cheese and keep it aside.
5. Whisk the salt, pepper, egg, egg yolks, and six tbsp parmesan cheese into the bowl.
6. Add pasta to the boiling water and cook for one minute.
7. Add spinach and peas and cook for one minute more until tender.
8. Save ¼ cup of the cooking water for your next use. Drain it and place it into the bowl.
9. Whisk the reserved cooking water into the egg mixture, add to the pasta, and toss to combine.
10. Top with breadcrumb mixture and serve!

NUTRITION FACTS:
Calories; 430kcal,carbs; 54.1g, protein; 20.2g, fat; 14.5g, fiber; 8.2g

457. SAUTÉED BROCCOLI WITH PEANUT SAUCE

Preparation time: 5 minutes

Cooking time: 10 minutes

Serving: 6

INGREDIENTS:
- Broccoli florets – eight cups
- Sesame oil – two tbsp, toasted
- Red bell pepper – one cup, sliced
- Yellow onion – half cup, sliced
- Garlic – three cloves, chopped
- Peanut butter – three tbsp
- Tamari – 2 ½ tbsp, low-sodium
- Rice vinegar – two tbsp
- Brown sugar – one tbsp
- Cornstarch – one tsp
- Sesame seeds – one tbsp, toasted

DIRECTIONS:
1. Add water into the pot and boil it. Then, add broccoli and cook for three to four minutes until tender.
2. During this, add oil into the skillet and cook over medium-high flame.
3. Add garlic, onion, and bell pepper and cook for three minutes.
4. Add steamed broccoli and cook for three minutes. Stir well.
5. Whisk the cornstarch, sugar, vinegar, tamari, and peanut butter into the bowl. Add vegetables and stir well.
6. Let cook for one minute. Top with sesame seeds.
7. Serve and enjoy!

NUTRITION FACTS:
Calories; 154kcal,carbs; 12g, protein; 6g, fat; 9.7g, fiber; 3.4g

458. EDAMAME LETTUCE WRAPS BURGERS

Preparation time: 5 minutes

Cooking time: 25 minutes

Serving: 4

INGREDIENTS:
- Carrots – one cup, julienned
- Lime juice – three tbsp
- Chili-garlic sauce – two tsp
- Shelled edamame – 1 ½ cups, thawed
- Cooked brown rice – one cup
- Peanut butter powder – half cup
- Scallions – ¼ cup, chopped
- Red Thai curry paste – one tbsp
- Peanut oil – three tbsp
- Tamari – two tbsp, low-sodium
- Bibb lettuce – four leaves
- Red onion – one cup, thinly sliced

DIRECTIONS:
1. Firstly, toss carrots with one tsp chili garlic sauce and two tbsp lime juice and keep it aside.
2. Add tamari, one tbsp oil, curry paste, scallions, edamame rice, and ¼ cup peanut butter powder into the blender and blend until smooth.
3. Shape the mixture into four burgers.
4. Add two tbsp oil into the skillet and cook over medium flame.
5. Add burgers and cook for three to four minutes per side.
6. When done, transfer it to the plate.
7. During this, whisk the one tsp chili garlic sauce, tamari, one tbsp lime juice, and ¼ cup peanut butter powder into the bowl until smooth.
8. Then, drain the carrots. Add marinade to the peanut sauce. Stir well.
9. Wrap burger in lettuce leaves and top with sauce, onions, and carrots.

NUTRITION FACTS:
Calories; 310kcal,carbs; 31.6g, protein; 14.6g, fat; 14.5g, fiber; 7.6g

459. PIZZA STUFFED SPAGHETTI SQUASH

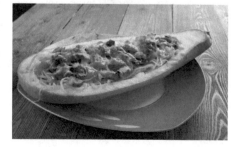

Preparation time: 10 minutes

Cooking time: 1 hour

Serving: 4

INGREDIENTS:
- Spaghetti squash – three pounds, halved lengthwise and seeded
- Water – ¼ cup
- Extra-virgin olive oil – two tbsp
- Onion – one cup, chopped
- Garlic – two cloves, minced
- Mushrooms – eight ounce, sliced
- Bell pepper – one cup, chopped
- No-salt-added crushed tomatoes – two cups
- Italian seasoning – one tsp
- Ground pepper – half tsp
- Crushed red pepper – ¼ tsp, crushed
- Salt – ¼ tsp
- Pepperoni – two ounce, halved
- Part-skim mozzarella cheese – one cup, shredded
- Parmesan cheese – two tbsp, grated

DIRECTIONS:
1. Preheat the oven to 450°F-230°C.
2. Add squash into the microwave-safe dish and then add water.
3. Let microwave it for ten to twelve minutes until tender.
4. Then, place it into the oven and bake for forty to fifty minutes at 400°F-200°C.
5. During this, add oil into the skillet and cook over medium flame.
6. Add garlic and onion and cook for three to four minutes.
7. Add bell pepper and mushrooms and cook for five minutes more until tender.
8. Add salt, crushed red pepper, pepper, Italian seasoning, and tomatoes and cook for two minutes.
9. When done, remove from the flame.
10. Add ten to twelve pepperoni halves and cover them with a lid.
11. Scrape the squash from the shells and place it into the bowl.
12. Add salt, pepper, mozzarella, and parmesan cheese and stir well.
13. Add tomato mixture to the bowl and stir well.
14. Place squash shells onto the rimmed baking sheet and divide the filling among the halves, and top with pepperoni and mozzarella cheese. Place it into the oven and bake for fifteen minutes.
15. Let broil it for one to two minutes.
16. Serve and enjoy!

NUTRITION FACTS:
Calories; 373kcal,carbs; 32.2g, protein; 16.4g, fat; 20.6g, fiber; 7.5g

 SPINACH AND ARTICHOKE DIP PASTA

Preparation time: 5 minutes

Cooking time: 15 minutes

Serving: 4

INGREDIENTS:

- Whole-wheat rotini – eight ounce
- Baby spinach – five ounce, chopped
- Cream cheese – four ounce, low-fat, cut into chunks
- Milk – ¾ cup, low-fat
- Parmesan cheese – half cup, grated
- Garlic powder – two tsp
- Ground pepper – ¼ tsp
- Artichoke hearts – 14 ounce, rinsed, squeezed dry and chopped

DIRECTIONS:

1. Add water into the saucepan and boil it. Add pasta and cook it. Then, drain it.
2. Mix the one tbsp water and spinach into the saucepan and cook over medium flame. Cook for two minutes until wilted.
3. Transfer it to the bowl. Add milk and cream to the pan and whisk it well.
4. Add pepper, garlic powder, and parmesan cheese and cook until thickened. Drain spinach and add to the sauce with pasta and artichoke. Cook it well.
5. Then, serve and enjoy!

NUTRITION FACTS:

Calories; 371kcal, carbs; 56.1g, protein; 16.6g, fat; 9.1g, fiber; 7.9g

 461. GRILLED EGGPLANT

Preparation time: 5 minutes

Cooking time: 40 minutes

Serving: 4

INGREDIENTS:

- Water – four cups
- Cornmeal – one cup
- Butter – one tbsp
- Salt – half tsp
- Plum tomatoes – 1lb, chopped
- Extra-virgin olive oil – four tbsp
- Fresh oregano – two tsp, chopped
- Garlic – one clove, grated
- Ground pepper – half tsp
- Crushed red pepper – ¼ tsp
- Eggplant – 1 ½ lbs, cut into half-inch-thick slices
- Feta cheese – ¼ cup, crumbled
- Fresh basil – half cup, chopped

DIRECTIONS:

1. Add water into the saucepan and boil it over high flame.
2. Add cornmeal and whisk it well. Then, lower the heat and cook for thirty-five minutes until tender.
3. When done, remove from the flame. Add salt and butter and stir well.
4. During this, preheat the grill over medium-high heat.
5. Add salt, crushed red pepper, pepper, garlic, oregano, three tbsp oil, and tomatoes into the bowl and toss to combine.
6. Rub eggplant with one tbsp oil and place onto the grill, and cook for four minutes per side. Let cool it for ten minutes.
7. Let chop it and add to the tomatoes.
8. Sprinkle with fresh basil leaves.
9. Place vegetable mixture over the polenta and top with cheese.

NUTRITION FACTS:

Calories; 354kcal, carbs; 39g, protein; 6.8g, fat; 20.6g, fiber; 8.4g

 462. STUFFED POTATOES WITH SALSA AND BEANS

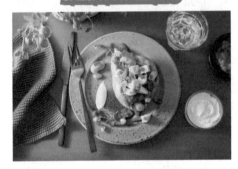

Preparation time: 5 minutes

Cooking time: 20 minutes

Serving: 4

INGREDIENTS:

- Russet potatoes – four
- Fresh salsa – half cup
- Avocado – one, sliced
- Pinto beans – 15 ounce, rinsed, warmed and mashed
- Jalapeños – four tsp, chopped, pickled

DIRECTIONS:

1. Firstly, pierce potatoes using a fork.
2. Let microwave for twenty minutes over medium heat.
3. Place onto the cutting board and let cool it.
4. Cut to open the potato lengthwise and pinch the ends to expose the flesh and top with jalapeno, beans, avocado, and salsa.
5. Serve and enjoy!

NUTRITION FACTS:

Calories; 324kcal, carbs; 56.7g, protein; 9.2g, fat; 8g, fiber; 11g

 463. MUSHROOM QUINOA VEGGIE BURGERS

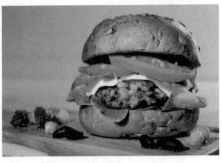

Preparation time: 5 minutes

Cooking time: 25 minutes

Chill time: 1 hour

Serving: 4

INGREDIENTS:

- Portobello mushroom – one, gills removed, chopped
- Black beans – one cup, rinsed, unsalted
- Almond butter – two tbsp, creamy and unsalted
- Canola mayonnaise – three tbsp
- Ground pepper – one tsp
- Smoked paprika – ¾ tsp
- Garlic powder – ¾ tsp
- Salt – half tsp
- Cooked quinoa – half cup
- Old-fashioned rolled oats – ¼ cup
- Ketchup – one tbsp
- Dijon mustard – one tsp
- Extra-virgin olive oil – one tbsp
- Whole-wheat hamburger buns – four, toasted
- Green-leaf lettuce – two leaves, halved
- Tomato – four sliced
- Red onion – four, thinly sliced

DIRECTIONS:

1. Add salt, half tsp garlic powder, paprika, pepper, one tbsp mayonnaise, almond butter, black beans, and mushrooms into the food processor. Blend until smooth.
2. Transfer it to the bowl. Add oats and quinoa and stir well.
3. Place it into the refrigerator for one hour.
4. During this, whisk the ¼ tsp garlic powder, two tbsp mayonnaise, mustard, and ketchup into the bowl until smooth.
5. Make the mixture into four patties.
6. Add oil into the non-stick skillet and cook over medium-high flame.
7. Fry patties for four to five minutes.
8. Flip and cook for two to four minutes until golden brown.
9. Top burger with onion, tomato, lettuce, and sauce.

NUTRITION FACTS:

Calories; 395kcal, carbs; 45.9g, protein; 11.6g, fat; 19.8g, fiber; 9.4g

 464. TURKEY MEATBALLS

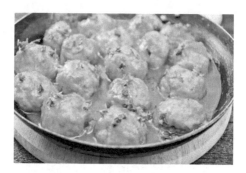

Preparation time: 15 minutes

Cooking time: 25 minutes

Serving: 4

INGREDIENTS:

- Olive oil – one tsp
- Button mushrooms – three cups, sliced
- Egg – one, beaten
- Quick-cooking rolled oats – 1/3 cup
- Parmesan cheese – 1/3 cup, grated
- Garlic – three cloves, minced
- Dried Italian seasoning – two tsp, crushed
- Salt – half tsp
- Ground pepper – ¼ tsp
- Lean ground turkey – 1 ¼ lbs

DIRECTIONS:

1. Preheat the oven to 400°F-200°C.
2. Line a baking pan with foil and coat it with cooking spray.
3. Add oil into the skillet and cook over medium flame.
4. Add mushroom and cook for eight to ten minutes.
5. Transfer it to the blender and blend until chopped.
6. Mix the pepper, salt, Italian seasoning, garlic, parmesan cheese, oats, and egg into the bowl. Add chopped mushrooms and turkey and combine well.
7. Place meat mixture onto the cutting board and cut into thirty squared.
8. Roll each square into the ball, place it onto the pan, and bake for twelve to fifteen minutes.
9. Serve and enjoy!

NUTRITION FACTS:

Calories; 467kcal,carbs; 49.2g, protein; 36.3g, fat; 16.1g, fiber; 7.6g

465. SWEET POTATO SOUP

Preparation time: 15 minutes

Cooking time: 30 minutes

Serving: 6

INGREDIENTS:

- Canola oil – ¼ cup
- Corn tortillas – four, halved and thinly sliced
- Salt – ¾ tsp
- Poblano pepper – one, seeded and chopped
- Onion – one, chopped
- Chili powder – two tbsp
- Chicken broth or vegetable broth – four cups
- Sweet potatoes – 1 ½ lbs, peeled and cut into half-inch pieces
- Tomatoes – 14 ounce, unsalted, pitted, diced
- Black beans – 15 ounce, low-sodium, rinsed
- Lime juice – three tbsp
- Radishes – three, halved and thinly sliced
- Pumpkin seeds – ¼ cup, roasted, unsalted
- Queso fresco – half cup, crumbled
- Avocado – one, chopped

DIRECTIONS:

1. Add oil into the pot and cook over medium flame.
2. Add tortilla strips and cook for five minutes until crispy.
3. Transfer it to the plate lined with a paper towel using a slotted spoon.
4. Sprinkle with ¼ tsp salt.
5. Add half tsp salt, chili powder, onion, and poblano, and cook for two minutes until softened.
6. Add tomatoes, beans, broth, and sweet potatoes and simmer for twenty minutes.
7. Add lime juice into the soup and top with tortilla strips, avocado, queso fresco, pepitas, and radish slices. Stir well.
8. Serve and enjoy!

NUTRITION FACTS:

Calories; 412kcal,carbs; 45g, protein; 13.5g, fat; 21.6g, fiber; 11.7g

466. MINESTRONE SOUP

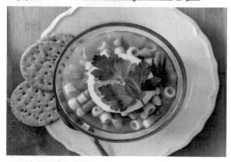

Preparation time: 5 minutes

Cooking time: 25 minutes

Serving: 6

INGREDIENTS:

- Garlic – five cloves, minced
- Extra-virgin olive oil – three tbsp
- Whole-grain rustic bread – one cup, cubed
- Leek – one cup, chopped, white and light green parts only
- Carrots – one cup, chopped
- Vegetable broth – three cups
- Water – three cups
- Kosher salt – ¾ tsp
- Ditalini pasta – one cup
- Zucchini – ten ounce, halved lengthwise and thinly sliced
- Cannellini beans – 15 ounce, unsalted, rinsed
- Kale – three cups, chopped
- Frozen peas – one cup, thawed
- Ground pepper – half tsp

DIRECTIONS:

1. Preheat the oven to 350°F-180°C.
2. Add two tbsp oil and garlic and cook over medium flame for three to four minutes.
3. Add bread and toss to combine. Place mixture onto the baking sheet and bake for eight to ten minutes.
4. During this, add one tbsp oil into the pot and cook over medium-high flame. Add carrots and leek and cook for five to six minutes.
5. Add salt, water, and broth and cover with a lid and boil it over high flame. Add pasta and lower the heat to medium-high and cook for five minutes. Add zucchini and cook for five minutes until al dente.
6. Add pepper, peas, kale, and beans and stir well. Let cook for two minutes.
7. Place soup into the six bowls. Top with croutons.

NUTRITION FACTS:

Calories; 267kcal,carbs; 38.7g, protein; 9.7g, fat; 8.6g, fiber; 7.2g

467. LENTIL SOUP

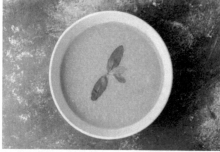

Preparation time: 5 minutes

Cooking time: 1 hour

Serving: 6

INGREDIENTS

- Onion – one, chopped
- Olive oil – ¼ cup
- Carrots – two, diced
- Celery – two stalks, chopped
- Garlic – two cloves, minced
- Dried oregano – one tsp
- Bay leaf – one
- Dried basil – one tsp
- Crushed tomatoes – 14.5 ounces

- Dry lentils – two cups
- Water – eight cups
- Spinach – half cup, rinsed and thinly sliced
- Vinegar – two tbsp
- Salt and ground black pepper – to taste

DIRECTIONS:
1. Add oil into the pot and cook over medium flame.
2. Add celery, carrots, and onions and cook until tender.
3. Add basil, oregano, bay leaf, garlic, and stir well and cook for two minutes.
4. Add tomatoes, water, and lentils and stir well. Let boil it.
5. Lower the heat and simmer for one hour.
6. Add spinach and cook until wilted.
7. Add pepper, salt, and vinegar and stir well.

NUTRITION FACTS:
Calories; 349kcal,carbs; 48.2g, protein; 18.3g, fat; 10g, fiber; 22.1g

 468. GRILLED CORN SALAD

Preparation time: 15 minutes

Cooking time: 10 minutes

Additional time: 45 minutes

Servings: 6

INGREDIENTS:
- Freshly shucked corn – six ears
- Green pepper – one, diced
- Tomatoes – two plum, diced
- Red onion – ¼ cup, diced
- Fresh cilantro – half bunch, chopped
- Olive oil – two tsp
- Salt and ground black pepper – to taste

DIRECTIONS:
1. Preheat the grill over medium heat. Oil the grate.
2. Place corn onto the grill and cook for ten minutes and keep it aside.
3. Let cool it. Cut the kernels off the cob and place them into the medium bowl.
4. Mix the olive oil, cilantro, onion, diced tomato, green pepper, and corn kernels and sprinkle with pepper and salt.
5. Toss to combine. Let stand for thirty minutes.
6. Serve and enjoy!

NUTRITION FACTS:
Calories; 103kcal,carbs; 19.7g, protein; 3.4g, fat; 2.8g, fiber; 3.3g

  469. KALE SOUP

Preparation time: 25 minutes

Cooking time: 30 minutes

Servings: 8

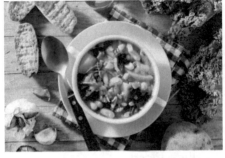

INGREDIENTS:
- Olive oil – two tbsp
- Yellow onion – one, chopped
- Garlic – two, tbsp
- Kale – one bunch, stems removed and leaves chopped
- Water – six cups
- Vegetable bouillon – six cubes
- Tomatoes – 15 ounce, diced
- White potatoes – six, peeled and cubed
- Cannellini beans – 30 ounce, drained
- Italian seasoning – one tbsp
- Dried parsley – two tbsp
- Salt and pepper – to taste

DIRECTIONS:
1. Add olive oil into the pot and heat it.
2. Add garlic and onion and cook until softened.
3. Add kale and stir, and cook for two minutes.
4. Add parsley, Italian seasoning, beans, potatoes, tomatoes, vegetable bouillon, and water and stir well. Let simmer for twenty-five minutes.
5. Sprinkle with pepper and salt.

NUTRITION FACTS:
Calories; 277kcal,carbs; 50.9g, protein; 9.6g, fat; 4.5g, fiber; 10.3g

470. PASTA FAGIOLI

Preparation time: 10 minutes

Cooking time: 30 minutes

Servings: 4

INGREDIENTS:
- Olive oil – one tbsp
- Carrot – one, diced
- Celery – one stalk, diced
- Onion – one, diced, thinly sliced
- Garlic – half tsp, chopped
- Tomato sauce – eight ounce
- Chicken broth – 14 ounce
- Ground black pepper – to taste
- Dried parsley – one tbsp
- Dried basil leaves – half tbsp
- Cannellini beans – 15 ounce, drained and rinsed
- Ditalini pasta – 1 ½ cups

DIRECTIONS:
1. Add olive oil into the saucepan and heat it over medium flame.
2. Add onion, celery, and carrot and cook until fragrant.
3. Add garlic and cook it well. Add basil, parsley, pepper, chicken broth, and tomato sauce and simmer for twenty minutes.
4. Add salt and water into the pot and boil it. Add ditalini pasta and cook for eight minutes until al dente. Let drain it.
5. Add beans to the sauce mixture and simmer for a few minutes.
6. When pasta is done, add bean mixture and sauce and stir well.
7. Serve and enjoy!

NUTRITION FACTS:
Calories; 338kcal,carbs; 60.7g, protein; 13.4g, fat; 5.1g, fiber; 9.4g

471. SWEET POTATO GNOCCHI

Preparation time: 30 minutes

Cooking time: 35 minutes

Servings: 4

INGREDIENTS:
- Sweet potatoes – eight ounce
- Garlic – one clove, pressed
- Salt – half tsp
- Ground nutmeg – half tsp
- Egg – one
- All-purpose flour – two cups

DIRECTIONS:
1. Preheat the oven to 350°F-180°C.
2. Let bake for thirty minutes until softened.
3. When done, remove it from the oven and keep it aside to cool.
4. When cooled, peel and mash them and add them to the bowl.
5. Add egg, nutmeg, salt, and garlic and mix it well.
6. Add flour and combine it well.
7. Add water and salt into the pot and boil it.
8. To prepare the gnocchi: Roll the dough onto the floured surface and cut it into sections.
9. Add pieces into the boiled water and cook until they floated on the surface.
10. When done, remove and serve!
11. Top with cream sauce or butter.

NUTRITION FACTS:
Calories; 346kcal,carbs; 71.1g, protein; 9.9g, fat; 2.1g, fiber; 5.2g

472. 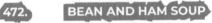 **BEAN AND HAM SOUP**

Preparation time: 25 minutes

Cooking time: 10 hours

Servings: 12

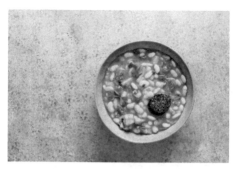

INGREDIENTS:
- Sweet potatoes – two
- Garlic – one clove, pressed
- Salt – half tsp
- Ground nutmeg – half tsp
- Egg – one
- All-purpose flour – two cups
- Bean mixture – 20 ounce, soaked overnight
- Ham bone – one
- Ham – 2 ½ cups, cubed
- Onion – one, chopped
- Celery – three stalks, chopped
- Carrots – five, chopped
- Tomatoes – 14.5 ounce, diced, with liquid
- Vegetable juice – 12 fluid ounce, low-sodium
- Vegetable broth – three cups
- Worcestershire sauce – two tbsp
- Dijon mustard – two tbsp
- Chili powder – one tbsp
- Bay leaves – three
- Ground black pepper – one tsp
- Dried parsley – one tbsp
- Lemon juice – three tbsp
- Chicken broth – seven cups, low-sodium
- Kosher salt – one tsp

DIRECTIONS:
1. Add soaked beans into the pot, and then add water until it covers the beans. Let boil it on low flame for thirty minutes. Then, drain it.
2. Add vegetable broth, vegetable juice, tomatoes, carrots, celery, onion, ham, and ham bone and sprinkle with lemon juice, parsley, pepper, bay leaf, chili powder, Dijon mustard, and Worcestershire sauce.
3. Add chicken broth and simmer on low flame for eight hours.
4. Add more chicken broth as required. Remove the ham bone and sprinkle with salt.
5. Let simmer for two hours more.
6. Discard bay leaves.

NUTRITION FACTS:
Calories; 260kcal, carbs; 37.9g, protein; 17.3g, fat; 3.6g, fiber; 14.8g

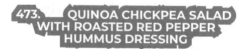

473. QUINOA CHICKPEA SALAD WITH ROASTED RED PEPPER HUMMUS DRESSING

Preparation Time: 10 minutes

Cooking Time: 0 minutes

Servings: 1

INGREDIENTS:
- 2 tablespoons hummus
- 1 tablespoon lemon juice
- 1 tablespoon chopped and roasted red pepper
- 2 cups mixed salad greens
- 1/2 cup cooked quinoa
- 1/2 cup chickpeas, rinsed
- 1 tablespoon unsalted sunflower seeds
- 1 tablespoon chopped fresh parsley
- A pinch of salt
- A pinch of ground pepper

DIRECTIONS:
1. In a small bowl, combine hummus, red peppers and lemon extract. To achieve the desired consistency, add enough water to thin.
2. In a large dish, place chickpeas, greens and quinoa. Flavor with salt and pepper to taste and garnish with parsley and sunflower seeds. Serve with dressing.

NUTRITION FACTS:
Calories: 379; Saturated Fat: 1 g Sodium: 607 mg Fiber: 13 g Cholesterol: 0 g Sugar: 3 g Protein: 16 g Fat: 10 Carbs: 59 g

474. RAINBOW BUDDHA BOWL WITH CASHEW TAHINI SAUCE

Preparation Time: 10 minutes

Cooking Time: 0 minutes

Servings: 2

INGREDIENTS:
- 3/4 cup unsalted cashews
- 1/2 cup water
- 1/4 cup packed parsley leaves
- 1 tablespoon lemon juice or cider vinegar
- 1 tablespoon extra-virgin olive oil
- 1/2 teaspoon reduced-sodium tamari or soy sauce
- 1/4 teaspoon salt
- 1/2 cup cooked lentils
- 1/2 cup cooked quinoa
- 1/2 cup shredded red cabbage
- 1/4 cup grated raw beet
- 1/4 cup chopped bell pepper
- 1/4 cup grated carrot
- 1/4 cup sliced cucumber
- Toasted chopped cashews for garnishing (optional)

DIRECTIONS:
1. In a blender, mix soy sauce or tamari, cashews, salt, water, oil, lemon juice or vinegar, and parsley until smooth.
2. In the middle of a serving bowl, put in quinoa and lentils; add cucumber, cabbage, carrot, pepper, and beet on top.
3. Ladle 2 tablespoons of cashew sauce over the vegetables; reserve the extra sauce for future use.
4. f desired, add cashews on top.

NUTRITION FACTS:
Calories: 361 Fat: 10 g Saturated Fat: 2 g Cholesterol: 0 g Sodium: 139 mg Fiber: 14 g Carbs: 54 g Sugar: 9 g Protein: 17 g

475. RICE BEAN FREEZER BURRITOS

Preparation Time: 10 minutes

Cooking Time: 0 minutes

Servings: 8

INGREDIENTS:
- 2 (15 ounces) cans low-sodium black or pinto beans, rinsed
- 4 teaspoons chili powder
- 1 teaspoon ground cumin
- 2 cups shredded sharp Cheddar cheese
- 1 cup chopped grape tomatoes
- 4 scallions, chopped
- 1/4 cup chopped pickled jalapeños
- 2 tablespoons chopped fresh cilantro
- 8 (8 inches) whole-wheat tortillas, at room temperature
- 2 cups cooked brown rice

DIRECTIONS:
1. In a big bowl, mash the beans with cumin and chili powder until it becomes almost smooth. Stir in cilantro, jalapeños, scallions, tomatoes and cheese then mix to blend.
2. On the bottom of every tortilla, put about 1/2 cup of the filling then spread, and put about 1/4 cup of rice on top.
3. Roll it up snugly and tuck the ends as you go. Use a foil to wrap each burrito. You can freeze it for up to 3 months.

Note: To warm your frozen burritos unwrap the foil and put it on a microwave-safe plate. Use a paper towel to cover it and heat for 1-2 minutes on high, until it becomes steaming hot.

NUTRITION FACTS:
Calories: 401 Fat: 13 g Saturated Fat: 6 g Cholesterol: 28 g Sodium: 646 mg Fiber: 8 g Carbs: 53 g Sugar: 4 g Protein: 17 g

476. ROASTED VEGGIE HUMMUS PITA POCKETS

Preparation Time: 10 minutes

Cooking Time: 0 minutes

Servings: 1

INGREDIENTS:
- 1 (6 ½ inches) whole-wheat pita bread
- 4 tablespoons hummus
- 1/2 cup mixed salad greens
- 1/2 cup Sheet-Pan Roasted Root Vegetables, roughly chopped (see associated recipe)
- 1 tablespoon crumbled Feta cheese

DIRECTIONS:
1. Halve the pita bread. Set the inside of each half of the pita pocket with 2 tablespoons of hummus.
2. Stuff with Feta, roasted vegetables and greens on each pita pocket.

NUTRITION FACTS:
Calories: 357 Sodium: 768 mg Cholesterol: 8 g Carbs: 54 g Sugar: 5 g Protein: 14 g Saturated Fat: 3 g Fiber: 10 g Fat: 12 g

 SALMON SUSHI BUDDHA BOWL

Preparation Time: *10 minutes*

Cooking Time: *0 minutes*

Servings: *1*

INGREDIENTS:
- 1/2 teaspoon rice vinegar
- 1/2 teaspoon honey
- 1/2 cup cooked short-grain brown rice
- 3 ounces sliced smoked salmon
- 1/2 avocado, sliced
- 1/2 cup cucumber
- 1 teaspoon reduced-sodium tamari or soy sauce
- 1 teaspoon toasted sesame oil
- 1/4 teaspoon wasabi paste
- Sesame seeds for garnishing (optional)

DIRECTIONS:
1. In a small-size bowl, mix honey and rice vinegar. Mix rice in. Into a shallow serving bowl, put the rice.
2. Place the smoked salmon, cucumber and avocado on top.
3. In a small-size bowl, mix sesame oil, wasabi and soy sauce or tamari; sprinkle on top of all. If wished, put sesame seeds on top.

NUTRITION FACTS:
Calories: 432 Sugar: 4 g Fiber: 9 g Saturated Fat: 4 g Sodium: 772 mg Cholesterol: 20 g Carbs: 37 g Protein: 20 g Fat: 24 g

 SAUSAGE PEPPERS BAKED ZITI

Preparation Time: *10 minutes*

Cooking Time: *30 minutes*

Servings: *4*

INGREDIENTS:
- 8 ounces whole-wheat penne or ziti pasta
- 1 (16 ounces) bag frozen pepper and onion mix
- 6 ounces turkey sausage crumbled
- 2 (8 ounces) cans no-salt-added tomato sauce
- 1 teaspoon garlic powder
- 1 teaspoon dried oregano
- 1/4 teaspoon salt
- 1/2 cup reduced-fat Cottage cheese
- 3/4 cup Italian blend shredded cheese

DIRECTIONS:
1. Following the package instructions, cook the pasta properly in a pot of boiling water. Strain.
2. Meanwhile, place a large ovenproof skillet on medium-high heat. Put in the sausage and frozen vegetables; cook while stirring occasionally for 10-15 minutes, till most of the liquid from the vegetables is evaporated.
3. Set a rack in the upper third of the oven; preheat the broiler.
4. Combine salt, oregano, garlic powder and tomato sauce into the skillet. Set the heat down to medium-low; mix in the pasta and Cottage cheese.
5. Cook while stirring for around 2 minutes, till heated through. Place shredded cheese on top.
6. Place the skillet under the preheated broiler; brown the cheese for 1-2 minutes.

NUTRITION FACTS:
Calories: 408 Fat: 10 g Sodium: 702 mg Fiber: 11 g Cholesterol: 48 g Carbs: 58 g Sugar: 9 g Saturated Fat: 4 g Protein: 27 g

 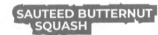 **SAUTEED BUTTERNUT SQUASH**

Preparation Time: *10 minutes*

Cooking Time: *15 minutes*

Servings: *7*

INGREDIENTS:
- 1 large butternut squash (2-3 pounds), peeled, seeded and cubed
- 1 tablespoon extra-virgin olive oil

DIRECTIONS:
1. In a big saucepan, heat oil on moderate fire.
2. Put in the squash and cook for 15 minutes while stirring often, until brown slightly and soften.

NUTRITION FACTS:
Calories: 75 Sugar: 3 g Protein: 1 g Fat: 2 g Saturated Fat: 0 g Sodium: 5 mg Fiber: 3 g Cholesterol: 0 g Carbs: 15 g

 SEARED SALMON WITH PESTO FETTUCCINE

Preparation Time: *10 minutes*

Cooking Time: *20 minutes*

Servings: *4*

INGREDIENTS:
- 8 ounces whole-wheat Fettuccine
- 2/3 cup pesto
- 1 ¼ pound wild salmon, skinned and cut into 4 portions
- 1/4 teaspoon salt
- 1/4 teaspoon ground pepper
- 1 tablespoon extra-virgin olive oil

DIRECTIONS:
1. Boil a large pot of water. Include in the Fettuccine; cook for around 9 minutes, or till just tender. Strain; transfer into a large bowl. Toss with pesto.
2. Meanwhile, season with pepper and salt on salmon. Set a large, non-stick, or cast-iron skillet on medium-high heat; heat oil. Include in the salmon; cook for 2-4 minutes per side, or till just opaque in the center, turning once.
3. Serve the salmon accompanied with the pasta.

NUTRITION FACTS:
Calories: 603 Protein: 44 g Fat: 28 g Saturated Fat: 7 g Sodium: 537 mg Fiber: 8 g Cholesterol: 80 g Carbs: 45 g Sugar: 2

 SESAME GINGER CHICKEN SALAD

Preparation Time: *10 minutes*

Cooking Time: *0 minutes*

Servings: *1*

INGREDIENTS:
- 4 cups chopped romaine lettuce
- 3 ounces shredded cooked chicken breast
- 1/2 cup fresh spinach
- 1/4 cup shredded carrot
- 1/4 cup sliced radishes
- 1 scallion, sliced
- 3 tablespoons prepared sesame-ginger dressing

DIRECTIONS:
1. In a medium bowl, mix scallion, radishes, carrot, spinach, chicken and lettuce, then put in the dressing and toss to coat well.

NUTRITION FACTS:

Calories: 331 Fat: 17 g Saturated Fat: 3 g Cholesterol: 72 g Carbs: 16 g Protein: 30 g Sodium: 378 mg Fiber: 6 g Sugar: 7 g

482. SKILLET GNOCCHI WITH CHARD WHITE BEANS

Preparation Time: 10 minutes

Cooking Time: 30 minutes

Servings: 6

INGREDIENTS:

- 1 tablespoon extra-virgin olive oil
- 1 (16 ounces) package shelf-stable gnocchi
- 1 teaspoon extra-virgin olive oil
- 1 medium yellow onion, thinly sliced
- 4 garlic cloves, minced
- 1/2 cup water
- 6 cups chopped chard leaves or spinach
- 1 can diced tomatoes with Italian seasonings
- 1 (15 ounces) can white beans, rinsed
- 1/4 teaspoon freshly ground pepper
- 1/2 cup shredded part-skim Mozzarella cheese
- 1/4 cup finely shredded Parmesan cheese

DIRECTIONS:

1. On medium heat, heat 1 tablespoon of oil in a big non-stick pan. Add and cook the gnocchi while stirring frequently for 5-7 minutes until it begins to brown and plump; move to a bowl.
2. Add the onion and the remaining teaspoon of oil into the pan.
3. On medium heat, cook and stir for 2 minutes. Mix in water and garlic; cover. Cook for 4-6 minutes until the onion is soft; put the chard or spinach in. Cook and stir for 1-2 minutes until it begins to wilt.
4. Mix in pepper, beans, and tomatoes; simmer. Combine in the gnocchi then scatter Parmesan and Mozzarella; cover. Cook for about 3 minutes until the sauce bubbles and the cheese melts.

NUTRITION FACTS:

Calories: 259 Sodium: 505 mg Carbs: 29.5 g Cholesterol: 23 g Protein: 9.7 g Fat: 11.1 g

483. SPAGHETTI GENOVESE

Preparation Time: 10 minutes

Cooking Time: 20 minutes

Servings: 5

INGREDIENTS:

- 2 cups packed baby spinach
- 8 ounces whole-wheat spaghetti
- 1 cup thinly sliced new or baby potatoes (about 4 ounces)
- 1 pound green beans
- 1/2 cup prepared pesto
- 1 teaspoon freshly ground pepper
- 1/2 teaspoon salt

DIRECTIONS:

1. Boil a big pot of water on medium-high heat. Put in the spinach and cook for about 45 seconds, just until it wilts.
2. Move the spinach to a blender using a fine sieve or a slotted spoon.
3. Bring the water back to a boil and put in potatoes and spaghetti.
4. Cook for 6-7 minutes until they are almost soft, only stirring 1-2 times.
5. Put in green beans and cook for another 3-4 minutes until they become soft.
6. When the vegetables and spaghetti are almost cooked, carefully take out 1 cup of the cooking liquid.
7. Pour 1/2 cup of the liquid into the blender; place in salt, pepper, and pesto. Merge until smooth, stop to scrape down the sides if you want.
8. Strain the vegetables and the spaghetti, set back to the pot; add the pesto mixture and stir. Set the heat and cook while gently stirring the pasta for 1-2 minutes until it is hot and the sauce is thickened. If you want a thinner sauce, you can add in more cooking liquid.

NUTRITION FACTS:

Calories: 333 Saturated Fat: 3 g Cholesterol: 8 g Fat: 12 g Carbs: 47 g Sugar: 3 g Protein: 14 g Sodium: 438 mg Fiber: 10 g

484. SPICED SWEET POTATO WEDGES

Preparation Time: 10 minutes

Cooking Time: 25-30 minutes

Servings: 4

INGREDIENTS:

- 2 (20 ounces) sweet potatoes, scrubbed
- 1 tablespoon olive oil
- 1 teaspoon packed brown sugar
- 1/4 teaspoon kosher salt
- 1/4 teaspoon smoked paprika
- 1/4 teaspoon black pepper
- 1/4 teaspoon pumpkin pie spice
- 1/4 teaspoon hot chili powder

DIRECTIONS:

1. Set an oven to preheat at 425°F-220°C.
2. Put a baking tray in the oven to preheat.
3. Halve each sweet potato lengthwise into 8 wedges or 16 wedges in total.
4. Drizzle olive oil on sweet potato wedges in a big bowl, then toss to coat well.
5. Stir the chili powder, pumpkin pie spice, pepper, smoked paprika, kosher salt, and brown sugar in a small bowl.
6. Sprinkle sweet potatoes with the spice mixture then toss to coat well.
7. On the hot baking tray, lay out the wedges in one layer. Roast until it turns brown and soft, or for 25-30 minutes, flipping the wedges once halfway through the roasting time.

NUTRITION FACTS:

Calories: 124 Cholesterol: 0 g Saturated Fat: 0 g Fiber: 3 g Carbs: 22 g Sugar: 5 g Protein: 2 g Fat: 3 g Sodium: 184 mg

485. STETSON CHOPPED SALAD

Preparation Time: 10 minutes

Cooking Time: 10 minutes

Servings: 1

INGREDIENTS:

- 3/4 cup water
- 1/2 cup Israeli couscous
- 6 cups baby arugula
- 1 cup fresh corn kernels
- 1 cup halved or quartered cherry tomatoes
- 1 firm-ripe avocado, diced
- 1/4 cup toasted pepitas
- 1/4 cup dried currants
- 1/2 cup chopped fresh basil
- 1/4 cup buttermilk
- 1/4 cup mayonnaise
- 1 tablespoon lemon juice
- 1 small clove garlic, peeled
- 1/4 teaspoon salt
- 1/4 teaspoon ground pepper

DIRECTIONS:

1. In a small saucepan, set water to a boil. Put in couscous and lower heat to keep a gentle simmer, then cover and cook for 8-10 minutes, until water is absorbed.
2. Move to a fine-mesh sieve and rinse under cold water, then drain well.
3. On a serving plate, spread the arugula. Put the arugula over the currants, pepitas, avocado, tomatoes, corn and couscous in decorative lines.
4. In a blender or mini food processor, mix pepper, salt, garlic, lemon juice, mayonnaise, buttermilk and basil, then pulse until smooth. Right before serving, drizzle the salad with the dressing.

NUTRITION FACTS:

Calories: 376 Carbs: 39 g Sugar: 11 g Saturated Fat: 4 g Fiber: 7 g Protein: 9 g Fat: 23 g Sodium: 266 mg Cholesterol: 7 g

486. STUFFED SWEET POTATO WITH HUMMUS DRESSING

Preparation Time: 10 minutes

Cooking Time: 15 minutes

Servings: 1

INGREDIENTS:
- 1 large sweet potato, scrubbed
- 3/4 cup chopped kale
- 1 cup canned black beans, rinsed
- 1/4 cup hummus
- 2 tablespoons water

DIRECTIONS:
1. Using a fork, stab the sweet potato all over then microwave on high for 7-10 minutes until completely cooked.
2. Rinse and drain the kale, let the water hold to the leaves. On medium-high heat, cook the kale in a medium saucepan, covered, until it wilts; stir 1-2 times.
3. Put in beans; pour 1-2 tablespoons of water if the pot dries.
4. Cook and stir occasionally without cover for 1-2 minutes until the mixture is steaming.
5. Break and open the sweet potato; add the beans and the kale mixture on top.
6. In a small dish, mix 2 tablespoons of water and hummus. If needed, pour in more water to reach the preferred thickness.
7. Spread the hummus dressing on top of the sweet potato.

NUTRITION FACTS:
Calories: 472 Fiber: 22 g Cholesterol: 0 g Carbs: 85 g Sugar: 20 g Sodium: 489 mg Protein: 21 g Fat: 7 g Saturated Fat: 1 g

487. SUMMER SQUASH WHITE BEAN SAUTE

Preparation Time: 10 minutes

Cooking Time: 20 minutes

Servings: 4

INGREDIENTS:
- 1 tablespoon olive oil
- 1 medium onion, halved and sliced
- 2 garlic cloves, minced
- 1 medium zucchini, halved lengthwise and sliced
- 1 medium yellow summer squash, halved lengthwise and sliced
- 1 tablespoon chopped fresh oregano
- 1/4 teaspoon salt
- 1/4 teaspoon ground pepper
- 1 (15-19 ounces) can cannellini or great northern beans, rinsed
- 2 medium tomatoes
- 1 tablespoon red-wine vinegar
- 1/3 cup finely shredded Parmesan cheese

DIRECTIONS:
1. In a big non-stick skillet, heat oil over medium heat. Add garlic and onion. Cook while stirring for 3 minutes until starting to get tender.
2. Add pepper, salt, oregano, summer squash, and zucchini; mix to blend.
3. Lower the heat to low; put a cover on and cook for 3-5 minutes until the vegetables are tender-crisp, stirring 1 time.
4. Mix in vinegar, tomatoes, and beans; raise the heat to medium and cook for 2 minutes until heated through.
5. Take away from the heat and sprinkle Parmesan cheese.

NUTRITION FACTS:
Calories: 193 Cholesterol: 5 g Protein: 10 g Fat: 6 g Saturated Fat: 2 g Sugar: 7 g Sodium: 599 mg Fiber: 7 g Carbs: 25 g

488. SWEET SAVORY HUMMUS PLATE

Preparation Time: 10 minutes

Cooking Time: 0 minutes

Servings: 4

INGREDIENTS:
- 3/4 cup white bean dip
- 1 cup green beans, stem ends trimmed
- 8 mini bell peppers
- 20 olives
- 8 small watermelon wedges or 2 cups cubed watermelon
- 1 cup red grapes
- 20 gluten-free crackers
- 1/2 cup salted roasted pepitas
- 8 coconut-date balls

DIRECTIONS:
1. Separate the items equally into 4 plates.
2. Serve with hard cider if desired.

NUTRITION FACTS:
Calories: 654 Cholesterol: 0 g Protein: 14 g Fat: 30 g Fiber: 11 g Sugar: 39 g Saturated Fat: 3 g Sodium: 568 mg Carbs: 84 mg

489. SWEET POTATO BLACK BEAN CHILI FOR TWO

Preparation Time: 10 minutes

Cooking Time: 20 minutes

Servings: 2

INGREDIENTS:
- 2 teaspoons virgin olive oil
- 1 small onion
- 1 small sweet potato
- 2 garlic cloves
- 1 tablespoon chili powder
- 2 teaspoons ground cumin
- 1/4 teaspoon ground chipotle chile
- 1/8 teaspoon salt, or to taste
- 1 1/3 cup water
- 1 (15 ounces) can black beans, rinsed
- 1 cup canned diced tomatoes
- 2 teaspoons lime juice
- 2 tablespoons chopped fresh cilantro

DIRECTIONS:
1. Heat a big pan with oil over medium-high heat, add potato and onion, then cook, stirring frequently, until the onion becomes slightly soft, roughly 4 minutes.
2. Add salt, chipotle, cumin, chili powder, and garlic, then cook, continuously stirring, for around 30 seconds until aromatic.
3. Attach the water and bring to a simmer, cover, turn the heat down to keep it gently simmering.
4. Cook until the potato becomes tender, around 10-12 minutes.
5. Add lime juice, tomatoes, and beans, then turn the heat up to high and simmer, stirring frequently.
6. Turn the heat down to keep at a simmer and cook until the mixture reduces slightly, roughly 4 minutes.

NUTRITION FACTS:
Calories: 365 Fat: 7 g Sodium: 629 mg Carbs: 67 g Sugar: 16 g Protein: 14 g Saturated Fat: 1 g Fiber: 18 g Cholesterol: 0 g

490. TABBOULEH, HUMMUS PITA PLATE

Preparation Time: 10 minutes

Cooking Time: 0 minutes

Servings: 4

INGREDIENTS:
- 2 cups tabbouleh
- 1 cup beet hummus
- 1 cup sugar snap peas, stem ends snapped off
- 4 radishes
- 1 cup mixed olives
- 1 cup raspberries
- 1 cup blackberries
- 4 whole-wheat pita bread
- 2/3 cup unsalted dry-roasted pistachios
- 4 vegan cookies

DIRECTIONS:

1. Distribute all the ingredients among 4 serving plates.

NUTRITION FACTS:

Calories: 537 Fat: 31 g Sugar: 12 g Protein: 13 g Saturated Fat: 5 g Sodium: 655 g Fiber: 14 g Cholesterol: 0 g Carbs: 55 g

491. PORK AND PENNE PASTA

Preparation Time: 20 mins.

Cooking Time: 30 mins.

Servings: 4

INGREDIENTS:

- whole wheat penne pasta (1 lb.)
- ground Pork lean (1 lb)
- extra virgin olive oil (2 tbs)
- onion (1 small, chopped)
- garlic cloves (2, minced)
- can tomatoes (1 (15 oz), diced, seeded)
- green zucchini (2 cups sliced to 1/4 cubes)
- baby spinach (8 oz., fresh, chopped)
- low fat parmesan cheese (1 cup, grated)

DIRECTIONS:

1. Bring a pot of water to a boil, ensure that the water is salted. Cook the pasta to an al dente consistency or according to package directions.
2. In a non-stick pan, cook the ground Pork over medium heat for 8 minutes or until it is browned, ensure to break up any large pieces in the pan.
3. Remove Pork and set aside. Discard drippings. Add in your oil on medium heat.
4. Cook onions and garlic for about 5 minutes or until soft. Add tomatoes and zucchini and continue cooking 5 minutes more.
5. Add spinach and cook until it just wilts, 2-3 minutes. Place the Pork back into the skillet and add 1/2 cup cheese; stir and heat through.
6. Plate your pasta then top with your meat mixture. Toss well and top evenly with cheese.

NUTRITION FACTS:

206 calories, 9 g fat, 24g carbs, 13 g fiber, 17 g protein

492. TOMATO ARTICHOKE GNOCCHI

Preparation Time: 10 minutes

Cooking Time: 20 minutes

Servings: 4

INGREDIENTS:

- 2 tablespoons extra-virgin olive oil
- 1 (16 ounces) package shelf-stable gnocchi
- 1 small onion, sliced
- 1 small red bell pepper
- 4 large garlic cloves
- 1 tablespoon chopped fresh oregano
- 1 (15 ounces) can chickpeas
- 1 (14 ounces) can no-salt-added diced tomatoes
- 1 (9 ounces) box frozen artichoke hearts
- 8 pitted Kalamata olives, sliced
- 1 tablespoon red-wine vinegar
- 1/4 teaspoon ground pepper

DIRECTIONS:

1. In a non-stick skillet, heat 1 tablespoon of oil over medium-high heat.
2. Put in the gnocchi; cook and stir often for about 5 minutes, until plumped and beginning to brown.
3. Place them in a bowl and cover
4. -up to keep warm.
5. Lower heat to medium. Attach in the onion and the remaining tablespoon of oil.
6. Cook for 2-3 minutes, stirring occasionally, until beginning to brown.
7. Add in bell pepper; cook for about 3 minutes, stirring occasionally, until crisp-tender.
8. Put in the oregano and garlic; cook for half a minute, stirring.
9. Set in artichokes, tomatoes and chickpeas; cook for about 3 minutes, stirring, until hot.
10. Mix in the gnocchi, pepper, vinegar and olives.
11. Sprinkle oregano on top, if desired.

NUTRITION FACTS:

Calories: 427 Fat: 11 g Sugar: 5 g Protein: 12 g Carbs: 71 g Saturated Fat: 1 g Sodium: 615 mg Fiber: 10 g Cholesterol: 0 g

493. VEGAN BUDDHA BOWL

Preparation Time: 10 minutes

Cooking Time: 20 minutes

Servings: 4

INGREDIENTS:

- 1 medium sweet potato
- 3 tablespoons extra-virgin olive oil
- 1/2 teaspoon salt
- 1/2 teaspoon ground pepper
- 2 tablespoons tahini
- 2 tablespoons water
- 1 tablespoon lemon juice
- 1 small clove garlic
- 2 cups cooked quinoa
- 1 (15 ounces) can chickpeas, rinsed
- 1 firm-ripe avocado, diced
- 1/4 cup cilantro or parsley

DIRECTIONS:

1. Set the oven temperature to 425°F -220°C to preheat.
2. In a medium bowl, mix the sweet potato with 1/4 teaspoon each of salt and pepper plus 1 tablespoon of oil.
3. Move to a rimmed baking sheet. For 15-18 minutes, roast, stir once, until tender.
4. In a small bowl, mix the leftover 2 tablespoons of oil, lemon juice, tahini, garlic, water, and the leftover 1/4 teaspoon each of salt and pepper.
5. Split the quinoa among 4 bowls to serve.
6. Garnish with equal amounts of chickpeas, sweet potato and avocado.
7. Drizzle with the tahini sauce.
8. Top with parsley or cilantro.

NUTRITION FACTS:

Calories: 455 Fat: 25 g Sodium: 472 mg Sugar: 3 g Protein: 11 g Carbs: 51 g Saturated Fat: 3 g Fiber: 11 g Cholesterol: 0 g

494. VEGAN CAULIFLOWER FRIED RICE

Preparation Time: 10 minutes

Cooking Time: 15 minutes

Servings: 4

INGREDIENTS:

- 3 tablespoons peanut oil, divided
- 3 scallions, sliced
- 1 tablespoon grated fresh ginger
- 1 tablespoon minced garlic
- 1/2 cup diced red bell pepper
- 1 cup trimmed and halved snow peas
- 1 cup shredded carrots
- 1 cup frozen shelled edamame, thawed
- 4 cups riced cauliflower
- 1/3 cup unsalted roasted cashews
- 3 tablespoons tamari or soy sauce
- 1 teaspoon toasted sesame oil

DIRECTIONS:

1. In a cooking pan or wok, heat 1 tablespoon of peanut oil over high heat.
2. Cook and stir the ginger, garlic, and scallions in the hot oil for 30-40 seconds until scallions have softened.
3. Add the snow peas, bell pepper, edamame, and carrots then cook while stirring for 2-4 minutes until just tender.
4. Move everything to a dish or plate.
5. Set the remaining 2 tablespoons of peanut oil into the pan.
6. Stir the cauliflower in the oil for about 2 minutes until it's mostly softened.
7. Put the vegetables back in the pan; add tamari or soy sauce, cashews and sesame oil.
8. Stir together until blended

properly.

NUTRITION FACTS:

Calories: 287 Fat: 19 g Saturated Fat: 3 g Fiber: 6 g Cholesterol: 0 g Carbs: 18 g Sodium: 451 mg Sugar: 6 g Protein: 10 g

495. OATMEAL BREAD TO LIVE FOR

Preparation Time: 10 minutes

Cooking Time: 30 minutes

Servings: 12

INGREDIENTS:

- 1 ¼ cup (295 ml) water
- 2 teaspoons (10 ml) canola oil
- 1 tablespoon (15 g) brown sugar
- 1 cup (80 g) quick-cooking oats
- 2 ¼ cups whole-wheat flour, divided
- 1 tablespoon vital wheat gluten
- 1 ¼ teaspoon yeast
- 1 tablespoon shelled sunflower seeds

DIRECTIONS:

1. Put water, oil, and sugar in the bread machine.
2. Add the oats and let them sit for 5 minutes.
3. Pour 2 cups (240 g) of flour and the gluten.
4. Set a well in the middle of the flour for the yeast.
5. Turn on the bread machine. (Use a setting for 1 ½-pound [680 g] loaf, dark if you have it). If the dough seems too sticky, attach additional flour as required.
6. Add the sunflower seeds to the beep.

NUTRITION FACTS:

Calories: 287 Fat: 19 g Saturated Fat: 3 g Fiber: 6 g Cholesterol: 0 g Carbs: 18 g

496. VERMICELLI PUTTANESCA

Preparation Time: 10 minutes

Cooking Time: 15 minutes

Servings: 6

INGREDIENTS:

- 4 large tomatoes
- 1/4 cup chopped flat-leaf parsley
- 16 large black olives
- 3 tablespoons capers
- 4 anchovy fillets
- 2 tablespoons olive oil
- 3 large garlic cloves
- 1/2 teaspoon ground pepper
- 1 pound whole-wheat vermicelli, or spaghettini
- 1/4 cup freshly grated Pecorino Romano

DIRECTIONS:

1. Combine pepper, garlic, oil, anchovies, capers, olives, parsley, and tomatoes in a large pasta serving bowl.
2. In the meantime, in a pot of boiling salted water, cook pasta for 8-10 minutes, until just tender, or following the package directions.
3. Drain the pasta and put it into the bowl with the sauce.
4. Next, toss well to combine.
5. Then taste and adjust seasonings.
6. Dust with cheese and immediately serve.

NUTRITION FACTS:

Calories: 379 Saturated Fat: 2 g Sodium: 379 mg Fiber: 11 g Sugar: 6 g Fat: 10 g Cholesterol: 5 g Carbs: 64 g Protein: 14 g

497. HEAVENLY TASTY STEW

Preparation Time: 15 minutes

Cooking Time: 35 minutes

Servings: 6

INGREDIENTS:

- ¼ C. olive oil
- 1 large yellow onion, chopped
- 8 oz. fresh shiitake mushrooms, sliced
- 2 large tomatoes, chopped
- 2 tbsp. garlic, chopped finely
- 2 bay leaves
- 2 tbsp. mixed Italian herbs (rosemary, thyme, basil), chopped
- 1 tsp. cayenne pepper
- 4 C. homemade vegetable broth
- 2 tbsp. apple cider vinegar
- 1 C. whole-wheat fusilli pasta
- 1/3 C. nutritional yeast
- 8 oz. fresh collard greens
- 1 (15-oz.) can cannellini beans, drained and rinsed
- Salt and freshly ground black pepper, to taste

DIRECTIONS:

1. In a large pan, heat the oil over medium heat and sauté the onion, mushrooms, potato and tomato for about 4-5 minutes.
2. Add the garlic, bay leaves, herbs and cayenne pepper and sauté for about 1 minute.
3. Add the broth and bring to a boil.
4. Stir in the vinegar, pasta and nutritional yeast and again bring to a boil.
5. Reduce the heat to medium-low and simmer, covered for about 20 minutes.
6. Uncover and stir in the greens and beans.
7. Simmer for about 4-5 minutes.
8. Stir in the salt and black pepper and remove from the heat.
9. Serve hot.

NUTRITION FACTS:

calories: 314; carbs: 46g; Protein: 14.4g; Fat: 10g; Sugar: 6.2g; Sodium: 489mg; Fiber: 12.3g

498. THANKSGIVING DINNER CHILI

Preparation Time: 15 minutes

Cooking Time: 45 minutes

Servings: 6

INGREDIENTS:

- 2 tbsp. olive oil
- 1 red bell pepper, seeded and chopped
- 1 onion, chopped
- 2 garlic cloves, chopped
- 1 lb. lean ground turkey
- 2 C. water
- 3 C. tomatoes, chopped finely
- 1 tsp. ground cumin
- ½ tsp. ground cinnamon
- 1 (15-oz.) can red kidney beans, rinsed and drained
- 1 (15-oz.) cans black beans, rinsed and drained
- ¼ C. scallion greens, chopped

DIRECTIONS:

1. In a large Dutch oven, heat the olive oil over medium-low heat and sauté bell pepper, onion and garlic for about 5 minutes.
2. Add the turkey and cook for about 5-6 minutes, breaking up the chunks with a wooden spoon.
3. Add the water, tomatoes and spices and bring to a boil over high heat.
4. Reduce the heat to medium-low and stir in beans and corn.
5. Simmer, covered for about 30 minutes, stirring occasionally.
6. Serve hot with the topping of scallion greens.

NUTRITION FACTS:

calories: 366; carbs: 40.6g; Protein: 28.7g; Fat: 11.2g; Sugar: 4.5g; Sodium: 100mg; Fiber: 13.4g

499. BEANS TRIO CHILI

Preparation Time: 15 minutes

Cooking Time: 1 hour

Servings: 6

INGREDIENTS:

- 2 tbsp. olive oil
- 1 green bell pepper, seeded and chopped
- 2 celery stalks, chopped
- 1 scallion, chopped
- 3 garlic cloves, minced
- 1 tsp. dried oregano, crushed
- 1 tbsp. red chili powder
- 2 tsp. ground cumin
- 1 tsp. red pepper flakes, crushed
- 1 tsp. ground turmeric
- 1 tsp. onion powder
- 1 tsp. garlic powder
- Salt and freshly ground black

- pepper, to taste
- 4½ C. tomatoes, peeled, seeded and chopped finely
- 4 C. water
- 1 (16-oz.) can red kidney beans, rinsed and drained
- 1 (16-oz.) can cannellini beans, rinsed and drained
- ½ of (16-oz.) can black beans, rinsed and drained

DIRECTIONS:

1. In a large pan, heat the oil over medium heat and cook the bell peppers, celery, scallion and garlic for about 8-10 minutes, stirring frequently.
2. Add the oregano, spices, salt, black pepper, tomatoes and water and bring to a boil.
3. Simmer for about 20 minutes.
4. Stir in the beans and simmer for about 30 minutes.
5. Serve hot.

NUTRITION FACTS:

calories: 342;carbs: 56g; Protein: 20.3g; Fat: 6.1g; Sugar: 6g; Sodium: 79mg; Fiber: 21.3g

 500. STAPLE VEGAN CURRY

Preparation Time: 15 minutes

Cooking Time: 40 minutes

Servings: 6

INGREDIENTS:

- 10 oz. whole-wheat pasta
- 1 tbsp. vegetable oil
- 1 medium white onion, chopped
- 3 garlic cloves, minced
- 1 tsp. dried basil, crushed
- 1 tbsp. curry powder
- ¼ tsp. red pepper flakes, crushed
- 2 lb. ripe tomatoes, peeled, seeded and chopped
- 4 C. cauliflower, cut into bite-sized pieces
- 1 medium red bell pepper, seeded and sliced thinly
- 1 C. water
- 1 (15-oz.) can chickpeas, drained and rinsed
- 1 C. fresh baby spinach
- ¼ C. fresh parsley, chopped
- Salt, to taste

DIRECTIONS:

1. In a pan of the salted boiling water, add the pasta and cook for about 8-10 minutes or according to package's directions.
2. Drain the pasta well and set aside.
3. Heat the oil in a large cast-iron skillet over medium heat and sauté the onion for about 4-5 minutes.
4. Add the garlic, basil, curry powder and red pepper flakes and sauté for 1 minute.
5. Stir in the tomatoes, cauliflower, bell pepper and water and bring to a gentle boil.
6. Reduce the heat to medium-low and simmer, covered for about 15-20 minutes.
7. Stir in the chickpeas and cook for about 5 minutes.
8. Add the spinach and cook for about 3-4 minutes.
9. Stir in the pasta and remove from the heat.
10. Serve hot.

NUTRITION FACTS:

calories: 338;carbs: 58.4g; Protein: 15.1g; Fat: 5.9g; Sugar: 10.9g; Sodium: 80mg; Fiber: 10.3g

 501. FRAGRANT VEGETARIAN CURRY

Preparation Time: 15 minutes

Cooking Time: 1½ hours

Servings: 8

INGREDIENTS:

- 8 C. water
- ½ tsp. ground turmeric
- 1 C. brown lentils
- 1 C. red lentils
- 1 tbsp. olive oil
- 1 large white onion, chopped
- 3 garlic cloves, minced
- 2 large tomatoes, peeled, seeded and chopped
- 1½ tbsp. curry powder
- ¼ tsp. ground cloves
- 2 tsp. ground cumin
- 3 carrots, peeled and chopped
- 3 C. pumpkin, peeled, seeded and cubed into 1-inch size
- 1 granny smith apple, cored and chopped
- 2 C. fresh spinach, chopped
- Salt and freshly ground black pepper, to taste

DIRECTIONS:

1. In a large pan, add the water, turmeric and lentils over high heat and bring to a boil.
2. Reduce the heat to medium-low and simmer, covered for about 30 minutes.
3. Drain the lentils, reserving 2½ C. of the cooking liquid.
4. Meanwhile, in another large pan, heat the oil over medium heat and sauté the onion for about 2-3 minutes.
5. Add in the garlic and sauté for about 1 minute.
6. Add the tomatoes and cook for about 5 minutes.
7. Stir in the curry powder and spices and cook for about 1 minute.
8. Add the carrots, potatoes, pumpkin, cooked lentils and reserved cooking liquid and bring to a gentle boil.
9. Reduce the heat to medium-low and simmer, covered for about 40-45 minutes or until desired doneness of the vegetables.
10. Stir in the apple and spinach and simmer for about 15 minutes.
11. Stir in the salt and black pepper and remove from the heat.
12. Serve hot.

NUTRITION FACTS:

calories: 263;carbs: 47g; Protein: 14.7g; Fat: 2.9g; Sugar: 9.7g; Sodium: 53mg; Fiber: 20g

502. OMEGA-3 RICH DINNER MEAL

Preparation Time: 15 minutes

Cooking Time: 40 minutes

Servings: 4

INGREDIENTS:

For Lentils:
- ½ lb. French green lentils
- 2 tbsp. extra-virgin olive oil
- 2 C. yellow onions, chopped
- 2 C. scallions, chopped
- 1 tsp. fresh parsley, chopped
- Salt and freshly ground black pepper, to taste
- 1 tbsp. garlic, minced
- 1½ C. carrots, peeled and chopped
- 1½ C. celery stalks, chopped
- 1 large tomato, peeled, seeded and crushed finely
- 1½ C. chicken bone broth
- 2 tbsp. balsamic vinegar

For Salmon:
- 2 (8-oz.) skinless salmon fillets
- 2 tbsp. extra-virgin olive oil
- Salt and freshly ground black pepper, to taste

DIRECTIONS:

1. In a heat-proof bowl, soak the lentils in boiling water for 15 minutes.
2. Drain the lentils completely.
3. In a Dutch oven, heat the oil in over medium heat and cook the onions, scallions, parsley, salt and black pepper for about 10 minutes, stirring frequently.
4. Add the garlic and cook for about 2 more minutes.
5. Add the drained lentils, carrots, celery, crushed tomato and broth and bring to a boil.
6. Reduce the heat to low and simmer, covered for about 20-25 minutes.
7. Stir in the vinegar, salt and black pepper and remove from the heat.
8. Meanwhile, for salmon: preheat your oven to 450 degrees F.
9. Rub the salmon fillets with oil and then, season with salt and black pepper generously.
10. Heat an oven-proof sauté pan over medium heat and cook the salmon fillets for about 2 minutes, without stirring.
11. Flip the fillets and immediately transfer the pan into the oven.

12. Bake for about 5-7 minutes or until desired doneness of salmon.
13. Remove from the oven and place the salmon fillets onto a cutting board.
14. Cut each fillet into 2 portions.
15. Divide the lentil mixture onto serving plates and top each with 1 salmon fillet.
16. Serve hot.

NUTRITION FACTS:

calories: 707;carbs: 50.2g; Protein: 16.1g; Fat: 29.8g; Sugar: 7.9g; Sodium: 496mg; Fiber: 16.2g

503. WEEKEND DINNER CASSEROLE

Preparation Time: 20 minutes

Cooking Time: 1 hour

Servings: 6

INGREDIENTS:

- 2½ C. water, divided
- 1 C. red lentils
- ½ C. wild rice
- 1 tsp. olive oil
- 1 small onion, chopped
- 3 garlic cloves, minced
- 1/3 C. zucchini, peeled, seeded and chopped
- 1/3 C. carrot, peeled and chopped
- 1/3 C. celery stalk, chopped
- 1 large tomato, peeled, seeded and chopped
- 8 oz. tomato sauce
- 1 tsp. ground cumin
- 1 tsp. dried oregano, crushed
- 1 tsp. dried basil, crushed
- Salt and freshly ground black pepper, to taste

DIRECTIONS:

1. In a pan, add 1 C. of the water and rice over medium-high heat and bring to a rolling boil.
2. Reduce the heat to low and simmer, covered for about 20 minutes.
3. Meanwhile, in another pan, add the remaining water and lentils over medium heat and bring to a rolling boil.
4. Reduce the heat to low and simmer, covered for about 15 minutes.
5. Transfer the cooked rice and lentils into a casserole dish and set aside.
6. Preheat your oven to 350 degrees F.
7. Heat the oil in a large skillet over medium heat and sauté the onion and garlic for about 4-5 minutes.
8. Add the zucchini, carrot, celery, tomato and tomato paste and cook for about 4-5 minutes.
9. Stir in the cumin, herbs, salt and black pepper and remove from the heat.
10. Transfer the vegetable mixture into the casserole dish with rice and lentils and stir to combine.
11. Bake for about 30 minutes.
12. Remove from the heat and set aside for about 5 minutes.
13. Cut into equal-sized 6 pieces and serve.

NUTRITION FACTS:

calories: 192;carbs: 34.5g; Protein: 11.3g; Fat: 1.5g; Sugar: 3.9g; Sodium: 239mg; Fiber: 12g

504. FAMILY DINNER PILAF

Preparation Time: 15 minutes

Cooking Time: 1 hour

Servings: 4

INGREDIENTS:

- 2 tbsp. olive oil
- 2 garlic cloves, minced
- 2 C. fresh mushrooms, sliced
- 1¼ C. brown rice, rinsed
- 2 C. homemade vegetable broth
- Salt and freshly ground black pepper, to taste
- 1 red bell pepper, seeded and chopped
- 4 scallions, chopped
- 1 (16-oz.) can red kidney beans, drained and rinsed
- 2 tbsp. fresh parsley, chopped

DIRECTIONS:

1. In a large pan, heat the oil over medium heat and sauté the onion for about 4-5 minutes.
2. Add the garlic and mushrooms and cook about 5-6 minutes.
3. Stir in the rice and cook for about 1-2 minutes, stirring continuously.
4. Stir in the broth, salt and black pepper and bring to a boil.
5. Reduce the heat to low and simmer, covered for about 35 minutes, stirring occasionally.
6. Add in the bell pepper and beans and cook for about 5-10 minutes or until all the liquid is absorbed.
7. Serve hot with the garnishing of parsley.

NUTRITION FACTS:

calories: 463;carbs: 76.7g; Protein: 18.5g; Fat: 10.1g; Sugar: 3.2g; Sodium: 431mg; Fiber: 11.6g

505. MEAT-FREE BOLOGNESE PASTA

Preparation Time: 20 minutes

Cooking Time: 2 hours

Servings: 5

INGREDIENTS:

For Bolognese Sauce:
- 5 tbsp. olive oil, divided
- 3 celery stalks, chopped finely
- 1 medium carrot, peeled and chopped finely
- 1 medium onion, chopped finely
- 1 C. quinoa, rinsed
- 3 C. fresh mushrooms, chopped
- 4 garlic cloves, chopped
- ¾ tsp. dried oregano
- ½ tsp. dried thyme
- ¼ tsp. dried rosemary
- ¼ tsp. dried sage
- 1/8 tsp. red pepper flakes
- 1½ C. homemade vegetable broth
- 2 cups tomatoes, peeled, seeded and crushed finely
- ½-1 C. water
- 1 tbsp. balsamic vinegar
- 4 bay leaves
- 2 tbsp. nutritional yeast
- ¼ C. oat milk
- Salt and freshly ground black pepper, to taste
- ¼ C. fresh basil leaves

For Pasta:
- 1 lb. whole-wheat pasta (of your choice)

DIRECTIONS:

1. Preheat your oven to 300°F-150°C.
2. In a large Dutch oven, heat 3 tbsp. of the olive oil over medium heat and cook the celery, carrots and onion for about 10 minutes, stirring frequently.
3. Stir in the quinoa and cook for about 3 minutes.
4. Add the remaining oil and mushrooms and stir to combine.
5. Increase the heat to medium-high and cook for about 5 minutes.
6. Add the garlic, dried herbs and red pepper flakes and cook for about 1-2 minutes.
7. Add the broth and cook for about 5 minutes.
8. Add the tomatoes, water, vinegar and bay leaves and bring to a boil.
9. Remove the Dutch oven from heat and transfer into the oven.
10. Bake, uncovered for about 1½ hours, stirring once after 1 hour.
11. Meanwhile, in a pan of the lightly salted boiling water, cook the pasta for about 8-10 minutes or according to package's instructions.
12. Drin the pasta well.
13. Remove the Dutch oven from oven and stir in the nutritional yeast and oat milk.
14. Divide the pasta onto serving plates and top with Bolognese sauce.
15. Garnish with basil leaves and serve.

NUTRITION FACTS:

calories: 510;carbs: 71g; Protein: 17.1g; Fat: 18.3g; Sugar: 5.9g; Sodium: 241mg; Fiber: 6.5g

506. PASTA WITH ESCAROLE, BEANS AND TURKEY

Preparation Time: 20 mins.

Cooking Time: 16mins.

Servings: 4

INGREDIENTS:
- whole-wheat bowtie pasta (3/4 pound)
- olive oil (1 tbs)
- onion (1/2 medium, chopped)
- cloves garlic (3, minced)
- turkey (6 oz, ground)
- head escarole (1 medium, rinsed, drained and chopped)
- cannellini beans (1(14oz) can, drained and rinsed)
- chicken broth (1 1/2 cups)
- rosemary (1 tbs, chopped)
- salt (1/2 tsp)
- Parmesan cheese (1/4 cup, grated)

DIRECTIONS:
1. Bring a salted water to boil in a pot. Add the pasta and follow the cooking instruction on the package.
2. Drain. In a large non-stick pan, heat olive oil over medium heat.
3. Add onion and cook until softened, add garlic and turkey and cook until it browns, about 5 minutes.
4. Add the escarole and cook it for 4 minutes. Add the beans, 1 cup of turkey stock, rosemary, and salt.
5. Simmer until the mixture is slightly thickened. Add the pasta and toss well, thin the sauce with the additional 1/2 cup stock if needed.
6. Top with parmesan cheese. Serve.

NUTRITION FACTS:
289 calories, 6 g fat, 36 g carbs, 16 g fiber, 24 g protein

507. RICE BOWL WITH SHRIMP AND PEAS

Preparation Time: 15 mins.

Cooking Time: 48 mins.

Servings: 4

INGREDIENTS:
- long-grain brown rice (1 cup)
- soy sauce (1/4 cup)
- fresh lemon juice (1/4 cup)
- rice vinegar (2 tbs)
- honey (2 tbs)
- olive oil (1 tbs)
- shrimp (1 lb, medium, cleaned, peeled, deveined)
- snow peas (8 oz, thawed if frozen, cut in halves)
- piece fresh ginger (1 (1-inch long) shredded)
- Hass avocado (1, chopped)

DIRECTIONS:
1. Boil 2 cups of water in a saucepan. Add the rice and cover and turn the heat down to simmer.
2. Cook the rice for about 35-45 minutes. In a bowl, fully combine soy sauce, lemon juice, honey, and vinegar.
3. Set your olive oil to get hot on medium heat in a non-stick pan.
4. Add in your shrimp, ginger and peas then cook for about 3 minutes (or until shrimp becomes pink).
5. Transfer rice to serving bowls, then top with avocado and shrimp mixture. Serve the sauce on the side.

NUTRITION FACTS:
143 calories, 4 g fat, 19g carbs, 2 g fiber, 7 g protein

508. ROASTED CHICKEN AND VEGETABLES

Preparation Time: 15 mins.

Cooking Time: 55 mins.

Servings: 4

INGREDIENTS:
- Roma tomatoes (6, seedless, quartered)
- Zucchini (3 medium, chopped coarsely)
- Potatoes (2 large, unpeeled, quartered)
- olive oil (3 tbs, divided)
- salt (3/4 tsp, divided)
- cloves garlic (4, finely minced)
- fresh rosemary (1 tbs, chopped)
- fresh thyme (1 tbs, leaves taken off sprig)
- lemon zest (1 tsp)
- lemon juice (1 tbs)
- chicken breast halves (4, skinless)

DIRECTIONS:
1. Preheat oven to 375°F-190°C.
2. Put tomatoes, zucchini and potatoes in a roasting pan, and toss with 2 tbs of oil and 1/4 tsp salt.
3. Combine lemon zest, thyme, rosemary, garlic, oil, salt and lemon juice. Pour this mixture over chicken.
4. Place chicken in pan with vegetables. Bake in oven for 30 minutes.
5. Stir chicken and vegetables and bake another 25 minutes, or until chicken is cooked through and vegetables are tender.

NUTRITION FACTS:
147 calories, 11 g fat, 13g carbs, 3 g fiber, 2 g protein

509. SOUTHWESTERN CHICKEN PITAS

Preparation Time: 15 mins.

Cooking Time: 0 mins.

Servings: 6

INGREDIENTS:
- black beans (1 (15 oz) can, drained, rinsed)
- red bell pepper (1/2 cup, chopped, seeded)
- fresh lime juice (3 tbs)
- fresh cilantro leaves (2 tbs, minced)
- canola oil (2 tbs)
- chicken breasts (4, boneless, halved, skinless)
- round whole wheat pita bread (4)
- low-fat provolone cheese (6 slices, cut in halves)

DIRECTIONS:
1. In a bowl, combine beans, bell pepper, lime juice, and cilantro. Set aside. In a pan, heat up the oil over medium heat.
2. Cook chicken in pan until golden brown. Set aside for 10 without cutting. Warm pita bread in oven.
3. Cut chicken into slices. Place half a slice of cheese in center of one pita bread.
4. Top off the sandwich with bean mixture the chicken breast slices. Roll up tightly. Cut in half and serve.

NUTRITION FACTS:
345 calories, 12 g fat, 22 g carbs, 5 g fiber, 35 g protein

510. SPAGHETTI WITH ZUCCHINI

Preparation Time: 10 mins.

Cooking Time: 12 mins.

Servings: 4

INGREDIENTS:
- whole wheat spaghetti (1 lb)
- zucchini (2 medium, grated, water, squeezed out)
- butter (2 tbs)
- olive oil (1 tbs)
- cloves garlic (2, minced)
- Parmesan cheese (1/2 cup, freshly grated)

DIRECTIONS:
1. Bring a salted water to boil in a pot. Add pasta and cook until it is al dente or follow the instructions on the package.
2. While pasta cooks, in a large non-stick pan, heat the oil and butter together. Add in the zucchini and allow cook for 3 minutes.
3. Add in your garlic and continue to cook for another minute, stirring constantly. Add in a half of your parmesan cheese.
4. Transfer past to a serving bowl. Add your zucchini mixture. Toss then garnish with remaining

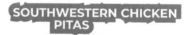

parmesan cheese. Enjoy!

NUTRITION FACTS:

156 calories, 11 g fat, 11 g carbs, 2 g fiber, 5 g protein

 511. SUMMER SPAGHETTI

Preparation Time: 15 mins.

Cooking Time: 8 mins.

Servings: 4

INGREDIENTS:

- whole wheat spaghetti (1 lb)
- olive oil (1/4 cup)
- shallot (1, minced)
- cloves garlic (2, minced)
- zucchini (1 medium, chopped)
- summer squash (1 medium, chopped)
- green beans (1/2 lb, ends cut)
- basil (1/4 cup, coarsely chopped)
- salt (1/2 tsp)
- lemon (1/2 medium, juiced)
- unsalted butter (2 tbs, room temperature)
- freshly grated lemon peel

DIRECTIONS:

1. Bring a salted water to boil in a pot. Add pasta and cook until it is al dente or follow the instructions on the package.
2. Heat up the oil over medium heat in a large pan. Add in your garlic and shallot, then stir frequently until fragrant (about 2 minutes).
3. Add the zucchini, squash, green beans, and basil. Continue to cook, stir occasionally, until all vegetables are tender.
4. Season vegetables with salt and lemon juice. In a large shallow pasta bowl, immediately place the sautéed vegetables with all their juices.
5. Add the butter and linguine, toss to mix well and serve immediately.

NUTRITION FACTS:

548 calories, 57 g fat, 14 g carbs, 3 g fiber, 3 g protein

 512. 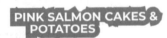 PINK SALMON CAKES & POTATOES

Preparation Time: 20 mins.

Cooking Time: 16 mins.

Servings: 4

INGREDIENTS:

- For Pink salmon Cakes:
- canola oil (3 tbs)
- pink salmon fish (2 (6 oz) cans, drained)
- egg (1, beaten)
- green onions (2 tablespoons, diced)
- mayonnaise (1/4 cup, non-fat)
- whole wheat bread (1/2 cup, cut into small pieces)
- Lemon juice, optional
- For Smashed Potatoes:
- Potatoes (2 large, unpeeled, chopped)
- salt (2 tsp)
- low fat milk (1/2 cup)
- unsalted butter (3 tablespoons)

DIRECTIONS:

1. Cook potatoes in a small saucepan until tender. Drain.
2. Place potatoes back in pan. Heat the butter and milk in microwave until hot.
3. Roughly smash the potatoes with a potato smasher while adding hot liquid until combined and set aside.
4. Combine egg, pink salmon, lemon juice, green onions, mayonnaise, breadcrumbs, and egg in a bowl.
5. Form into patties. Allow to refrigerate and become firm for 10 minutes.
6. Heat oil over medium heat, cook patties until golden brown, about 2 minutes on each side. Serve with potatoes.

NUTRITION FACTS:

432 calories, 34 g fat, 29 g carbs, 2 g fiber, 6 g protein

 513. TURKEY AND BARLEY CASSEROLE

Preparation Time: 15 mins.

Cooking Time: 1 hr. 10 mins.

Servings: 4

INGREDIENTS:

- ground turkey (3/4 lb)
- salt (1/2 tsp)
- onion (1, chopped finely)
- carrots (2, chopped)
- stalks celery (2, chopped)
- green bell pepper (1, seeded and chopped)
- button mushrooms (12, quartered)
- chicken stock (2 1/2 cups)
- barley (1 cup)
- poultry seasoning (1 tsp)
- bay leaf (1)

DIRECTIONS:

1. Preheat oven to 375°F-190°C.
2. Over medium heat, cook ground turkey with salt until browned, about 5 minutes, in a pan.
3. Add green peppers, celery, carrots and onions. Cook until tender, about 5 minutes.
4. Add bay leaf, poultry seasoning, barley, stock and mushrooms.
5. Mix together and place the mixture in a baking dish. Cover and bake in the preheated oven for 1 hour. Serve.

NUTRITION FACTS:

361 calories, 11 g fat, 42 g carbs, 10 g fiber, 30 g pr

514. BEEF WITH ZUCCHINI NOODLES

Preparation Time: 15 minutes

Cooking Time: 9 minutes

Servings: 4

INGREDIENTS:

- 1 teaspoon fresh ginger, grated
- 2 medium garlic cloves, minced
- 1/4 cup coconut aminos
- 2 tablespoons fresh lime juice
- 1 ½ pound NY strip steak, trimmed and sliced thinly
- 2 medium zucchini, spiralized with blade C
- Salt to taste
- 3 tablespoons essential olive oil
- 2 medium scallions, sliced
- 1 teaspoon red pepper flakes, crushed
- 2 tablespoons fresh cilantro, chopped

DIRECTIONS:

1. In a big bowl, merge ginger, garlic, coconut aminos and lime juice. Add the beef and coat with the marinade generously. Refrigerate to soak for approximately 10 minutes.
2. Set zucchini noodles over a large paper towel and sprinkle with salt.
3. Keep aside for around 10 minutes.
4. In a big skillet, heat oil on medium-high heat. Attach the scallions and red pepper flakes then saute for about 1 minute.
5. Attach the beef with the marinade and stir fry for around 3-4 minutes or till browned.
6. Stir in the fresh cilantro, then add the zucchini and cook for approximately 3-4 minutes.
7. Serve hot.

NUTRITION FACTS:

Calories: 366 Carbs: 5 g Cholesterol: 60 mg Fat: 30 g Protein: 21 g Fiber: 9 g

 515. 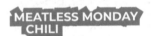 MEATLESS MONDAY CHILI

Preparation Time: 15 minutes

Cooking Time: 1 hour 25 minutes

Servings: 4

INGREDIENTS:

- 2 tbsp. avocado oil
- 1 medium onion, chopped
- 1 carrot, peeled and chopped
- 1 small bell pepper, seeded and chopped
- 1 lb. fresh mushrooms, sliced
- 2 garlic cloves, minced

- 2 tsp. dried oregano
- 1 tbsp. red chili powder
- 1 tbsp. ground cumin
- Salt and freshly ground black pepper, to taste
- 8 oz. canned red kidney beans, rinsed and drained
- 8 oz. canned white kidney beans, rinsed and drained
- 2 C. tomatoes, peeled, seeded and chopped finely
- 1½ C. homemade vegetable broth

DIRECTIONS:

1. In a large Dutch oven, heat the oil over medium-low heat and cook the onions, carrot and bell pepper for about 10 minutes, stirring frequently.
2. Increase the heat to medium-high.
3. Stir in the mushrooms and garlic and cook for about 5-6 minutes, stirring frequently.
4. Add the oregano, spices, salt and black pepper and cook for about chili 1-2 minutes.
5. Stir in the beans, tomatoes and broth and bring to a boil.
6. Reduce the heat to low and simmer, covered for about 1 hour, stirring occasionally.
7. Serve hot.

NUTRITION FACTS:
calories: 346;carbs: 59.9g; Protein: 23.4g; Fat:3.7g; Sugar: 10.5g; Sodium: 545mg; Fiber: 16.7g

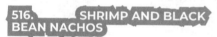

516. SHRIMP AND BLACK BEAN NACHOS

Preparation Time: 25 mins.

Cooking Time: 0 mins.

Servings: 4

INGREDIENTS:

- Cilantro (3/4 cup, fresh chopped)
- red onion (1/2 cup, diced)
- lime juice (2 tbs)
- olive oil (1 tbs)
- Worcestershire sauce (1 tsp)
- salt (1/2 tsp)
- shrimp (3/4 lb medium, peeled, cooked, and chopped)
- tomatoes (2 cups, seeded, diced)
- avocado (1/2 cup, diced)
- black bean (1 (15 oz) can, rinsed and drained)
- ground cumin (1/2 tsp)
- baked tortilla chips (4 cup)

DIRECTIONS:

1. In a bowl combine cilantro, onion, lime juice, oil, Worcestershire sauce, shrimp and salt. Cover and refrigerate for 30 minutes.
2. Add tomato and avocado; stir well. Place the cumin and beans in a food processor, and process until smooth.
3. Spread 1-teaspoon black-bean mixture on each chip. Top with 1-tablespoon shrimp mixture. Serve.

NUTRITION FACTS:
172 calories, 14 g fat, 12 g carbs, 5 g fiber, 4 g protein

 517 **HEALTHY VEGAN BROWNIES**

INGREDIENTS:

- 4 tablespoon ground flax
- ⅔ cup warm water
- 1 cup date sugar or coconut sugar
- 1 cup cacao powder
- ½ cup white whole wheat flour
- ½ tablespoon salt
- 1 tablespoon baking powder
- ½ cup unsweetened applesauce or pumpkin puree
- 1 tablespoon vanilla extract
- ¼ cup unsweetened almond milk optional

DIRECTIONS:

1. Preheat the oven to 325*F-160°C. In a small dish, combine ground flax and warm water. Allow for a 15-minute resting period.
2. In a medium mixing bowl, combine the dry ingredients (date sugar, cacao powder, white whole wheat flour, baking powder, and salt) while the flax egg is setting.
3. 8n the middle of the dry ingredients, make a well. Combine the wet and dry components (flax egg, applesauce/or pumpkin puree, and vanilla extract). Stir until well mixed. If the batter appears to be too dry, add the unsweetened almond milk.
4. Pour the batter into an 8-inch square baking dish lined with parchment paper. Distribute evenly.
5. 30–35 minutes in the oven, or until a toothpick inserted in the middle comes out clean. Allow cooling fully in the pan before removing and cutting into squares.

NUTRITION FACTS:
calories: 126 |carbs: 28 g | protein: 3 g | fat: 1 g | cholesterol: 172 mg

518. GREEN RISOTTO RECIPE

Preparation Time: 10 minutes

Cooking Time: 40 minutes

Total time: 50 minutes

Servings: 8

INGREDIENTS:

- Two cups arborio rice
- Three tablespoons butter
- Three tablespoons olive oil
- Six scallions, greens and whites chopped
- Two and a half cups fresh packed spinach leaves
- One cup packed fresh parsley
- 12 fresh basil leaves
- Three garlic cloves
- Six cups chicken broth, room temperature (vegetable broth for vegetarians)
- One cup of white wine
- One cup of shredded parmesan cheese
- Salt

DIRECTIONS:

1. In a blender, combine spinach, parsley, basil, and garlic. Add 4 cups broth and purée until completely smooth.
2. In a large sauté pan, combine the butter and oil. In a medium saucepan over medium heat, melt the butter. Add the scallions once the butter has melted and cooked for 2 minutes. After adding the rice, cook for another 2 minutes. Then stir in the wine, 1 1/2 teaspoons of salt, and 1/2 teaspoon ground.
3. Simmer, occasionally stirring, until the wine has been absorbed. Start with the 2 cups of liquid that was not put into the blender and add one cup of broth at a time to the rice. Stir the rice after each addition of liquid and let it boil until the broth is absorbed before adding more. Ensure that all of the green herb broth is included in the blender. This procedure will take approximately 25 minutes.
4. Stir in the grated parmesan cheese after you've poured the rest of the green liquid and the rice is cooked but still firm. Turn off the heat before the last round of stock has been completely absorbed, leaving the risotto a bit soupy. As it cools, it will stiffen up. Season to taste with salt and serve warm.

NUTRITION FACTS:
calories: 283 |carbs: 36 g | protein: 1 g | fat: 1 g | cholesterol: 53 mg

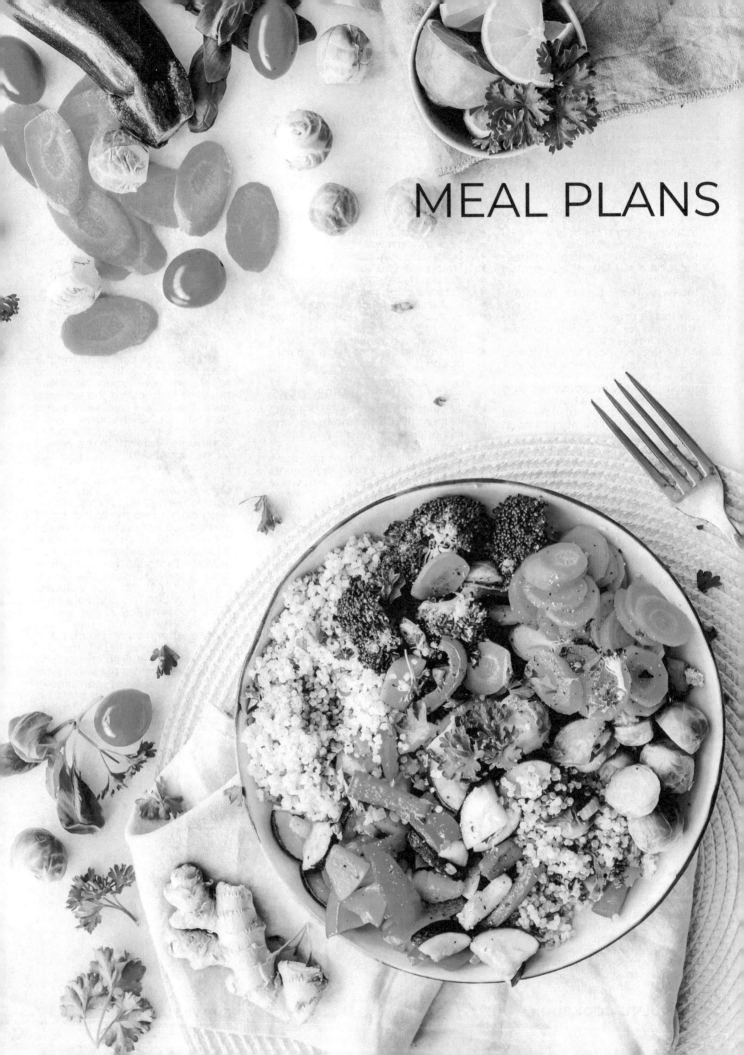

MEAL PLANS

CLEAR LIQUID

MEAL PLAN

DAYS	Breakfast	Lunch	Dinner
1	Banana breakfast smoothie	Healthier apple juice Best hommade broth	Chicken bone broth Chicken Vegetal Soup
2	Ginger peach smoothie	Citrus apple juice Fish broth	Homemade beef stock Kulfi indian ice cream
3	Lemon cheesecake smoothielemon cheesecake smoothie	Richly fruity juice Clear pumpkin broth	Three-ingredient sugar-free gelatin Healthy 5-minute strawberry pineapple sherbet
4	Chocolate smoothie	Delish grape juice Slow cooker pork bone broth	Cranberry-kombucha jell-o Healthy watermelon smoothie
5	Persimmon smoothie	Lemony grape juice Mineral rich broth	Strawberry gummies Coconut milk ice cream
6	Cranberry smoothie	Holiday special juice Citrus realish	Fruity jell-o stars Peach cobbler
7	Kale apple smoothie	Vitamin c rich juice Healing broth	Sugar-free cinnamon jelly Pineapple orange creamsicle
8	Glowing skin smoothie	Incredible fresh juice Clean testing broth	Homey clear chicken broth Hummus
9	Cranberry sauce	Favorite summer lemonade Banana apple smoothie	Oxtail bone broth Carrot ginger soup
10	Chocolate tahini pumpkin smoothie	Ultimate fruity punch Berrylicious smoothie	Chicken bone broth with ginger and lemon Eggplant paste

LOW RESIDUE

MEAL PLAN

DAYS	Breakfast	Lunch	Dinner
1	Lemon baked eggs	Barbecue beef stir-fry	Italian styled stuffed zucchini boats
2	Banana pancakes	Chicken saffron rice pilaf	Chicken cutlets
3	Deviled egg	Stir-fry ground chicken and green beans	Slow cooker salsa turkey
4	Basil zoodle frittata	Stewed lamb	Sriracha lime chicken and apple salad
5	Pear and muesli muffins	Pulled chicken salad	Pan-seared scallops with lemon-ginger vinaigrette
6	Green omelet with portobello fries	Lemongrass beef	Roasted salmon and asparagus
7	Shakshuka	Beetroot carrot salad	Orange and maple-glazed salmon
8	Salmon fritter	Crunchy maple sweet potatoes	Cod with ginger and black beans
9	Vanilla almond hot chocolate	Veggie bowl	Halibut curry
10	Banana and pear pita pockets	Pomegranate salad	Chicken cacciatore
11	Ripe plantain bran muffins	Dijon orange summer salad	Chicken and bell pepper saute
12	Easy breakfast bran muffins	Pulao rice prawns	Chicken salad sandwiches

DAYS	Breakfast	Lunch	Dinner
13	Apple oatmeal	White radish crunch salad	Rosemary chicken
14	Breakfast burrito wrap	Apple and mushroom soup	Gingered turkey meatballs
15	Zucchini omelet	Spring watercress soup	Turkey and kale saute
16	Coconut chia seed pudding	Oyster sauce tofu	Turkey with bell peppers and rosemary
17	Spiced oatmeal	Potato and rosemary risotto	Mustard and rosemary pork tenderloin
18	Breakfast cereal	Cheesy baked tortillas	Thin-cut pork chops with mustardy kale
19	Sweet potato hash with sausage and spinach	Smoky rice	Beef tenderloin with savory blueberry sauce
20	Cajun omelet	Zucchini lasagna	Ground beef chili with tomatoes

HIGH FIBER

MEAL PLAN

DAYS	Breakfast	Lunch	Dinner
1	Cherry spinach smoothie	Pea soup	Grilled pear cheddar pockets
2	Banana cacao smoothie	Guacamole	Chicken and apple kale wraps
3	Spinach and egg scramble with raspberries	Cauliflower and potato curry soup	Cauliflower rice pilaf
4	Blackberry smoothie	Sweet potato and black bean chili	Fresh herb and lemon bulgur pilaf
5	Veggie frittata	White bean chili	Corn chowder
6	Chocolate banana protein smoothie	Chickpea stew	Strawberry and rhubarb soup
7	Cocoa almond french toast	Veggie sandwich	Chicken sandwiches
8	Muesli with raspberries	Bean and veggie taco bowl	Tex-mex bean tostadas
9	Mocha overnight oats	Cobb salad	Fish tacos
10	Baked banana-nut oatmeal cups	Asparagus soup	Cucumber almond gazpacho
11	Pineapple green smoothie	Creamy carrot soup	Pea and spinach carbonara
12	Pumpkin bread	Lentil soup	Sautéed broccoli with peanut sauce

DAYS	Breakfast	Lunch	Dinner
13	Banana-bran muffins	Mushroom barley soup	Edamame lettuce wraps burgers
14	Banana bread	Broccoli soup	Pizza stuffed spaghetti squash
15	Chocolate-raspberry oatmeal	Chicken and asparagus pasta	Spinach and artichoke dip pasta
16	Chai chia pudding	Red beans and rice	Grilled eggplant
17	Apple cinnamon oatmeal	Beef stir fry	Stuffed potatoes with salsa and beans
18	Apple butter bran muffins	Black bean nacho soup	Mushroom quinoa veggie burgers
19	Pineapple raspberry parfaits	Butternut squash soup	Turkey meatballs
20	Berry chia pudding	Broccoli salad	Sweet potato soup
21	Spinach avocado smoothie	Beef and bean sloppy joes	Minestrone soup
22	Strawberry pineapple smoothie	Sweet potato and peanut soup	Lentil soup
23	Peach blueberry parfaits	Beet salad	Grilled corn salad
24	Raspberry yogurt cereal bowl	Broccoli casserole	Kale soup
25	Avocado toast	Chicken fajita bowls	Pasta fagioli
26	Loaded pita pockets	Pumpkin soup	Sweet potato gnocchi
27	Homestyle pancake mix	High-fiber dumplings	Bean and ham soup
28	Multigrain pancakes	Pizza made with bamboo fibers	Quinoa chickpea salad with roasted red pepper hummus dressing

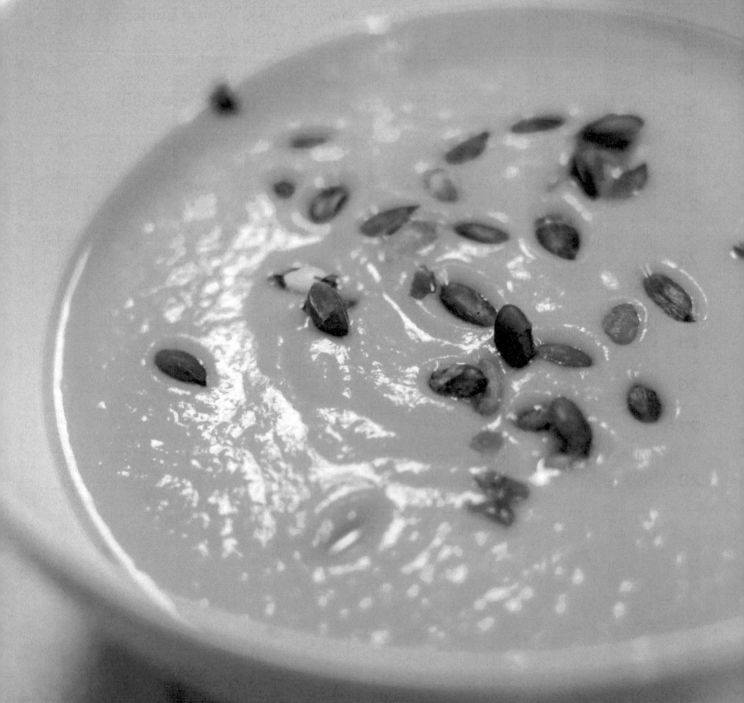

CONCLUSION

A high-fiber, high-water diet is usually recommended for diverticulitis. It will ensure that your gastrointestinal tract and system get enough rest, allowing you to recuperate. As soon as you start eating properly, you should see results in a few days.

Water intake is equally important; the usual guideline is that your body will need 1/2 of your weight in oz per day so that a 150-pound person will require 75 oz of water each day. Water coupled with a high fiber diet is required to keep your colon moving properly and reduce the risk of an attack or the formation of further diverticula.

Seeds and nuts should be avoided like the plague! Anything with a husk, such as sesame seeds, should be avoided at all costs. In essence, they will irritate the lining of your colon once again, resulting in the formation of diverticula.

Maize is another item to avoid if at all possible, including any corn-based products such as popcorn or corn flour and tortillas. Chili peppers and other hot and spicy foods are thought to be very hazardous to diverticulitis sufferers.

If your diverticulitis diet plan allows it, try to consume fruits and vegetables that you like. If you don't like greens, consider eating more fresh fruit instead, and vice versa. Vegetable and fruit seeds are safe to eat for most patients, such as those found in cucumbers and tomatoes.

Foods that are high in fiber. Whole-wheat bread and other whole-grain items are high in dietary fiber. You may also add bran to your food. Uncooked or just lightly cooked legumes, as well as fermented greens (e.g., sauerkraut). Fresh fruit and vegetables should not be peeled; they should be consumed naturally (juices are devoid of fiber). Dried fruit, such as raisins, plums, apricots, and dates, are an excellent source.

Naturally, just as we don't all consume the same kind of meals throughout life, diverticulitis foods to avoid will vary from case to instance. Our unhealthy eating habits and poor nutrition and the poisons that arise from them are the root reasons. It's an excellent time to become interested in health and nutrition if you haven't already guessed.

If you wish to reduce or perhaps eliminate future episodes of diverticulitis, you need to eat the right foods. While antibiotics may frequently alleviate severe pain and suffering in the short term, taking them for an extended length of time can be nearly as hazardous as the illness itself, not to mention that your body will ultimately become resistant to their effects.

Consequently, it is often essential to undergo a hazardous and invasive operation, which may result in a decrease in life quality.

Most people would agree that prevention is preferable to treatment. So, to avoid this illness from infecting your stomach, and in light of the current economic climate, we should pay close attention to our health and take appropriate action. Because it is nearly completely due to a lack of dietary fiber, the best course of treatment is to consume the appropriate meals.

Appendix 1

RECIPE INDEX

1. Ginger peach smoothie 18
2. Persimmon smoothie 18
3. Cranberry smoothie 18
4. Kale apple smoothie 19
5. Glowing skin smoothie 19
6. Cranberry sauce 19
7. Chocolate tahini pumpkin smoothie 19
8. Caramel sauce 20
9. Lemon cheesecake smoothie 20
10. Brandy java ice 20
11. Chocolate smoothie 20
12. Banana breakfast smoothie 20
13. Spinach vegetable barley bean soup 21
14. Chocolate nice cream 21
15. Healthy watermelon popsicles 21
16. Spinach mango vegan popsicles 21
17. Mango banana smoothie 21
18. Spinach blueberry smoothie 22
19. Snowman christmas smoothie 22
20. Clean green shamrock shake 22
21. Pumpkin smoothiePumpkin smoothie 22
22. Citrus Sports Drink 22
23. Homemade Orange Gelatin 22
24. Raspberry Lemonade Ice Pops 22
25. Homemade No Pulp Orange Juice 23
26. Apple Orange Juice 23
27. Pineapple Mint Juice 23
28. Celery Apple Juice 23
29. Homemade Banana Apple Juice 23
30. Sweet Detox Juice 23
31. Pineapple Ginger Juice 24
32. Carrot Orange Juice 24
33. Strawberry Apple Juice 24
34. Autumn Energizer Juice 24
35. Asian Inspired Wonton Broth 24
36. Mushroom, Cauliflower and Cabbage Broth 24
37. Indian Inspired Vegetable stock 25
38. Beef Bone Broth 25
39. Ginger, Mushroom and Cauliflower Broth 25
40. Fish Broth 25
41. Clear Pumpkin Broth 25
42. Pork Stock 25
43. Slow Cooker Pork Bone Broth 26
44. Healthier Apple Juice 28
45. Citrus Apple Juice 28
46. Richly Fruity Juice 28
47. Delish Grape Juice 28
48. Lemony Grape Juice 28
49. Holiday Special Juice 28
50. Vitamin C Rich Juice 29
51. Incredible Fresh Juice 29
52. Favorite Summer Lemonade 29
53. Ultimate Fruity Punch 29
54. Thirst Quencher Sports Drink 29
55. Refreshing Sports Drink 29
56. Perfect Sunny Day Tea 29
57. Nutritious Green Tea 30
58. Simple Black Tea 30
59. Lemony Black Tea 30
60. Metabolism Booster Coffee 30
61. Best Homemade Broth 30
62. Clean Testing Broth 30
63. Healing Broth 31
64. Veggie Lover's Broth 31
65. Brain Healthy Broth 31
66. Minerals Rich Broth 31
67. Holiday Favorite Gelatin 31
68. Banana-apple smoothie 32
69. Berrylicious smoothie 32
70. Buttermilk herb ranch dressing 32
71. Citrus relish 32
72. Red wine sangria recipe 32
73. Salty dog cocktail recipe 33
74. Simple syrup 33
75. Rose sangria recipe 33
76. Champagne holiday punch 33
77. White sangria 33
78. Raspberry mojitos with basil 33
79. Margarita 34
80. Grapefruit basil sorbet 34

- 81. Bruleed grapefruit (pamplemousse brûlé) 34
- 82. Frozen beeritas recipe 34
- 83. Spicy pineapple habanero margaritas 35
- 84. Cranberry pomegranate margarita with spiced rim 35
- 85. Peach milkshake (copycat chik-fil-a peach shake recipe!) 35
- 86. Jugo verde (green juice) 35
- 87. Perfect manhattan recipe 35
- 88. Frozen coconut mojito 35
- 89. Mulled lemonade recipe 36
- 90. Cucumber rose aperol spritz 36
- 91. Pink grapefruit margarita 36
- 92. Strawberry margarita 36
- 93. Large-batch goombay smash caribbean cocktails 36
- 94. Green chicken soup 36
- 95. Vegetable Beef Stock 37
- 96. Fishy Tomato Broth 37
- 97. Chicken Bone Broth 38
- 98. Homemade Beef Stock 38
- 99. Three-Ingredient Sugar-Free Gelatin 38
- 100. Cranberry-Kombucha Jell-O 38
- 101. Strawberry Gummies 39
- 102. Fruity Jell-O Stars 39
- 103. Sugar-Free Cinnamon Jelly 39
- 104. Homey Clear Chicken Broth 39
- 105. Oxtail Bone Broth 39
- 106. Chicken Bone Broth with Ginger and Lemon 39
- 107. Vegetable Stock 40
- 108. Chicken Vegetable Soup 40
- 109. Carrot Ginger Soup 40
- 110. Tomato Cashew Pesto 40
- 111. Sweet Potato Aioli 40
- 112. Eggplant paste 40
- 113. Kulfi indian ice cream 41
- 114. Dark Chocolate with Pomegranate Seeds 41
- 115. Covered Bananas 41
- 116. Hummus with Tahini and Turmeric 41
- 117. Pineapple orange creamsicle 41
- 118. Easy peach cobbler recipe with bisquick 41
- 119. Healthy 5-minute strawberry pineapple sherbet 42
- 120. Best coconut milk ice cream (dairy-free!) 42
- 121. Lemon crinkle cookies recipe 42
- 122. The best no-bake chocolate lasagna 43
- 123. Easiest healthy watermelon smoothie recipe 43
- 124. Watermelon 43
- 125. Best orange julius 43
- 126. Lemon Baked Eggs 46
- 127. Banana Pancakes 46
- 128. Deviled egg 46
- 129. Basil Zoodle Frittata 46
- 130. Pear and Muesli Muffins 47
- 131. Green Omelet with Portobello fries 47
- 132. Shakshuka 47
- 133. Salmon Fritter 47
- 134. Vanilla Almond Hot Chocolate 47
- 135. Banana and Pear Pita Pockets 48
- 136. Ripe Plantain Bran Muffins 48
- 137. Easy Breakfast Bran Muffins 48
- 138. Apple Oatmeal 48
- 139. Breakfast Burrito Wrap 48
- 140. Zucchini Omelet 48
- 141. Spiced Oatmeal 49
- 142. Breakfast Cereal 49
- 143. Sweet Potato Hash with Sausage and Spinach 49
- 144. Cajun Omelet 49
- 145. Peanut Butter Banana Oatmeal 49
- 146. Overnight Peach Oatmeal 49
- 147. Mediterranean Salmon and Potato Salad 49
- 148. Celery Soup 50
- 149. Pea Tuna Salad 50
- 150. Vegetable Soup 50
- 151. Carrot and Turkey Soup 50
- 152. Creamy Pumpkin Soup 50
- 153. Chicken Pea Soup 51
- 154. Spinach Frittata 51
- 155. Almond Peanut Butter Fudge 51
- 156. Quick Cocoa Mousse 51
- 157. Cinnamon Pear Chips 51
- 158. Chocolate Yogurt Cream & Roasted Bananas 51
- 159. Coconut Celery Smoothie 52
- 160. Apple Spinach Smoothie 52
- 161. Barbecue Beef Stir-Fry 53
- 162. Chicken Saffron Rice Pilaf 53
- 163. Stir-Fry Ground Chicken and Green Beans 53
- 164. Stewed Lamb 54
- 165. Pulled Chicken Salad 54
- 166. Lemongrass Beef 54
- 167. Beetroot Carrot Salad 54
- 168. Crunchy Maple Sweet Potatoes 54
- 169. Veggie Bowl 55
- 170. Pomegranate Salad 55
- 171. Dijon Orange Summer Salad 55

172. Pulao Rice Prawns 55	195. Liver with Onion and Parsley One 60	218. Greek Inspired Cucumber Salad 65	241. Gingered Turkey Meatballs 70
173. White Radish Crunch Salad 55	196. Egg and Avocado Wraps 61	219. Light Veggie Salad 65	242. Turkey and Kale Saute 70
174. Apple and mushroom Soup 56	197. Creamy Sweet Potato Pasta with Pancetta 61	220. Eastern European Soup 65	243. Turkey with Bell Peppers and Rosemary 71
175. Spring Watercress Soup 56	198. Roasted Beet Pasta with Kale and Pesto 61	221. Citrus Glazed Carrots 66	244. Mustard and Rosemary Pork Tenderloin 71
176. Oyster Sauce Tofu 56	199. Veggies and Apple with Orange Sauce 61	222. Braised Asparagus 66	245. Thin-Cut Pork Chops with Mustardy Kale 71
177. Potato and Rosemary Risotto 56	200. Cauliflower Rice with Prawns and Veggies 62	223. Spring Flavored Pasta 66	246. Beef Tenderloin with Savory Blueberry Sauce 71
178. Cheesy Baked Tortillas 56	201. Lentils with Tomatoes and Turmeric 62	224. Versatile Mac 'n Cheese 66	247. Ground Beef Chili with Tomatoes 72
179. Smoky Rice 57	202. Fried Rice with Kale 62	225. Gluten-Free Curry 66	248. Fish Taco Salad with Strawberry Avocado Salsa 72
180. Zucchini Lasagna 57	203. Tofu and Red Pepper Stir-Fry 62	226. New Year's Luncheon Meal 66	249. Beef and Bell Pepper Stir-Fry 72
181. Greek Chicken Skewers 57	204. Sweet Potato and Bell Pepper Hash with a Fried Egg 62	227. Entertaining Wraps 67	250. Veggie Pizza with Cauliflower-Yam Crust 72
182. Roast Beef 57	205. Quinoa Florentine 63	228. Italian Styled Stuffed Zucchini Boats 68	251. Toasted Pecan Quinoa Burgers 73
183. Banana Cake 58	206. Tomato Asparagus Frittata 63	229. Chicken Cutlets 68	252. Sizzling Salmon and Quinoa 73
184. Grilled Fish Steaks 58	207. Tofu Sloppy Joes 63	230. Slow Cooker Salsa Turkey 68	253. Papaya-Mango Smoothie 73
185. Apple Pudding 58	208. Broccoli and Egg "Muffins" 63	231. Sriracha Lime Chicken and Apple Salad 69	254. Cantaloupe Smoothie 73
58	209. Shrimp Scampi 63	232. Pan-Seared Scallops with Lemon-Ginger Vinaigrette 69	255. Cantaloupe-Mix Smoothie 73
186. Lamb Chops 58	210. Shrimp with Cinnamon Sauce 64	233. Roasted Salmon and Asparagus 69	256. Applesauce-Avocado Smoothie 74
187. Eggplant Croquettes 58	211. Super-Food Scramble 64	234. Orange and Maple-Glazed Salmon 69	257. Pina Colada Smoothie 74
188. Cucumber Egg Salad 59	212. Family Favorite Scramble 64	235. Cod with Ginger and Black Beans 69	258. Diced FruitsDiced Fruits 74
189. Shrimp and Mango Salsa Lettuce Wraps 59	213. Tasty Veggie Omelet 64	236. Halibut Curry 69	Applesauce 74
190. Bacon-Wrapped Asparagus 59	214. Garden Veggies Quiche 64	237. Chicken Cacciatore 70	259. Avocado Dip 74
191. Zucchini Pasta with Shrimp 59	215. Fluffy Pumpkin Pancakes 64	238. Chicken and Bell Pepper Saute 70	260. Homemade Hummus 74
192. Sweet Potato Buns Sandwich 60	216. Sper-Tasty Chicken Muffins 65	239. Chicken Salad Sandwiches 70	261. Tofu 74
193. Shrimp, Sausage and Veggie Skillet 60	217. Classic Zucchini Bread 65	240. Rosemary Chicken 70	262. Almond Butter Sandwich 75
194. Sea Scallops with Spinach and Bacon 60			

- 263. Gluten-Free Muffins 75
- 264. Outdoor Chicken Kabobs 75
- 265. Flavorful Shrimp Kabobs 75
- 266. Pan-Seared Scallops 75
- 267. Mediteranean Shrimp Salad 76
- 268. Helth Conscious People's Salad 76
- 269. Italian Pasta Soup 76
- 270. Pure Comfort Soup 76
- 271. Goof-for-You Stew 76
- 272. Zero-Fiber Chicken Dish 76
- 273. Amazing Chicken Platter 77
- 274. Colorful Chicken Dinner 77
- 275. Easiest Tuna Salad 77
- 276. Lemony Salmon 77
- 277. Herbed Salmon 77
- 278. Delicious Combo Dinner 78
- 279. Turkey Sweet Potato Hash 78
- 280. Chicken Tenders with Honey Mustard Sauce 78
- 281. Chicken Breasts with Cabbage and Mushrooms 78
- 282. Duck with Bok Choy 78
- 283. Beef with Mushroom and Broccoli 79
- 284. Ground Beef with Veggies 79
- 285. Ground Beef with Greens and Tomatoes 79
- 286. Roasted Carrot Sticks in a Honey Garlic Marinade 79
- 287. Apple and Pistachio Salad on Spinach 79
- 288. Catalan Style Spinach 80
- 289. Energy Balls 80
- 290. Cherry Spinach Smoothie 82
- 291. Banana cacao smoothie 82
- 292. Spinach and Egg Scramble with Raspberries 82
- 293. Blackberry Smoothie 82
- 294. Veggie Frittata 83
- 295. Chocolate Banana Protein Smoothie 83
- 296. Cocoa Almond French toast 83
- 297. Muesli with Raspberries 83
- 298. Mocha Overnight Oats 83
- 299. Baked Banana-Nut Oatmeal Cups 84
- 300. Pineapple Green Smoothie 84
- 301. Pumpkin BreadPumpkin Bread 84
- 302. Banana-Bran Muffins 84
- 303. Banana Bread 85
- 304. Chocolate-Raspberry Oatmeal 85
- 305. Chai Chia Pudding 85
- 306. Apple Cinnamon Oatmeal 85
- 307. Apple Butter Bran Muffins 86
- 308. Pineapple Raspberry Parfaits 86
- 309. Berry Chia Pudding 86
- 310. Spinach avocado smoothie 86
- 311. Strawberry pineapple smoothie 86
- 312. Peach Blueberry Parfaits 87
- 313. Raspberry Yogurt Cereal Bowl 87
- 314. Avocado toast 87
- 315. Loaded Pita Pockets 87
- 316. Homestyle Pancake Mix 87
- 317. Multigrain Pancakes 88
- 318. Cinnamon–Oat Bran Pancakes 88
- 319. Whole-Wheat Buttermilk Pancakes 88
- 320. Cornmeal Pancakes 88
- 321. Oven-Baked Pancake 88
- 322. Baked Pancake 88
- 323. Wheat Waffles 89
- 324. Oatmeal Waffles 89
- 325. Bran Applesauce Muffins 89
- 326. Oat Bran Muffins 89
- 327. Orange Bran Muffins 89
- 328. Pasta Fritters 89
- 329. Cinnamon Honey Scones 90
- 330. Oatmeal Raisin Scones 90
- 331. Whole Grain Scones 90
- Granola 90
- 332. Toasty Nut Granola 90
- 333. Breakfast Bars 91
- 334. Whole-Wheat Coffee Cake 91
- 335. Crunchy Breakfast Topping 91
- 336. Pear pancakes 91
- 337. Almond pancakes 91
- 338. Avocado pancakes 91
- 339. Strawberry pancakes 92
- 340. Carambola pancakes 92
- 341. Ginger muffins 92
- 342. Carrot muffinsC 92
- 343. Blueberry muffins 92
- 345. Raisin muffin 93
- 346. Parmesan omelete 93
- 347. Asparagus omelet 93
- 348. Onion omelet 93
- 349. Olive omelete 93
- 350. Tomato omelet 93
- 351. Morning bagel 93
- 352. Oatmeal custard 94
- 353. Scrambled eggs 94
- 354. French toast 94
- 355. Simple pizza recipe 94
- 356. Zucchini pizza

357. Leeks fritatta 94
358. Mushroom fritatta 94
359. Peas fritatta 94
360. Vitamins Packed Green Juice 95
361. Healthier Breakfast Juice 95
362. Summer Perfect Smoothie 95
363. Filling Breakfast Smoothie 95
364. Bright Green Breakfast Bowl 95
365. Quickest Breakfast Porridge 95
366. Halloween Morning Oatmeal 96
367. Authentic Bulgur Porridge 96
368. 2-Grains Porridge 96
369. Savory Crepes 96
370. Egg-Free Omelet 96
371. Summer Treat Salad 96
372. Secretly Amazing Salad 97
373. Double chocolate scones 97
374. Banana and blueberry fritters 97
375. Strawberry overnight oats 97
376. Strawberry banana peanut butter smoothie 98
377. Pea soup 99
378. Guacamole 99
379. Cauliflower and Potato Curry Soup 100
380. Sweet Potato and Black Bean Chili 100
381. White Bean Chili 100
382. Chickpea Stew 100
383. Veggie Sandwich 101
384. Bean and Veggie Taco Bowl 101
385. Cobb Salad 101
386. Asparagus Soup 101
387. Creamy Carrot Soup 101
388. Mushroom Barley Soup 101
389. Broccoli Soup 102
390. Chicken and Asparagus Pasta 102
391. Red Beans and Rice 102
392. Beef Stir Fry 102
393. South Western Salad 102
394. Vegan-Friendly Platter 103
395. Broccoli Salad 103
396. Beef and Bean Sloppy Joes 103
397. Sweet Potato and Peanut Soup 103
398. Beet Salad 103
399. Broccoli Casserole 104
400. Chicken Fajita Bowls 104
401. Pumpkin Soup 104
402. High-Fiber Dumplings 104
403. Pizza Made with Bamboo Fibers 105
404. Vegetarian Hamburgers 105
405. Pork Steaks with Avocado 105
406. Chicken with Asparagus Salad 105
407. Hot Pepper and Lamb Salmon 106
408. Pork rolls à la Ratatouille 106
409. Pepper Fillet with Leek 107
410. Lamb Chops with Beans 107
411. Fillet of Beef on Spring Vegetables 107
412. Bolognese with Zucchini Noodles 108
413. Chicken with Chickpeas 108
414. Ham with Chicory 108
415. Pork medallions with asparagus and coconut curry 109
416. Lamb with Carrot and Brussels Sprouts Spaghetti 109
417. Cabbage Wrap 109
418. Veal with Asparagus 109
419. Salmon with Sesame Seeds and Mushrooms 110
420. Stuffed Trout with Mushrooms 110
421. Salmon with Basil and Avocado 110
422. Leek Quiche with Olives 110
423. Fried Egg on Onions with Sage 111
424. Quinoa Mushroom Risotto 111
425. Vegetarian Lentil Stew 111
426. Lemon Chicken Soup with Beans 112
427. Crowd Pleasing Salad 112
428. Great Luncheon Salad 112
429. Flavors Powerhouse Lunch Meal 112
430. Eye-Catching Sweet Potato Boats 112
431. Mexican Enchiladas 113
432. Unique Banana Curry 113
433. Armenian Style Chickpeas 113
434. Protein-Packed Soup 113
435. One-Pot Dinner Soup 114
436. 3-Beans Soup 114
437. Chicken and Quinoa Pita 114
438. Turkey Florentine 114
439. Chicken Lettuce Wraps 114
440. Couscous with Turkey 115
441. Easy Turkey Chili 115
442. Ham, Bean and Cabbage Stew 115
443. Grilled Fish Tacos 115
444. Pasta with Turkey and Olives 115
445. Banana oat shakeBanana oat shake 116
446. Grilled Pear Cheddar Pockets 118
447. Chicken and Apple Kale Wraps 118
448. Cauliflower Rice Pilaf 118

APPENDIX

449. Fresh Herb and Lemon Bulgur Pilaf 118
450. Corn Chowder 119
451. Strawberry and Rhubarb Soup 119
452. Chicken Sandwiches 119
453. Tex-Mex Bean Tostadas 120
454. Fish Tacos 120
455. Cucumber Almond Gazpacho 120
456. Pea and Spinach Carbonara 120
457. Sautéed Broccoli with Peanut Sauce 121
458. Edamame lettuce wraps burgers 121
459. Pizza stuffed Spaghetti Squash 121
460. Spinach and Artichoke Dip Pasta 121
461. Grilled Eggplant 122
462. Stuffed potatoes with salsa and beans 122
463. Mushroom quinoa veggie Burgers 122
464. Turkey Meatballs 122
465. Sweet Potato Soup 123
466. Minestrone Soup 123
467. Lentil Soup 123
468. Grilled Corn Salad 124
469. Kale Soup 124
470. Pasta Fagioli 124
471. Sweet Potato Gnocchi 124
472. Bean and Ham Soup 124
473. Quinoa Chickpea Salad with Roasted Red Pepper Hummus Dressing 125
474. Rainbow Buddha Bowl with Cashew Tahini Sauce 125
475. Rice Bean Freezer Burritos 125
476. Roasted Veggie Hummus Pita Pockets 125
477. Salmon Sushi Buddha Bowl 126
478. Sausage Peppers Baked Ziti 126
479. Sauteed Butternut Squash 126
480. Seared Salmon with Pesto Fettuccine 126
481. Sesame Ginger Chicken Salad 126
482. Skillet Gnocchi with Chard White Beans 127
483. Spaghetti Genovese 127
484. Spiced Sweet Potato Wedges 127
485. Stetson Chopped Salad 127
486. Stuffed Sweet Potato with Hummus Dressing 128
487. Summer Squash White Bean Saute 128
488. Sweet Savory Hummus Plate 128
489. Sweet Potato Black Bean Chili for Two 128
490. Tabbouleh, Hummus Pita Plate 128
491. Pork and Penne Pasta 129
492. Tomato Artichoke Gnocchi 129
493. Vegan Buddha Bowl 129
494. Vegan Cauliflower Fried Rice 129
495. Oatmeal Bread to Live for 130
496. Vermicelli Puttanesca 130
497. Heavenly Tasty Stew 130
498. Thanksgiving Dinner Chili 130
499. Beans Trio Chili 130
500. Staple Vegan Curry 131
501. Fragrant Vegetarian Curry 131
502. Omega-3 Rich Dinner Meal 131
503. Weekend Dinner Casserole 132
504. Family Dinner Pilaf 132
505. Meat-Free Bolognese Pasta 132
506. Pasta with Escarole, Beans and Turkey 132
507. Rice Bowl with Shrimp and Peas 133
508. Roasted Chicken and Vegetables 133
509. Southwestern Chicken Pitas 133
510. Spaghetti with Zucchini 133
511. Summer Spaghetti 134
512. Pink Salmon Cakes & Potatoes 134
513. Turkey and Barley Casserole 134
514. Beef with Zucchini Noodles 134
515. Meatless Monday Chili 134
517 Healthy vegan brownies 135
518. Green risotto recipe 135

Appendix 2

MEASUREMENT CONVERSION CHART

Volume Equivalents (Dry)

US Standard	Metric (Approximate)
⅛ teaspoon	0.5 mL
¼ teaspoon	1 mL
½ teaspoon	2 mL
¾ teaspoon	4 mL
1 teaspoon	5 mL
1 tablespoon	15 mL
¼ cup	59 mL
⅓ cup	79 mL
½ cup	118 mL
⅔ cup	156 mL
¾ cup	177 mL
1 cup	235 mL
2 cups or 1 pint	475 mL
3 cups	700 mL
4 cups	1 L

Volume Equivalents (Liquid)

US Standard	US Standard (Ounces)	Metric (Approximate)
2 tablespoons	1 fl. oz.	30 ml
¼ cup	2 fl. oz.	60 ml
½ cup	4 fl. oz.	120 ml
1 cup	8 fl. oz.	240 ml
1½ cups	12 fl. oz.	355 ml
2 cups or 1 pint	16 fl. oz.	475 ml
4 cups or 1 quart	32 fl. oz.	1 L
1 gallon	128 fl. oz.	4 L

Weight Equivalents

US Standard	Metric (Approximate)
1 ounce	28 g
2 ounces	57 g
5 ounces	142 g
10 ounces	284 g
15 ounces	425 g
16 ounces or 1 pound	455 g
1.5 pounds	680 g
2 pounds	907 g

Temperature Equivalents

Fahrenheit (F)	Celsius (C) (Approximate)
225°F	107°C
250°F	120°C
300°F	150°C
325°F	165°C
350°F	180°C
375°F	190°C
400°F	200°C
425°F	220°C
450°F	230°C
475°F	245°C
500°F	260°C

Made in United States
Troutdale, OR
04/23/2025